Cancer and Pregnancy

Springer
London
Berlin
Heidelberg
New York
Barcelona
Hong Kong
Milan
Paris
Singapore
Tokyo

Eytan R. Barnea, Eric Jauniaux
and Peter E. Schwartz (Eds)

Cancer and Pregnancy

Springer

Eytan R. Barnea, MD, FACOG
Society for the Investigation of Early Pregnancy, 1697 Lark Lane, Cherry Hill, NJ 08003-3157, USA

Eric Jauniaux, MD, PhD
Department of Obstetric and Gynaecology, University College London Medical School, 86-96 Chenies Mews, London, WC1E 6HX

Peter E. Schwartz, MD, FACOG
Department of Obstetrics and Gynaecology, Yale University School of Medicine, 333 Cedar Street, New Haven, CT 06510, USA

British Library Cataloguing in Publication Data
Cancer and pregnancy
1. Cancer in pregnancy
I. Barnea, E. R. II. Jauniaux, E. III. Schwartz, Peter E.
618.3
ISBN-13:978-1-4471-1184-9

Library of Congress Cataloging-in-Publication Data
Cancer and pregnancy
Cancer in pregnancy / Eytan R. Barnea, Eric Jauniaux and Peter E. Schwartz (eds.).
p. ; cm
Includes bibliographical references and index.
ISBN-13:978-1-4471-1184-9 e-ISBN-13:978-1-4471-0707-1
DOI:10.1007/978-1-4471-0707-1

1. Cancer in pregnancy. 2. Pregnancy–Complications. I. Barnea, E. R. II. Jauniaux, E. III. Schwartz, Peter E.
[DNLM: 1. Pregnancy Complications, Neoplastic. WQ 240 C2147 2001]
RG580.C3 C35 2001
618.3–dc21 00–049240

ISBN-13:978-1-4471-1184-9 Springer-Verlag London Berlin Heidelberg
a member of BertelsmannSpringer Science+Business Media GmbH
http://www.springer.co.uk

Softcover reprint of the hardcover 1st edition 2001

Typeset by Bookcraft Ltd, Stroud, Gloucestershire
28/3830-543210 Printed on acid-free paper SPIN 10779570

Contents

Contributors

George Aboagye-Mathiesen, PhD
Institute of Medical Biochemistry
University of Aarhus
Ole Worms Alle, Building 170
8000 Aarhus C, Denmark

Matthew L. Anderson, MD, PhD
Department of Obstetrics and Gynecology
and Divisions of Maternal-Fetal Medicine
Yale University School of Medicine
New Haven, Connecticut USA

Eytan R. Barnea, MD, FACOG
Chairman
The Society for the Investigation of Early Pregnancy (SIEP)
1697 Lark Lane
Cherry Hill, NJ 08003-3157, USA

Frank A. Chervenak, MD
Professor and Acting Chairman
Department of Obstetrics and Gynecology
New York Weill Cornell Medical Center
525 East 68th Street, Room J130
New York, NY 10021, USA

Carolyn B. Coulam, MD
Sher Institute for Reproductive Medicine of Chicago
233 E Erie, Suite 500
Chicago, IL 60611, USA

Orna Diav-Citrin, MD
Department of Pediatrics
The Hebrew University
Hadassah Medical School
P.O. Box 12272
Jerusalem 91120, Israel

Tuan A Dinh, MD
Departmenet of Obstetrics and Gynecology
Cooper Hospital / University Medical Center
1 Cooper Plaza, suite 623
Camden NJ 08103, USA

Russell Foulk, MD, FACOG
University of Nevada School of Medicine
Medical Director
The Nevada and Idaho Center for Reproductive Medicine
6630 S. McCarran Blvd, Suite 9
Reno, NV 89509, USA

Olga Genbacev, PhD
Department of Stomatology
University of California, San Francisco
513 Parnassus Avenue HSW 604
San Francisco, CA 94143-0512, USA

Yves Gillerot, MD, PhD
Institut de Morphologie
Pathologique Loverval (IMPL)
Allée des Templiers 41
6280 Gerpinnes (Loveral), Belgium

Jack Goldberg, MD
Department of Medicine
Division of Hematology/Medical Oncology
Cooper Hospital/University Medical Center
3 Cooper Plaza, Suite 220
Camden, NJ 08103, USA

Alexandre Hageboutros, MD
Department of Medicine
Division of Hematology/Medical Oncology
Cooper Hospital/University Medical Center
3 Cooper Plaza, Suite 220
Camden, NJ 08103, USA

Seth P. Harlow, MD
Assistant Professor of Surgery
Division of Surgical Oncology
University of Vermont
Given Building, Room 309
Burlington, VT 05405, USA

William C. Hatch, PhD
Boston Biomedical Research Institute
64 Grove Street
Watertown, MA 02472-2829, USA

Jean Hustin, MD, PhD
Institut de Morphologie
Pathologique Loverval (IMPL)
Allée des Templiers 41
6280 Gerpinnes (Loveral), Belgium

Eric Jauniaux, MD, PhD
Reader in Obstetrics and Maternofoetal Medicine
Academic Departments of Obstetrics and Gynaecology
University College London Medical School
86-96 Chenies Mews
London WC1E 6HX, UK

Sanja Kupesic, MD, PhD
Department of Obstetrics and Gynecology
Medical School University of Zagreb
Sveti Duh Jospital
Sveti Duh 64
10000 Zagreb, Croatia

Asim Kurjak, MD, PhD
Department of Obstetrics and Gynecology
Medical School University of Zagreb
Sveti Duh Jospital
Sveti Duh 64
10000 Zagreb, Croatia

Richard G. Lea, PhD
Senior Research Scientist
Division of Nutrition and Development
The Rowett Research Institute
Greenburn Road, Bucksburn
Aberdeen AB21 9SB, UK

Paul C. Leavis, PhD
Boston Biomedical Research Institute
64 Grove Street
Watertown, MA 02472-2829, USA

Z. M. Lei, PhD
Division of Basic Science Research
Department of Obstetrics and Gynecology
University of Louisville Health Sciences Center
Louisville, Kentucky, USA

Giancarlo Mari, MD
Department of Obstetrics and Gynecology
and Divisions of Maternal-Fetal Medicine
Yale University School of Medicine
New Haven, Connecticut, USA

Takeshi Maruo, MD
Department of Obstetrics and Gynecology
Kobe University School of Medicine
Kusunoki-Cho, Chuo-Ku
Kobe 650-0017, Japan

Laurence B. McCullough, PhD
Professor of Medicine and Medical Ethics
Center for Medical Ethics and Health Policy
Baylor College of Medicine
1 Baylor Plaza
Houston, TX 77030, USA

Richard K. Miller, PhD
Professor and Director
Department of Obstetrics and Gynecology
Division of Research/PEDECS
University of Rochester Medical Center
601 Elmwood Avenue, Box 668
Rochester, NY 14642-8668, USA

Muhammad Muslim, MD
Department of Medicine
Division of Hematology/Medical Oncology
Cooper Hospital, University Medical Center
3 Cooper Plaza, Suite 220
Camden NJ 08103, USA

Kunle Odunsi, MD, PhD
Department of Gynecological Oncology
Roswell Park Cancer Institute
Elm and Carlton Streets
Buffalo, NY 14263, USA

Asher Ornoy, MD
Department of Anatomy and Cell Biology
The Hebrew University
Hadassah Medical School
P.O. Box 12272
Jerusalem 91120, Israel

Tetsuo Otani, MD
Department of Obstetrics and Gynecology
Kobe University School of Medicine
Kusunoki-Cho, Chuo-Ku
Kobe 650-0017, Japan

Tanja Pejovic, MD, PhD
Department of Obstetrics and Gynecology
Yale University School of Medicine
333 Cedar Street
New Haven, CT 06520, USA

Ch. V. Rao, PhD
Division of Basic Science Research
Department of Obstetrics and Gynecology
University of Louisville Health Sciences Center
438 Medical-Dental Building
511 South Floyd Street
Louisville, KY 40292, USA

Daniel Rukavina, MD, DSc
Professor and Chairman
Department of Physiology and Immunology
Medical Faculty, University of Rijeka
B. Branchetta 20
51000 Rijeka, Croatia

Mrinal K. Sanyal, PhD
Departments of Obstetrics and Gynecology and Molecular, Cellular and Developmental Biology
Yale University School of Medicine
333 Cedar Street
New Haven, CT 06510, USA

Christobel Saunders, FRCS
Department of Surgery
Charles Bell House
Riding House Street
London, UK

Elizabeth F. Shah, MSc, FRCS
Department of Surgery
Charles Bell House
Riding House Street
London, UK

Peter E. Schwartz, MD, FACOG
Vice Chair/Director of Gynecologic Oncology
Department of Obstetrics and Gynecology
Yale University School of Medicine
333 Cedar Street
New Haven, CT 06510, USA

Shlomo Marc Stemmer, MD, MS, FACOG
Crispin Square
230 N Maple Ave
Marlton, NJ 08053, USA

David P. Warshal, MD
Department of Obstetrics and Gynecology
Cooper Hospital / University Medical Center
3 Cooper Plaza, suite 221
Camden, NJ 08103, USA

Tina Zodan, MD
Opca Bolnica
Sveti Duh 64
10000 Zagreb, Croatia

Marek Zygmunt, MD
Department of Obstetrics and Gynecology
University of Giessen
Klinikstr. 32
Giessen, 35385, Germany

Part I

Clinical Aspects: Diagnosis and Management

1. The Epidemiology of Cancer in Pregnancy

Tuan A. Dinh and David P. Warshal

Cancer in pregnancy presents a unique challenge to clinicians. Many diagnostic and therapeutic procedures routinely used in the care of patients with cancer are contraindicated in the presence of pregnancy. Definitive therapy, which may require either sacrificing the pregnancy or incurring significant risk to the fetus, may be unacceptable to some patients and therefore result in a delay in treatment until after delivery. In addition, fears are often raised regarding the possible biologic effect of the pregnancy on the cancer or the cancer's effect on the fetus. Guidelines for the evaluation and treatment of pregnant cancer patients must consider the gestational age of the pregnancy and include alternatives to accommodate the individual patient's wishes regarding her pregnancy. A relative paucity of experience with cancer in pregnancy among clinicians further complicates the situation. It is difficult to imagine circumstances that are more stressful to the patient or more challenging to her physician.

The incidence of cancer in pregnancy is unclear but is estimated to be 1/1000[1]. This estimate is derived from historical case series collected at a variety of referral institutions (see Table 1.1). From these series, many have concluded that cervical cancer is the most frequent cancer occurring in pregnancy. However, with the steady decline in the overall incidence of cervical cancer in the United States over the last several decades, this finding is likely to be inaccurate. Unfortunately, the current large cancer databases within the United States such as SEER (Surveillance, Epidemiology, and End Result) do not collect this information.

In a 1984 population-based study, Haas[2] reviewed the National Cancer Registry of the German Democratic Republic for the years between 1970 and 1979. Out of a total of 31,353 cancer cases and 2,103,112 live births among women between the ages of 15 and 44, 355 pregnant women were diagnosed with a malignancy. The incidence of cancer in pregnancy per 1000 live births rose from 0.02 for women aged 15–19 to 2.3 for women aged 40–44. The most frequent sites diagnosed during pregnancy, in order of decreasing frequency, were cervix, breast, ovary, lymphoma, melanoma, brain and leukemia. However, the current applicability of this data to the United States, in regard to population and screening practices, is questionable.

For most cancers, the peak incidence occurs well beyond the reproductive years. The median age at which a woman is diagnosed with cancer in the United States is 67. Above the age of 70, the age-specific rate of cancer in women reaches a plateau (see Fig. 1.1).

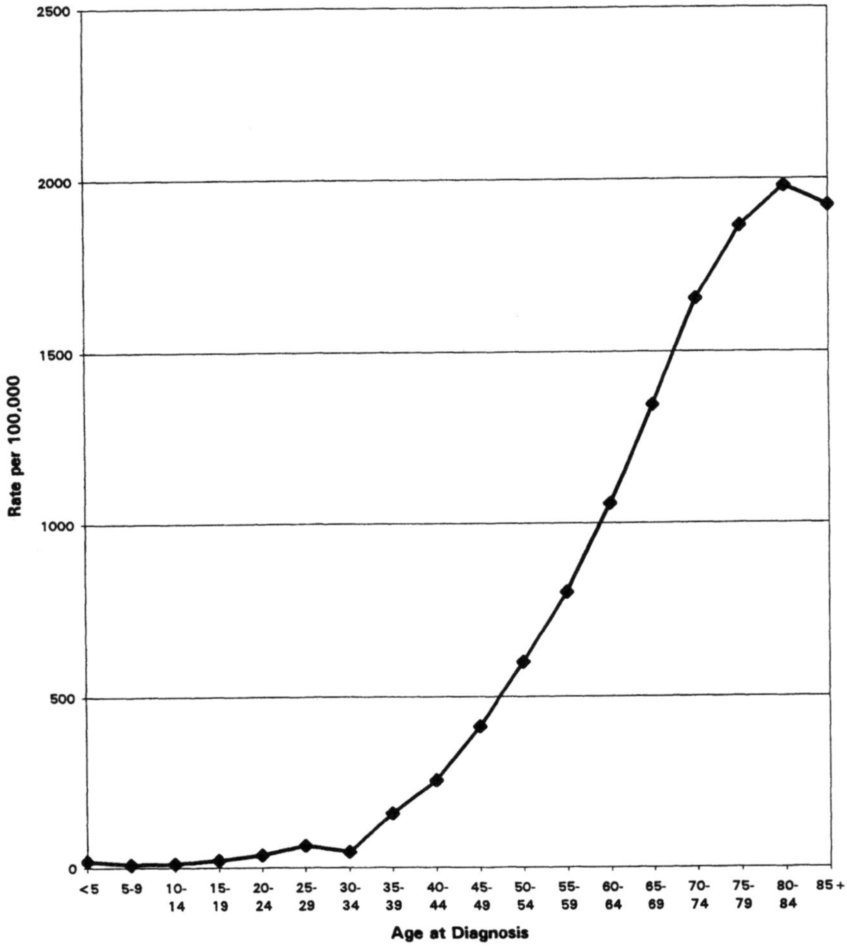

Fig. 1.1. Age-specific incidence of cancer in women.

According to estimates derived from SEER data (1992–1996), the most frequent cancer sites in women aged 15–44 are, in order of decreasing frequency, breast, melanoma, thyroid, cervix, lymphoma and ovary[3]. Over half of all thyroid cancers and more than a third of cervical cancers and melanomas occur in this age group (Table 1.2). During the reproductive years, the incidence of cancer rises rapidly with increasing age (Fig. 1.2), with cancer closely following injury as the leading cause of death in the United States.[4]

Additional population-based studies examining the epidemiology of cancer in pregnancy are needed. A comparison of the observed to expected rates and stages of cancer at specific primary sites will help to define the effect of pregnancy on the diagnosis and development of cancer. An excellent example is breast cancer. Surveillance of women who seek medical care only because they are pregnant and the frequency of their antepartum visits may increase the rate of breast cancer detection during pregnancy. The potential for accelerated tumor growth due to high intrapartum hormone

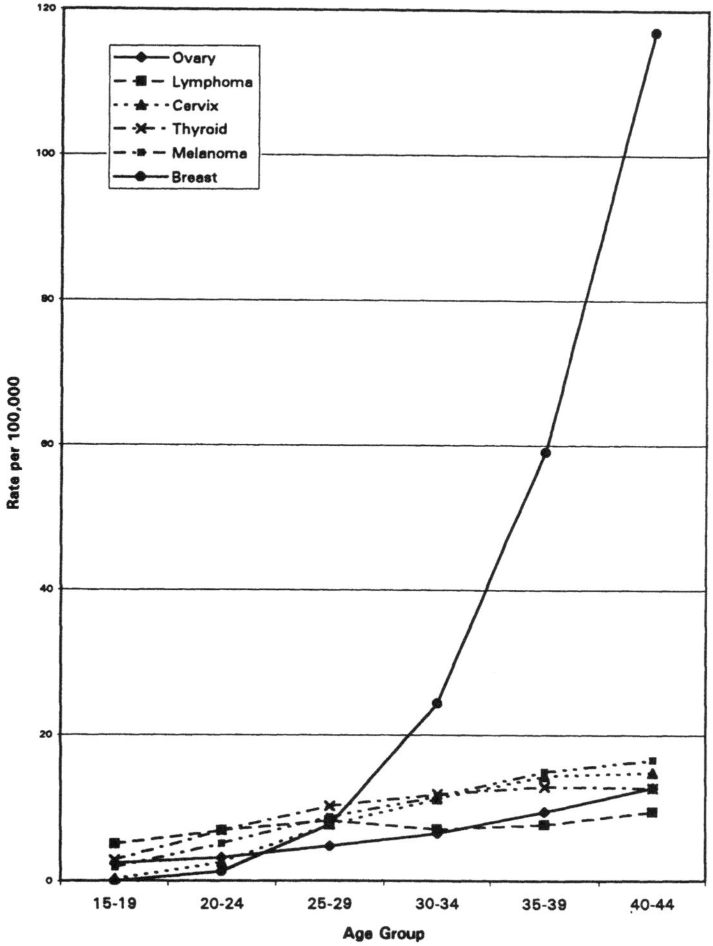

Fig. 1.2. Age-specific incidence of specific cancers in reproductive-age women.

levels or to altered immunity during pregnancy may also increase the detection rate. Conversely, physiologic changes associated with pregnancy such as breast swelling and tenderness and the contraindication to mammography could delay the diagnosis. Accelerated growth of malignancies or delays in diagnosis may also result in higher stages of disease at the time of detection.

Recently reported data from the Centers for Disease Control and Prevention highlight the trends in pregnancies in the United States over the past quarter century. The live birth rate in 1996 was 65.3 per 1000 women aged 15 to 44 years, 8% lower than the high of 70.9 in 1990 and the lowest recorded since 1976 (65.0). Changes in the pattern of births by maternal age are clearly evident. While the birth rate for women under the age of 30 rose slowly until the early 1990s, it has steadily declined since then. In contrast, as of 1996, the birth rate for women age 30 and above rose steadily over the 20-year period by an average of 67%. Preliminary data from 1998 show persistence of these trends.[5] This dramatic rise in births among 'reproductively' older women has

Table 1.1. Estimates of cancer during pregnancy.

Site	Estimated Incidence	Authors
Cervix invasive	1:2,000–2,500	Hacker et al.[6]
Breast	1:3,500–10,000	Parente, JT et al[8]
Ovary	1:12,000–25,000	Chung and Birnbaum.[9]
Leukemia	1:75,000	Yahia, C et al.[7]
Hodgkin's lymphoma	1:1,000–6,000	Stewart and Monto[10]
Melanoma	2.8:1,000	Smith and Randal[11]
Thyroid	unknown	

Table 1.2. Age distribution of cancer in women.

Site	Total cases	% Occuring between 15–44 years of age
Breast	81,769	12
Melanoma	8,113	36
Thyroid	5,417	54
Cervix	5,971	43
Lymphoma	11,337	19
Ovary	10,822	18

Source: SEER Data

been attributed to the changing attitudes regarding the role of women in the workplace. As these career women continue in greater numbers to delay childbearing, the incidence of cancer in pregnancy will surely rise.

With this delay in childbearing, clinicians will need to address questions regarding the advisability of pregnancy in patients with a history of cancer. What is the appropriate disease-free interval before attempting to become pregnant? Could pregnancy stimulate a recurrence of the cancer or could it be protective? How may the pregnancy be affected if the malignancy recurs? Current data provide few answers to these questions. In fact, a recent report describing the vertical transmission of maternal natural-killer-cell lymphoma to the fetus challenges many of our basic concepts regarding the relative immunity of the fetus.[12] Future studies in this area will be essential to answer many of these questions.

Recent advances in molecular genetics are beginning to play a major role in the evaluation and management of patients who appear to be at increased risk for cancer. A variety of genes have been identified whose germline mutations are associated with hereditary cancer syndromes; they include BRCA1 and BRCA2 for breast and/or ovarian cancer and MSH2, MLH1, PMS1 and PMS2 for hereditary nonpolyposis colorectal cancer (HNPCC). With the completion of the Human Genome Project, the number of genes associated with hereditary syndromes will rise exponentially. As younger asymptomatic individuals undergo testing, issues regarding screening practices and prophylactic measures for affected patients come to the fore. We anticipate that the complex strategies which often evolve for these patients will include consideration for their reproductive desires and an attempt to minimize the risk of cancer in pregnancy.

Clearly, these are exciting times with many significant discoveries just around the corner. The following chapters represent the most up-to-date information, both clinical and scientific, about cancer in pregnancy. You will encounter, on a site-by-site basis, a variety of ideas and recommendations which will challenge your basic knowledge of cancer in pregnancy and prepare you for the advances to come.

References

1. Waalen J. Pregnancy poses tough questions for cancer treatment. J Nat Cancer Inst 1991; 83:900
2. Haas JF. Pregnancy in association with a newly diagnosed cancer: A population-based epidemiologic assessment. Int J Cancer 1984; 34:229–35
3. Ries LAG, Kosary CL, Hankey BF, Miller BA, Clegg L, Edwards BK (eds). SEER Cancer Statistics Review, 1973–1996, National Cancer Institute. Bethesda, MD, 1999
4. Landis SH, Taylor M, Bolden S, et al. Cancer Statistics, 1999. CA Cancer J Clin 1999; 49, 8-31
5. Smith BL, Martin JA, Ventura SJ. Births and Deaths. Preliminary Data for July 97–June 98. National Center for Health Statistics. Vital Health Stat Series No. 22 (477), 1999
6. Hacker NF, Berek JS, Lagasse LD, et al. Carcinoma of the cervix associated with pregnancy. Obstet Gynecol 1982; 59: 735
7. Yahia C, Hyman GA, Phillips LL. Acute leukemia and pregnancy. Obstet Gynecol Surv 1958; 13:1–21
8. Parente JL, Amsel M, Lerner R, et al. Breast cancer associated with pregnancy. Obstet Gynecol 1988; 71:861–4
9. Chung A, Birnbaum SJ. Ovarian cancer associated with pregnancy. Obstet Gynecol 1973; 41–211
10. Stewart HL Jr, Monto RW. Hodgkin's disease and pregnancy. Am J Obstet Gynecol 1952; 63:570–8
11. Smith RS, Randall P. Melanoma during pregnancy. Obstet Gynecol 1969; 34:825–9
12. Catlin EA, Roberts JD, Erana R, et al. Transplacental transmission of natural-killer-cell lymphoma. N Engl J Med 1999; 341: 85–91.

2. Placental and Fetal Cancers

Eric Jauniaux, Yves Gillerot and Jean Hustin

Introduction

Placental and fetal cancers are rare complications of pregnancy but when they occur they are a real challenge for the perinatologists in terms of antenatal differential diagnosis and management. The main differences between placental and fetal cancers are at the level of incidence and potential effect on the mother during pregnancy or after delivery. Overall, placental cancers are more common than fetal cancers but are less often diagnosed before or immediately after delivery. Some types of placental cancer can have a lethal effect on the pregnancy, such as the placental choriocarcinoma-in-situ, and most placental cancers will continue to proliferate after delivery. Fetal cancers, however, are now often diagnosed before delivery and they only exceptionally spread beyond the placental barrier and thus are of little or no consequence to the mother. These unusual cancers are the basis of this chapter, in which the focus is on the role of non-invasive investigation in the diagnosis, follow-up and management of pregnancies presenting with a placental or fetal cancer.

Placental Cancer

The group of placental cancerous tumours includes a wide range of placental trophoblastic disorders involving the proliferation of one or more trophoblastic cellular types. Depending on their origin and anatomical characteristics, these tumours have different fetal and maternal consequences. Thus an early and accurate diagnosis is pivotal in patient counselling and perinatal management. In most cases, prenatal differential diagnosis is possible, based on specific clinical symptoms, ultrasound features and biological markers.

Molar Pregnancies and Persistent Trophoblastic Tumor (PTT)

The distinction between complete and partial mole was made in the late 1970s on the basis of gross morphological, histological and cytogenetic criteria. The complete or classical hydatidiform mole has been defined as a conceptus with a placenta showing generalized swelling of the villi (Fig. 2.1) and diffuse trophoblastic hyperplasia in the

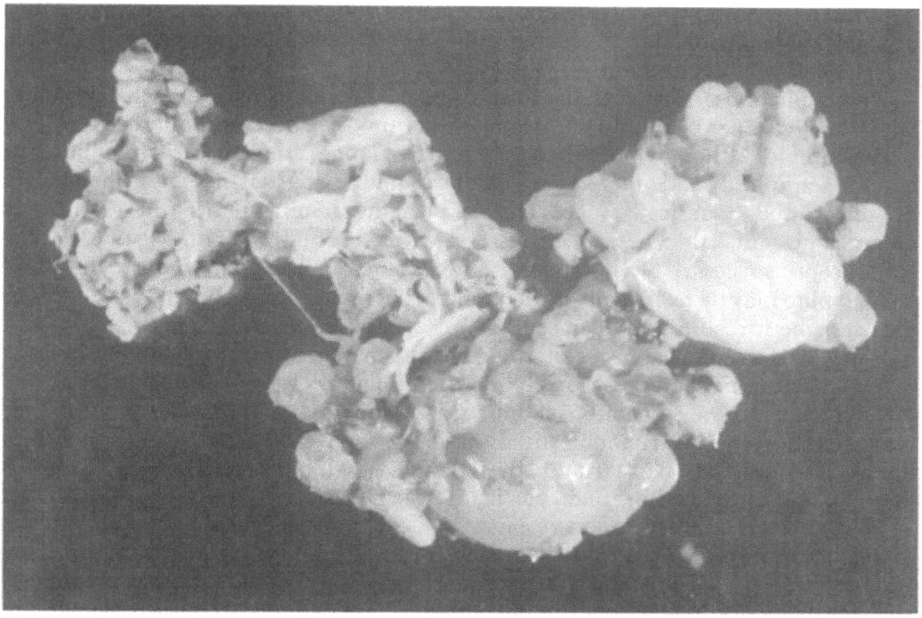

Fig. 2.1. Macroscopic view of a 12 weeks (menstrual age) CHM showing multiple hydatidiform vesicles of various shapes and sizes.

absence of an ascertainable fetus.[1] The partial hydatidiform mole has been characterized by focal trophoblastic hyperplasia with focal villous hydrops and identifiable embryonic or fetal tissue[2,3]. The clinico-pathologic picture of the two molar syndromes overlap to a degree since both the phenotype and natural history of the partial mole seem to represent a mild version of those of the complete mole.

The estimated incidence of partial mole is 1 per 700 pregnancies whereas the incidence of complete mole is around 1 per 1500–2000 pregnancies.[4,5] The vast majority of complete and partial moles abort spontaneously during the first three to four months of pregnancy resulting in an incidence of molar placenta of 1 per 41 miscarriages.[4] Complete moles have a diploid chromosomal constitution totally derived from the paternal genome usually resulting from the fertilization of an oocyte by a diploid spermatozoon.[6] Partial moles are usually triploid and of diandric origin, having two sets of chromosomes from paternal origin and one from maternal origin.[7,8] Most have a 69,XXX or 69,XXY genotype derived from a haploid ovum with either reduplication of the paternal haploid set from a single sperm, or less frequently, from dispermic fertilization. Triploidy of digynic origin due to a double maternal contribution are not associated with placental hydatidiform changes.[9]

Arteriography was the first method used for the diagnosis in utero of molar pregnancy. Due to the cost, maternal discomfort and morbidity it was rapidly replaced by ultrasound imaging in the 1960s.[10] Molar changes can now be detected from the second month of pregnancy by ultrasound which typically reveals a uterine cavity filled with multiple sonolucent areas of varying size and shape ("snowstorm" appearance) without an associated embryonic or fetal structure.[11] A classical mole may coexist with a normal fetus and placenta in cases of molar transformation of one ovum in a dizygotic twin pregnancy.[12,13] Mothers with this condition are at a higher risk of PTT, requiring multiple sessions of chemotherapy, than patients with classical mole (50–60% compared to 10–15%).

Prenatally, the presence of any form of placental villous hydropic changes and a coexistent fetus has been, and unfortunately continues to be, commonly referred to as a partial mole. Although more than 90% of partial mole are diandric triploidies, rare cases of tetraploidy and other aneuploidies can mimic a partial mole morphologically on ultrasound. Classically, partial mole present on ultrasound (Fig. 2.2) as an enlarged placenta (thickness > 4cm at 18–22 weeks) containing multicystic avascular sonolucent spaces ("Swiss cheese" appearance). Placental biopsy for fetal karyotyping may be technically difficult in partial mole because of villous edema and the cytogenetic results may be obscured, however infrequently, by confined placental mosaicism. If the fetus appears anatomically normal on ultrasound another invasive test, such as amniocentesis or fetal blood sampling, may be more appropriate.[14,15,16]

Following uterine evacuation, about 20% of patients with a complete mole develop persistent gestational trophoblastic disease.[17] Evidence of persisting trophoblastic disease after evacuation of a triploid partial mole was first reported in 1978.[18] The incidence of this complication after a partial mole is now stated to be between 1 and 11% [5,19,20] but in fact it appears lower since many partial moles escape diagnosis. Estimates of the incidence of PTT also vary because few countries have registries and complete and partial mole have often been treated as a single entity in epidemiological studies.

If the incidence of maternal complication has been reduced by early diagnosis, the reported incidence of PTT has remained unchanged despite the introduction of routine ultrasound examination during pregnancy.[17] This suggests there is a similar risk of PTT following either a first-trimester spontaneous molar abortion or after therapeutic abortion in a second-trimester molar pregnancy. Serial reading of hCG

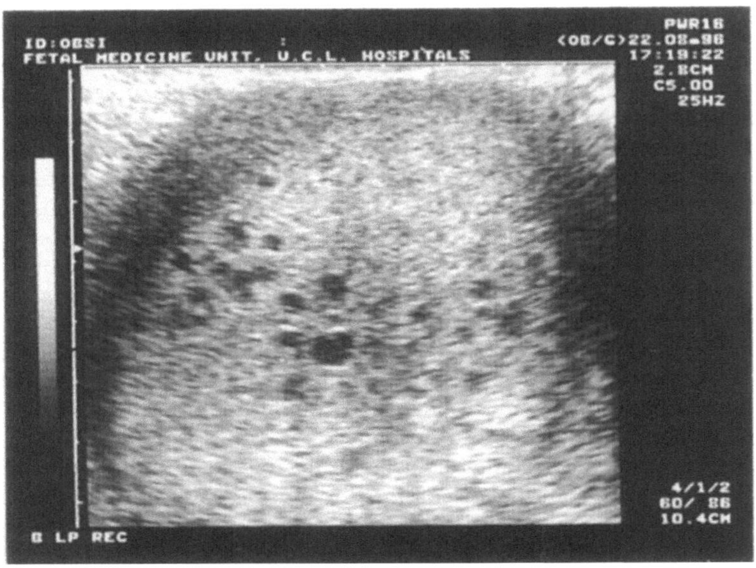

Fig 2.2. Ultrasound scan of the placenta in a triploid PHM at 20 weeks of gestation showing several echopoor "cystic" areas ("Swiss cheese" appearance) corresponding histologically to areas of villous hydrops.

levels is the gold standard for the diagnosis and monitoring of the therapeutic response of PTT. After evacuation of a molar pregnancy, the hCG level should be monitored weekly until undetectable, followed by monthly monitoring for 6–24 months.[17] In women with PTT or with chemotherapy-resistant disease, angiography has proved to be of great value in the diagnostic approach of myometrial invasion and surgical management.[21] Before the development of transvaginal sonography (TVS), transabdominal sonography (TAS) was used for the assessment of uterine involvement in patient with non-metastastic PTT[22] and is still used in some centres.[23]

TAS is only capable of detecting massive uterine involvement. All studies have shown that TVS is a more accurate method for the assessment of the depth of myometrial invasion than TAS.[24-31] The use of colour Doppler imaging (CDI) with its added capability of displaying blood flow data throughout an area of interest has improved the accuracy of TVS.[27-32] The colour maps produced by TVS-CDI can now be considered to be of similar diagnostic value to pelvic angiogram films in assessing the location and extent of a non-metastatic trophoblastic tumor. Ultrasound which is a non-invasive, painfree and safe imaging technique should, therefore, replace angiography which is invasive and associated with complications such as bleeding and sensitivity to contrast medium.

Nodules of residual trophoblatic tumor are surrounded by newly formed blood vessels with frequent arteriovenous anastomosis which produce a characteristic ultrasound pattern (Fig. 2.3). The most frequent feature is hypoechoic areas (blood lacunae) surrounded by irregular echogenic areas (trophoblastic nodules) and numerous intramyometrial signals (vascular shunts). In these cases, Doppler investigations of the uterine vasculature and of small intra-tumoral vessels have consistently shown a low resistance to flow and high peak systolic velocities.[33,34,35] Small nodules may not be detected by CDI. Hysteroscopy[36] and possibly sonohysterography may be

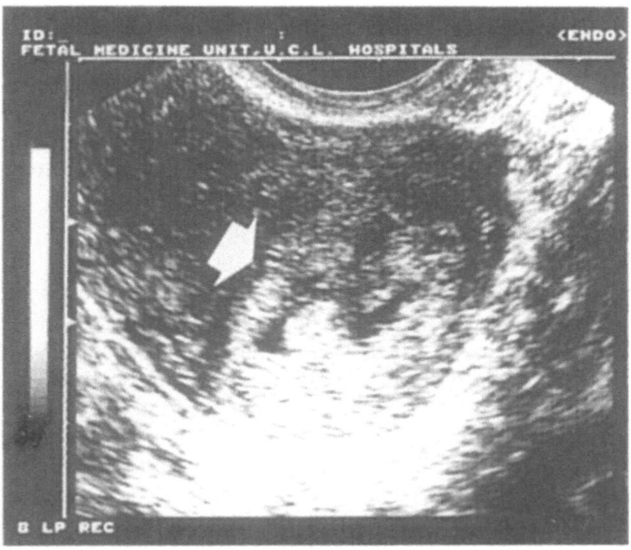

Fig. 2.3. Transvaginal ultrasound scan, 12 weeks after a spontaneous vaginal delivery at term in a patient with chronic vaginal bleeding and elevated hCG level, showing an heterogeneous uterine lesion (arrow), hypoechoic areas surrounded by irregular echogenic areas and numerous intramyometrial vascular signals on Doppler.

of clinical use in patients with an hCG level suggestive of PTT although negative on ultrasound examination.

TVS and Doppler are increasingly used to monitor the regression of the tumor after uterine evacuation and to follow up patients receiving chemotherapy. The changes in resistance to flow seem to parallel the gradual decrease in ßhCG levels, and patients with the lowest resistance to flow are more likely to develop drug resistance. This feature reflects a more severe destruction to the uterine vasculature, with more blood lacunae and shunts. The vascular changes associated with PTT may remain long after the disappearance of the tumor. The long-term follow up with sonography or angiography of PTT which has been successfully treated is thus of limited clinical interest.

Invasive Hydatidiform Mole

An invasive mole is defined as the penetration of molar villi into the myometrium or the uterine vasculature.[1] Both complete and partial moles can become invasive but the invasive capacity of a mole is not an indication that it is neoplastic. Trophoblasts enter the maternal circulation in every normal pregnancy and the fact that a molar trophoblast may be transported to an extrauterine site is not an indication of its malignancy. Rarely, the mole can penetrate the whole thickness of the myometrium (percreta) leading to uterine perforation and/or local pelvic extension. In contrast to choriocarcinoma, an invasive mole contains villous structures with a variable degree of trophoblastic proliferation and produces lower level of hCG.

An invasive mole usually becomes clinically apparent after the evacuation of a molar pregnancy, the patient usually presenting with heavy vaginal bleeding. The tumor appears sonographically as a focal area of increased echogenicity within the myometrium. These nodules usually appear several weeks after evacuation of a mole but may occur concurrently with a mole. The sonographic features of these nodules are similar to the lesions found in cases of placental site trophoblastic tumor.[37] In both these types of placental tumors, the lesions are usually heterogeneous, often containing fluid-filled cavities. Doppler colour flow mapping of the abnormal area can be used to evaluate the extent of the lesion and its subsequent response to chemotherapy.[38,39,40] An early diagnosis allowing an immediate treatment may, in some cases, prevent uterine perforation and the need to perform a hysterectomy.

Placental Site Trophoblastic Tumor (PSTT)

This rare variant of malignant trophoblastic tumor is composed of intermediate trophoblastic cells from the extravillous trophoblast of the placental bed (Fig. 2.4). In more than 90% of the cases, PSTT develops after a normal pregnancy. Rare cases have been reported after a diploid or triploid mole or in postmenopausal women. Amenorrhea of up to 1 year or irregular vaginal bleeding of varying duration are common presenting symptoms.[1] PSTT invade the myometrium by separating muscle bundles and fibres and about 15–20% behave in a malignant manner with metastases to the lungs, liver, abdominal cavity and brain. PSTT cells are capable of producing hCG but, in less than one third of the cases, the MShCG level is only moderately elevated. The principal protein produced by the intermediate trophoblast is human placental lactogen (hPL). Thus a relatively low hCG level and high hPL level should be found in the serum of patients with PSTT. Maternal biology can be an important parameter in the differential diagnosis since PSTT appear ultrasonographically as

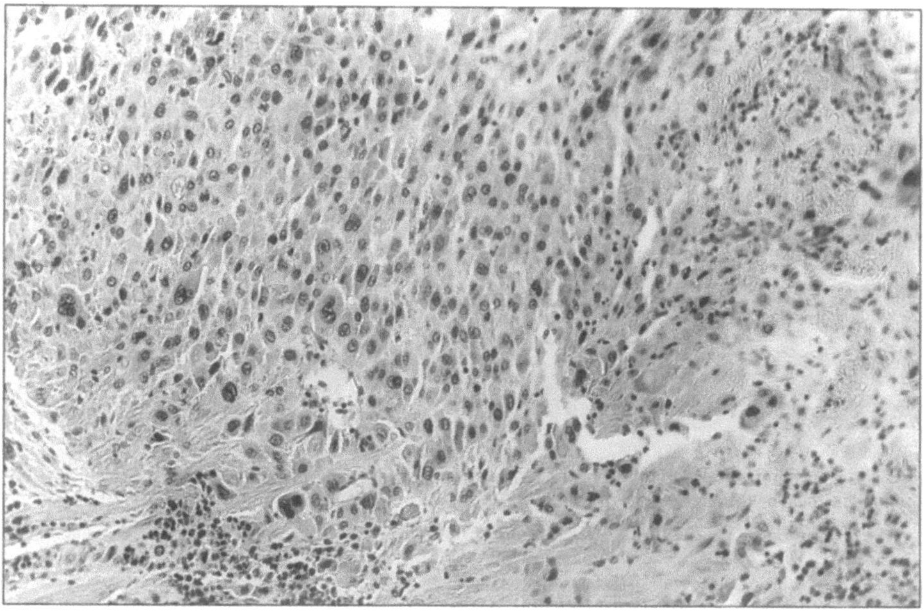

Fig 2.4. Placental site trophoblastic tumors typically composed intermediate trophoblastic cells from the extravillous trophoblast of the placental bed (HE ×250).

small heterogeneous echogenic areas with fluid-filled cystic lesions[37,41] representing hemorrhagic areas (Fig. 2.8), similar in appearance to an invasive mole or PTT. PSTT can also appear on scan as a solid tumor invading the myometrial wall.[42]

Choriocarcinoma

Choriocarcinoma is a highly malignant tumor that arises from the trophoblastic epithelium and metastasises readily to the lungs, liver and brain.[43] The primary symptoms of choriocarcinoma are gynecological, that is, vaginal bleeding, in only 50–60% of the cases. Women can present with dyspnoea, neurological symptoms and abdominal pain, a few weeks or months and sometimes up to 10–15 years after their last pregnancy.[1,43] Necrosis and hemorrhage are often present inside choriocarcinomas (Fig. 2.5) and the corresponding metastasis produces a sonographic picture of a semi-solid echogenic mass.[44] These lesions are often better evaluated using computerized tomography or magnetic resonance imaging. The serum hCG level must be measured and an appropriate histological examination should be performed in any women of reproductive age presenting with widespread lesions, metastasis of unknown origin or cerebral or intra-abdominal bleeding.[43]

Around 50% of choriocarcinomas follow a molar pregnancy, 30% occur after a miscarriage and 20% after an apparently normal pregnancy.[1] Exceptionally, choriocarcinomas can occur after an extrauterine pregnancy and will present with signs and symptoms similar to those classically outlined for ectopic pregnancy.[45] There have been a few well-documented examples of choriocarcinoma arising from

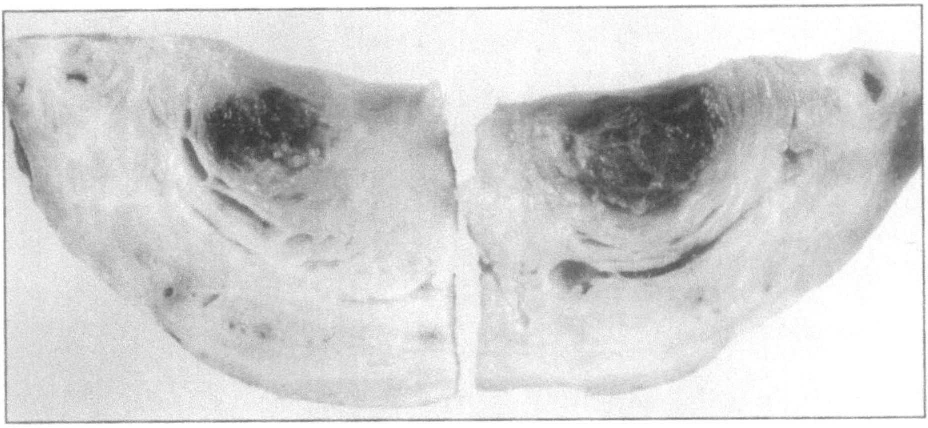

Fig. 2.5. Hysterectomy specimen showing necrotic tumor protruding into the uterine cavity which corresponded histologically to a choriocarcinoma.

villous tissue in an otherwise normally developed placenta (Fig. 2.6). This suggests that most or maybe all choriocarcinomas that follow an apparently normal pregnancy are in reality metastases from a small intraplacental choriocarcinoma.[1] The primary tumor is usually small in size ranging from 2.5 to 8 mm and an extensive search of the entire placenta is often required to find the lesion.[46,47,48] In most cases of intraplacental choriocarcinoma, the mother presents with multiple metastases during the course of pregnancy but the fetus is only rarely involved in the disease. In situ choriocarcinomas can also arise inside a triploid partial mole[49] or in association with a chorioangioma.[50,51] The latter tumor is often large (Fig. 2.7) and detectable by ultrasound but so far not one of the different types of intraplacental choriocarcinoma has been described sonographically.

Placental Metastasis

Metastases to the placenta are invariably blood-borne and occur mainly in the mother or fetus with widely disseminated malignant disease. Malignant melanomas, which are prone to develop in a young individual and spread extensively via the vascular system, are the most common maternal neoplasms involving the placenta.[1] Carcinomas of the breast and bronchus are increasingly common in young women due to changes in smoking habits. Other carcinomas involving the placenta are rare.[1] In the vast majority of cases, the metastases are microscopic, multifocal and remain inside the intervillous space, adjacent to intact villi. Metastasis from maternal melanomas are often macroscopic and can infiltrate the villous tissue and rarely pass over to the fetus. Similarly, fetal neuroblastomas can spread to the placenta and pass over to the mother. The main sonographic feature reported in cases of macroscopic metastasis to the villous tissue is an increased thickness in the placenta.[52]

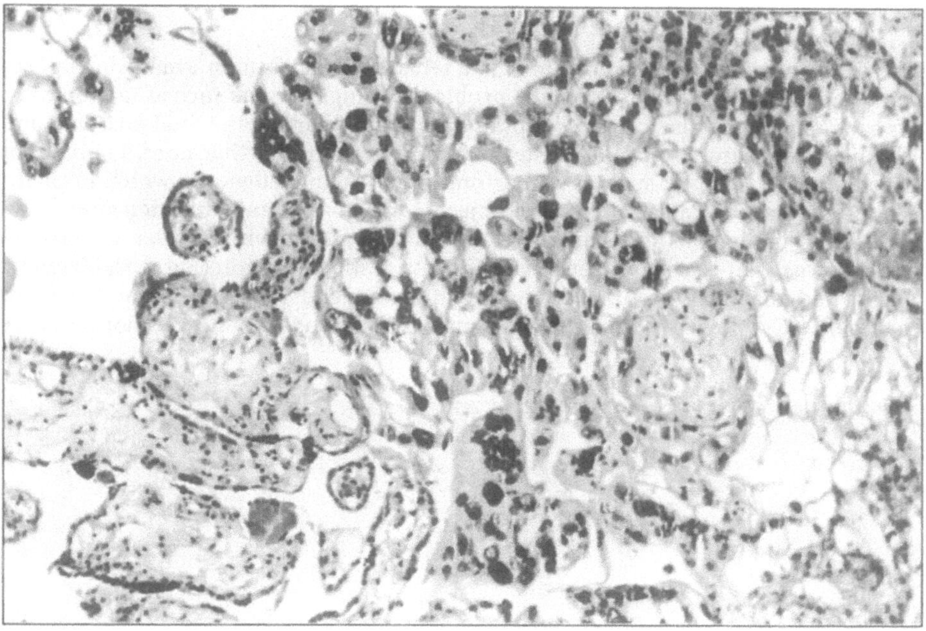

Fig. 2.6. Choriocarcinoma nodule inside a placenta at term in a pregnancy complicated by intrauterine fetal death and pulmonary metastasis in both maternal lungs (HE ×250).

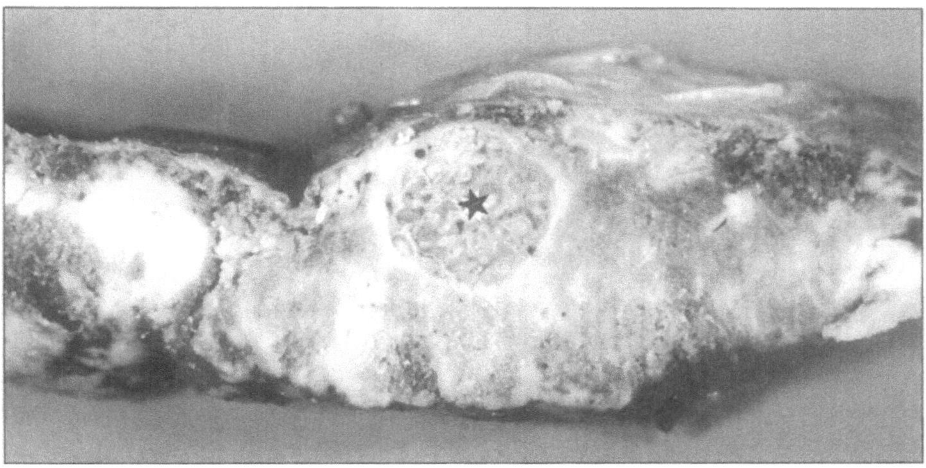

Fig. 2.7. Chorangiocarcinoma (star). (Modified from Ref. 50).

Fetal Cancer

The development of cancerous tumor in a fetus is an uncommon event which poses numerous diagnostic and therapeutic problems. Benign tumors such as teratomas or lyphangiomas may also progress rapidly in utero, distorting the fetal anatomy and leading to comparable fetal and obstetrical complications. Furthermore, a number of developmental tumors, such as hamartomas and vaginal adenosis, which in themselves are not malignant in utero, are subject to malignant transformation after delivery. Many malignant and benign fetal tumors present with similar ultrasound appearances, that is, a heterogeneous mass with cystic formation (Fig. 2.8). Magnetic ultrasound imaging is useful in evaluating the extent and the tissue characteristics of the lesion.[53] Cytology of fluid aspirated from cystic lesions, or of needle biopsies, may

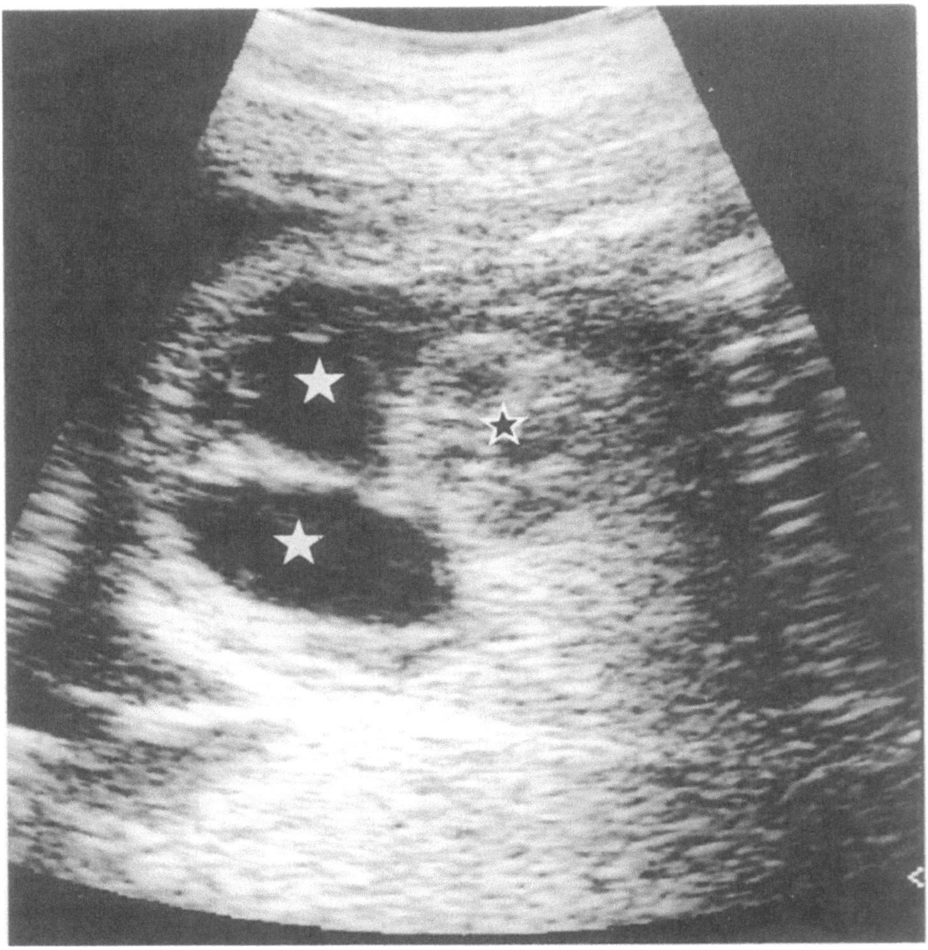

Fig. 2.8. Transverse ultrasound scan of the fetal upper abdomen at 29 weeks' gestation showing a septated cystic mass (stars) behind the right kidney (star).

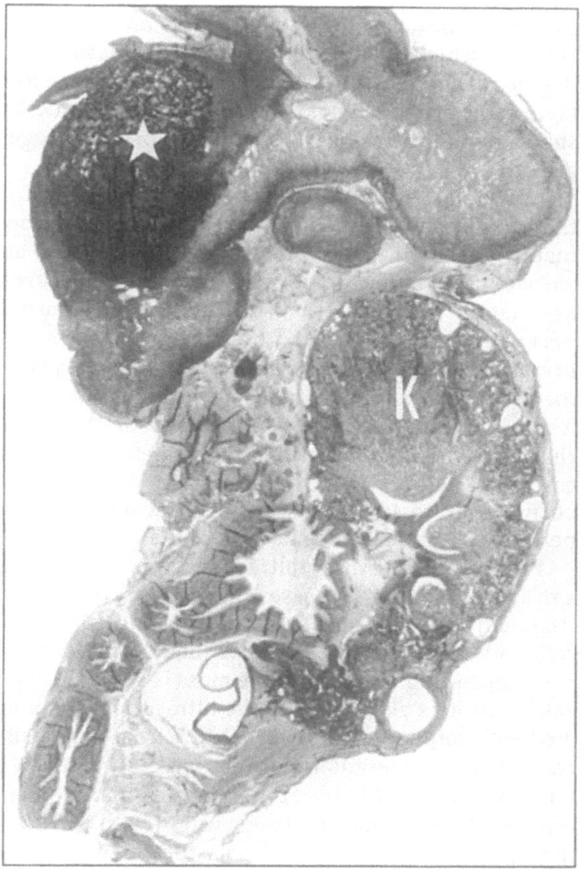

Fig. 2.9. Neuroblastoma of the adrenal medula (star). The tumor is growing above a small dyspastic kidney (K). Syndrome of Frazer or "cryptophtalmos syndrome".

guide the diagnosis and clarify the benefit to be gained from expectant management.[53] Overall, the success of surgical intervention and chemotherapy, and thus the neonatal outcome, depends on the size of the tumor and fetal lung maturation. Expectant management is, therefore, the first step. Serial ultrasound examinations should be performed to detect rapid enlargement, metastasis or secondary fetal complications, such as non-immune hydrops.

Congenital neuroblastoma

Neuroblastoma is an unconventional cancer of neuronal lineage that may occur in all sites of sympathetic ganglia from the neck to the ganglion impair in the presacral region, and including the adrenal medullae.[54,55] A genetic defect, characterised by the loss of a critical region (locus p36) in chromosome 1, is involved in the etiology.[56] The simplest "cellular" neuroblastoma is composed of a monomorphous population of hyperchromatic nuclei and scant, small, round cells. Macroscopically they appear as dark-red or purple tumors, often described as "hemorrhagic" because of their abundant sinusoidal blood supply (Fig. 2.9). Most neuroblastomas develop cell processes, and progressively Schwann cells appear, first perivascularly and then diffusely, to produce a stromal component. Mature neuroblastomas are pale and firm and often calcified producing in parts grittiness and a yellow-speckled appearance to the cut surfaces which is diagnostic of a neuroblastoma, macroscopically. All stages and degrees of aggressiveness may be present at, or before, birth. A neuroblastoma with a favourable prognosis has a low staging and mitotic-karyorrhexis index, is triploid and shows no amplification of the N-*myc* proto-oncogene, which plays a role in tumor growth.[55]

Neuroblastomas represent between 30 and 40% of all congenital tumors and are the most common malignant tumor in the newborn.[57] Their clinical features are mainly based on their size, location and humoral activity, that is, catecholamine or vasoactive intestinal polypeptide production. Neuroblastomas have been reported in association with genetic disorders such as neurofibromatosis, tuberous sclerosis, Beckwith–Wiedeman syndrome and DiGeorge syndrome.[55] The most common presentation is a microscopic, or barely visible, nodule of neuroblast in the adrenal medulla. This explains why most neuroblastomas are diagnosed after delivery. Larger lesions show degenerative features of cystic changes, hemosiderin deposition, hemorrhage and calcification, which can be detected in utero. The survival rate is higher in cases detected prenatally than in cases detected in infants. Spontaneous regression occurs in up to 40% of cases and surgical excision of the tumor during the neonatal period is curative in the majority of the cases.[57]

Prenatal diagnosis by ultrasound was first reported in 1983 by Feňart et al[58] and since then, about 60 cases have been published.[57,59] Fetal neuroblastomas are frequently well encapsulated and displace the kidney inferiorly and laterally. The right side appears to be more frequently affected. The sonographic appearance may vary depending on whether the mass is solid, purely cystic or mixed. The presence of calcification is also useful to the ultrasonographer and its presence has been associated with improved survival.[55] Differential diagnosis includes other adrenal tumors, renal, hepatic, mesenteric or ovarian cyst, cystic Wilms' tumor and retroperitoneal teratoma, hemangioma or lymphangioma. Non-immune fetal hydrops has been reported to occur in hemorragic tumor with chronic fetal anaemia or in massive liver invasion by the tumor.[60] Neuroblastoma cells may also infiltrate the placenta beyond the fetal capillaries and villous trophoblast with metastasis to maternal tissue. In tumors producing catecholamine, prepartum effects such as sweating, flushing, palpitations and hypertension can be observed in the mother.[57]

Congenital Leukemia

Acute congenital leukemia is the second most common fetal cancer with an incidence of 4.7 per million live births per year.[61] The diagnosis of congenital leukemia includes the proliferation of blast cells together with anaemia, thrombocytopenia and leucocytosis. The true neoplastic process has to be separated from a transient myeloproliferative disorder, associated congenital infection such as cytomegalovirus, rubella and toxoplasmosis. A greater than expected frequency of congenital leukemia has been reported in association with various genetic disorders including, trisomy 21, trisomy 13, monosomy X, Bloom syndrome, Ellis–Van Creveld syndrome and Klinefelter syndrome.[62] It probably represents a transient leukemoid reaction secondary to ineffective regulation of hematopoiesis. In utero, hepatosplenomegaly and non-immune fetal hydrops is common at presentation.[60]

Rare Congenital Cancers

Sporadic heritable retinoblastoma is a rare cancerous tumor of the retina which is inherited in an autosomal dominant manner and which arises from a de novo mutation in the retinoblastoma gene (*Rb*). This mutant *Rb* gene is known to be mainly derived from the father and it may be related to exposure of paternal germ cells to carcinogens and mutagens.[63]

Primary hepatic malignant neoplasms are extremely rare in the fetus and newborns. The presence of an abdominal mass is the most frequent mode of presentation and an association with fetal hydrops has been reported.[64] Serum levels of alpha-fetoprotein are markedly elevated in the majority of the cases of hepatoblastoma and can be followed for tumor progression.

Rhabdomyosarcoma is the most common soft-tissue sarcoma in children, making up 5% of all cancer under the age of 15 years. It originates from the embryonic mesenchyme, that also gives rise to striated muscle, it is most commonly located at the level of the head and neck (Fig. 2.10) and is characterized by the loss of heterozygosity of the short arm of chromosome 11. It is very rare for these tumors to occur before one month of age and only a few cases have been described during pregnancy.[66,67,68] In these cases, the tumor appears as rapidly growing masses of irregular contour and fibroid-like appearance.[68]

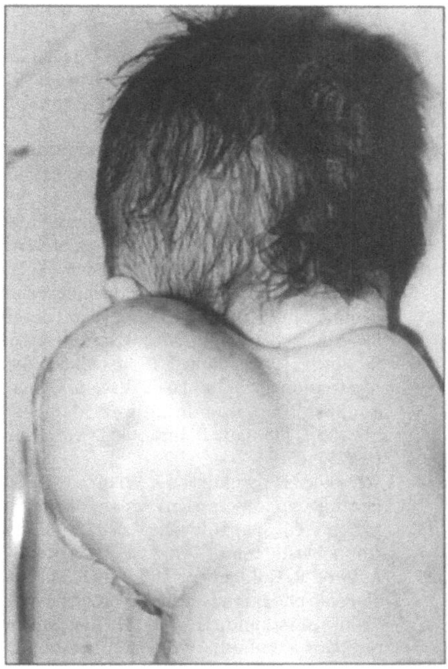

Fig. 2.10. Rhabdomyosarcoma of the fetal neck.

References

1. Fox H. Pathology of the placenta. 2nd edition. Saunders, London, 1997.
2. Szulman AE, Surti U. The syndromes of hydatidiform mole. I. Cytogenetic and morphologic correlations. Am J Obstet Gynecol 978;131:665–71.
3. Szulman AE, Surti U. The syndromes of hydatidiform mole. II. Morphologic evolution of the complete and partial mole. Am J Obstet Gynecol 1978;132:22–7.
4. Jeffers MD, O'Dwyer P, Curran B, Leader M, Gillian JE. Partial hydatidiform mole: A common but underdiagnosed condition. Int J Gynecol Pathol 1993;12:315–23.
5. Palmer JR. Advances in the epidemiology of gestational trophoblastic tumors. J Reprod Med 1994;39:155–62.
6. Kajii T, Ohama K. Androgenic origin of hydatidiform mole. Nature 1977;268:633–4.
7. Jacobs PA, Szulman AE, Funkhouser J, Matsuura JS, Wilson CC. Human triploidy: relationship between parental origin of the additional haploid complement and development of partial hydatidiform mole. Ann Hum Genet 1982;46:223–31.
8. McFadden DE, Kwong LC, Yam IYL, Langlois S. Parental origin of triploidy in human fetuses: evidence from genomic imprinting. Hum Genet 1993;92:465–9.
9. Jauniaux E. Partial moles: from postnatal to prenatal diagnosis. Placenta 1999;20:379–88.
10. Kohorn EI, Blackwell RJ. The diagnosis of hydatidiform mole by ultrasonic B-scanning. J Obstet Gynaec Brit Cwlth 1968;75:1014–8.
11. Jauniaux E. Ultrasound diagnosis and follow-up of gestational trophoblastic disease. Ultrasound Obstet Gynecol 1998;11:367–77
12. Steller MA, Genest DR, Bernstein MR, Lage JM, Goldstein DP, Berkowitz RS. Natural history of twin pregnancy with complete hydatidiform mole and coexisting fetus. Obstet Gynecol 1994;83:35–42.
13. Jauniaux E, Nicolaides KH. Early ultrasound diagnosis and follow-up of molar pregnancies. Ultrasound Obstet Gynecol 1997;9:17–21.
14. Jauniaux E, Campbell S. Ultrasonographic assessment of placental abnormalities. Am J Obstet Gynecol 1990;163:1650–8.
15. Jauniaux E, Brown R, Rodeck C, Nicolaides KH. Prenatal diagnosis of triploidy during the second trimester of pregnancy. Obstet Gynecol 1996;88:983–9.
16. Jauniaux E, Brown R, Snijders RJM, Noble P, Nicolaides K. Early renatal diagnosis of triploidy. Am J Obstet Gynecol 1997;176, 550–4.
17. Berkowitz RS, Goldstein DP. Chorionic tumors. N Eng J Med 1996;335:1740–8.
18. Szulman AE, Surti U, Bernan M. Patient with partial mole requiring chemotherapy. Lancet 1978;2:1099.
19. Bagshave KD, Lawler SD, Paradinas FJ, Dent J, Brown P, Boxer GM. Gestational trophoblastic tumours following initial diagnosis of partial hydatidiform mole. Lancet 1990;335:1074–6.
20. Chen RJ, Huang SC, Chow SN, Hsieh CY, Hsu HC. Persistent gestational trophoblastic tumour with partial hydatidiform mole as the antecedent pregnancy. Brit J Obstet Gynaecol 1994;101:330–4.
21. Flam F, Lundstrom V. Twenty years' experience of treating gestational trophoblastic neoplasia in Sweden. Acta Obstet Gynecol Scand 1989;68:65–9.
22. Berkowitz RS, Birnholz J, Goldstein DP, Berstein MR. Pelvic ultrasonography and the management of gestational trophoblastic disease. Gynecol Oncol 1983;15:403–12.
23. Boultbee JE, Newlands ES. New therapeutic approaches of gestational trophoblastic tumors. In Bourne T, Jauniaux E, Jurkovic D, eds. Transvaginal Colour Doppler. Heidelberg. Springer-Verlag, 1995:57–68.
24. Schneider DF, Bukovsky I, Weinraub Z, Golan A, Caspi E. Transvaginal ultrasound diagnosis and treatment follow-up of invasive gestational trophoblastic disease. J Clin Ultrasound 1990;18:110–3.
25. Mangili G, Spagnolo D, Valsecchi L, Maggi R. Transvaginal ultrasonography in persistent trophoblastic tumor. Am J Obstet Gynecol 1993;169:1218–23.
26. Achiron R, Goldenberg M, Lipitz S, Mashiach S. Transvaginal duplex Doppler ultrasonography in bleeding patients suspected of having residual trophoblastic tissue. Obstet Gynecol 1993;81:507–11.
27. Flam F, Lindholm H, Bui TH, Lundstrom-Lindstedt V. Color Doppler studies in trophoblastic tumours: a prelininary report. Ultrasound Obstet Gynecol 1991;1:249–52.
28. Tepper R, Shulman A, Altaras M, Goldberger S, Maymon R, Holzinger M, Beyth Y. The role of color Doppler flow in the management of nonmetastatic gestational trophoblastic disease. Gynecol Obstet Invest 1994;38:14–7.
29. Chan FY, Chau MT, Pun TC, Lam C, Ngan HYS, Wong RLC. A comparison of colour Doppler sonography and the pelvic arteriogram in assessment of patients with gestational trophoblastic disease. Brit J Obstet Gynecol 1995;102:720–5.

30. Maymon R, Schneider D, Shulman A, Bukovsky I, Weinraub Z. Serial color Doppler flow of uterine vasculature combined with serum β-hCG measurements for improved monitoring of patients with gestational trophoblastic disease. Gynecol Obstet Invest 1996;42:201–205.
31. Zanetta G, Lissoni A, Colombo M, Marzola M, Cappellini A, Mangioni C. Detection of abnormal intrauterine vascularization by color Doppler imaging: a possible additional aid for the follow up of patients with gestational trophoblastic tumors. Ultrasound Obstet Gynecol 1996;7:32–7.
32. Kawano M, Masuzaki H, Ishimaru T. Transvaginal color Doppler studies in gestational trophoblastic disease. Ultrasound Obstet Gynecol 1996;7:197–200.
33. Long MG, Boultbee JE, Begent RH, Hanson ME, Bagshawe KD. Preliminary Doppler studies on the uterine artery and myometrium in trophoblastic tumours requiring chemotherapy. Brit J Obstet Gynecol 1990;97:686–9.
34. Long MG, Boultbee JE, Langley R, Newlands ES, Begent RH, Bagshawe KD. Doppler assessment of the uterine circulation and the clinical behaviour of gestational trophoblastic tumors requiring chemotherapy. Br J Cancer 1992;66:883–7.
35. Hsieh FJ, Wu CC, Chen CA, Chen TM, Hsieh CY, Chen HY. Correlation of uterine hemodynamics with chemotherapy response in gestational trophoblastic tumors. Obstet Gynecol 1994;83:1021–5.
36. Lindholm H, Radestad A, Flam F. Hysteroscopy provides proof of trophoblastic tumors in three cases with negative color Doppler images. Ultrasound Obstet Gynecol 1997;9:59–61.
37. Caspi B, Elchalal U, Dgani R, Ben-Hur H, Rozenman D, Nissim F. Invasive mole and placental site trophoblastic tumor. Two entities of gestational trophoblastic disease with a common ultrasonographic appearance. J Ultrasound Med 1991;10:517–9.
38. Aoki S, Hata T, Hata K, Senoh D, Miyakado J, Takamiya O, Iwanari O, Kitao M. Doppler color flow mapping of an invasive mole. Gynecol Obstet Invest 1989;27:52–4.
39. Desai RK, Desberg AL. Diagnosis of gestational trophoblastic disease: Value of endovaginal color flow Doppler sonography. AJR 1991;157:787–8.
40. Chau MT, Chan FY, Pun TC, Leong L. Perforation of the uterus by an invasive mole using color Doppler ultrasound: case report. Ultrasound Obstet Gynecol 1993;3:51–3.
41. Sakamoto C, Oikawa K, Kashimura M, Egashira K. Sonographic appearance of placental site tumor. J Ultrasound Med 1990;9:533–5.
42. Abulafia O, Sherer D, Fultz P, Sternberg LB, Angel C. Unusual endovaginal ultrasonography and magnetic resonance imaging of placental site trophoblastic tumor. Am J Obstet Gynecol 1993;170:750–2.
43. Todd A, Newlands E, Palazzo M. Unusual case of choriocarcinoma ocurring 12 months after delivery. B M J 1998;316:532–4.
44. Fleischer AC, James AE, Krause DA, Mills JB. Sonographic patterns in trophoblastic disease. Radiology 1978;126:215–20.
45. Lurain JR, Sand PK, Brewer JI. Choriocarcinoma associated with ectopic pregnancy. Obstet Gynecol 1986;68:286–7.
46. Brewer JL, Mazur MT. Gestational choriocarcinoma: its origin in the placenta during seemingly normal pregnancy. Am J Surg Pathol 1981;5:267–77.
47. Hallam LA, McLaren KM, El-jabbour JN, Helm CW, Smart GE. Intraplacental choriocarcinoma: a case report. Placenta 1990;11:247–51.
48. Christopherson WA, Kanbour A, Szulman AE. Choriocarcinoma in a term placenta with maternal metastases. Gynecol Oncol 1992;46:239–45.
49. Heifetz SA, Czaja J. In situ choriocarcinoma arising in partial hydatidiform mole: Implications for the risk of persistent trophoblastic disease. Pediat Pathol 1992;12:601–11.
50. Jauniaux E, Zucker M, Meuris S, Verhest A, Wilkin P, Hustin J. Chorangiocarcinoma: An unusual tumour of the placenta. The missing link? Placenta 1988;9:607–13.
51. Trask C, Lage J, Roberts DJ. A second case of "Chorangiocarcinoma" presenting in a term asymptomatic twin pregnancy: Choriocarcinoma in situ with associated villous vascular proliferation. Int J Gynecol Pathol 1994;13:87–91.
52. Campbell WA, Storlazzi E, Vintzileos AM, Wu A, Schneiderman H, Nochinson DJ. Fetal malignant melanoma: Ultrasound presentation and review of the literature. Obsetet Gynecol 1987;70:434–9.
53. Kaminopetros P, Jauniaux E, Kane P, Weston M, Nicolaides KH, Campbell DJ. Prenatal diagnosis of an extensive fetal lymphangioma using ultrasonography, magnetic resonance imaging and cytology. Br J Radiol 1997;70:750–3.
54. Dehnerr LP. Primitive neuroectodermal tumor and Ewing's sarcoma. Am J Surg Pathol. 1993;17:1–13.
55. Chatten J. Neuroblastoma. Diseases of the fetus and newborn. In: Reed GB, Clairaux AE, Cockburn F (eds). Chapman & Hall, London. 1995.
56. Brodeur G. Neuroblastoma: clinical significance of genetic abnormality. Cancer Surv 1990;4:673–88.

57. Acharya S, Jayabose S, Kogan S, Tugal O, Beneck D, Leslie D, Slim M. Prenatally diagnosed neuroblastoma. Cancer 1997;80:304–10.
58. Fenart D, Deville A, Donzeau M, Bruneton J. Neuroblastome rétropéritoneal diagnostiqué in utero. A propos d'un cas. J Radiol 1983;64:359–61.
59. Kesrouani A, Duchatel F, Seilanian M, Murray JM. Prenatal diagnosis of adrenal neuroblastoma by ultrasound: a report of two cases and review of the literature. Ultrasound Obstet Gynecol 1999;13:446–9.
60. Jauniaux E, Kaminopetros P, Rodeck C. Hydrops fetalis. In: Brace RA, Hanson M, Rodeck C (eds). Body fluids and kidney function, Cambridge: University Press, 1997:207–30.
61. Badder JL, Miller RW. US cancer incidence and mortality in the first year of life. Am J Dis Child 1979;133:157–9.
62. Rosner F, Lee SL. Downs' syndrome and acute leukemia: myeloblastic or lymphoblastic. Am J Med 1972;53:203–18.
63. DerKinderen DJ, Koten JW, Tan KE. Parental age in sporadic hereditary retinoblastoma. Am J Ophtalmol 1990;110:605–9.
64. Kazzi NJ, Chang CH, Roberts EC, Shankaran S. Fetal hepatoblastoma presenting as nonimmune hydrops. Am J Perinatol 1989;66:278–80.
65. Pharham DM. The molecular biology of childhood rhabdomyosarcoma. Semin Diagn Pathol 1994;11:39–46.
66. Hart PS, Boudurtha J, McCall JB, Brown JA. Prenatal detection of non-cardiac rhabdomyosarcoma. Prenat Diagn 1990;10:169–73.
67. Pautard B, Canarelli JP, Gontier MF, Risbourg B, Puissant C, Flamant F. Embryonal rhabdomyosarcoma diagnosed antenatally. Arch Fr Pediatr 1990;47:433–5.
68. Onderoglu LS, Yucel A, Yuce K. Prenatal sonographic features of embryonal rhabdomyosarcoma. Ultrasound Obstet Gynecol 1999;13:210–2.

3. Breast Cancer and Pregnancy

Elizabeth Shah and Christobel Saunders

"...in the face of general enthusiasm for terminating the pregnancy we believe the evidence is that the cancer should be terminated." *B. F. Byrd, 1962*

Introduction

Traditionally "gestational breast cancer" is defined as breast cancer diagnosed during pregnancy or lactation and up to a year post-partum (Prosperi Porta et al. 1998). However it is unlikely that this narrow definition is biologically sound as it does not take into account the prolonged subclinical period in the natural history of breast cancer. In young women, this subclinical or preclinical phase may be from as long as 3 to 5 years based on current knowledge of growth rates (Moolgavkar et al. 1980). Moreover, should we be defining "gestational breast cancer" at all? By defining it we raise it to the status of a special disease entity in its own right, whereas recently it has been suggested that breast cancer and pregnancy should be considered two entirely separate conditions with none of the traditional interactions jointly attributed to them (Merkel 1996).

Breast cancer is a disease of older women. In the UK one in twelve women will develop breast cancer, but of these only 15% will be in women of reproductive age, that is, below 50 years old (Fig. 3.1). It has been reported that 3% of women who develop breast cancer will be pregnant or lactating (White 1955; Bunker and Peters 1963) and the incidence in the young pregnant female is the same as that in the young non-pregnant woman. Between one and three per hundred thousand pregnancies are complicated by breast cancer, making this the second commonest pregnancy-related cancer after cervical cancer (Shivvers and Miller 1997). The incidence of pregnancy-related breast cancer may increase as more women delay their pregnancies until a later age (Ventura 1989) in accordance with present trends. Breast cancer associated with pregnancy is currently seen mainly in the age group of 32 to 38 years (Gallenberg and Loprinzi 1989), but of course as the age at which women conceive does increase this is also likely to rise.

Pregnancy following treatment for breast cancer is said to occur in about 7% of patients who retain fertility after adjuvant systemic therapy. It is not yet known if the

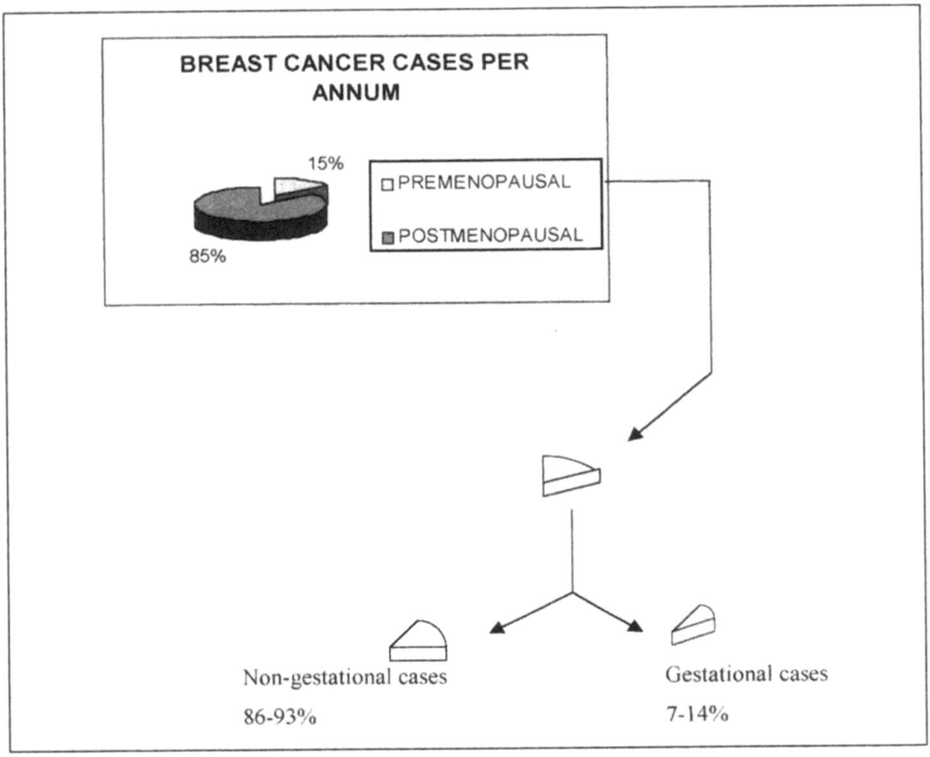

Fig. 3.1. Incidence of gestational breast cancer.

improving survival rates following breast cancer treatment (Hermon and Beral 1996) will lead to an increase in the number of women who subsequently conceive.

The combination of breast cancer and pregnancy provides a challenge both in terms of medical management of the mother and foetus, and in the management of the psychological and social issues that are invariably involved. Physicians are faced with an inadequate amount of evidence so advice offered to patients is often anecdotal. Although rare, this situation is perhaps one of the most difficult to be encountered by the breast multi-disciplinary team and presents complex dilemmas to the obstetric team: it is vital that we collect more facts.

Pathology

The pathology of pregnancy-associated breast cancer in many ways resembles that of non-pregnant premenopausal women. Although one recent study (Bonnier et al. 1997) reports an excess of inflammatory breast cancer, most other studies report the incidence of the inflammatory type of tumour as 2 to 3% (Clark and Reid 1978). There is a relatively high proportion of oestrogen receptor (ER) negative and progesterone receptor (PR) negative tumours (Nugent and O'Connell 1985), as may be expected in this young cohort of patients.

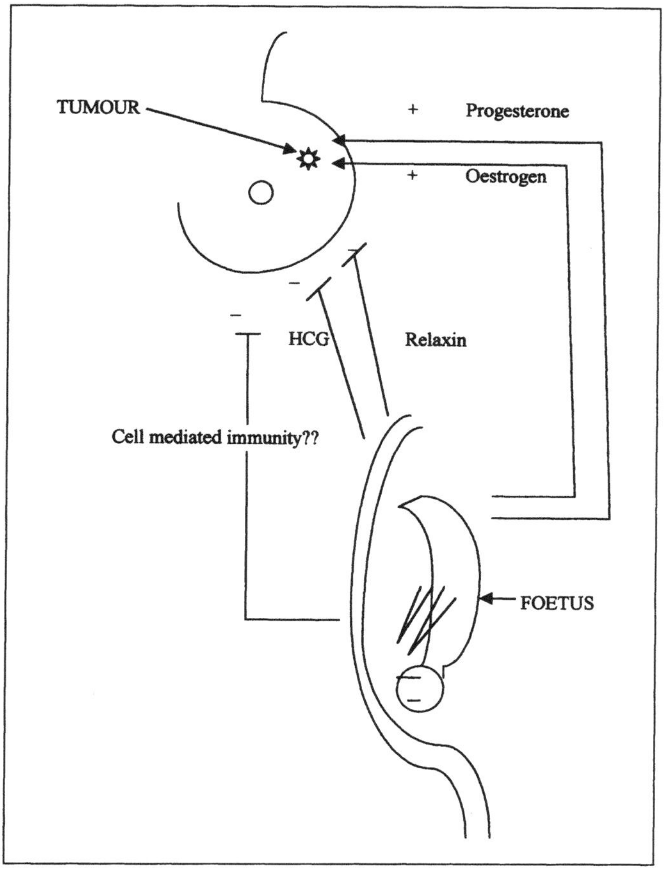

Fig. 3.2. Host–tumour interaction during pregnancy.

There are a number of host factors during pregnancy that would appear to support accelerated tumour growth (Fig.3.2). For instance, the rise in maternal serum oestrogens and progesterone and placental hormones are known to stimulate breast epithelial cell turnover and may promote tumour growth as well (McManus and Welsch 1984). The serum levels of prolactin, a hormone that promotes mammary tumourigenesis in experimental models, is also raised during pregnancy and lactation (Nagasawe 1989).

On the other hand some pregnancy-related hormones, e.g. human chorionic gonadotrophin (Meduri et al. 1997) and relaxin (Bani et al. 1995), may inhibit breast tumour growth (Fig.3.2). There is also some experimental evidence to suggest a role for pregnancy in immunising against breast cancer. Experiments testing the foetal antigen hypothesis have shown the presence of MUC1, a tumour-specific antigen, on foetal and breast cancer tissues, and multiparous women produce anti-MUC1 MHC-restricted cytotoxic T cell cytolytic activity against MUC1-bearing cancer cell lines (Botelho and Clark 1998). This is in contrast to previous hypotheses that pregnancy might have an immunosuppressive effect on the host (Purtillo 1972) and thus promote tumour growth (van der Vange and van Dongen 1991).

Diagnosis

The diagnosis of breast cancer during pregnancy is often delayed, leading to more advanced stage at presentation. Williams and Bitran quoted an average delay of 2 to 7 months (Williams and Bitran 1985). Another study demonstrated a mean delay of 10 months (Ribeiro 1986). This delay is usually caused by either patient or physician failing to notice a lump because its presence is masked by the physiological changes in the breast or by assuming that the presence of any lump can be explained by the effects of lactation rather than sinister pathology (Table 3.1). It may also be missed at antenatal checks for the same reasons.

Once a breast symptom or sign has been noted the methods of investigation are similar to those followed in the non-pregnant woman. A thorough clinical history and examination should be followed by tissue sampling by means of fine needle aspiration cytology (Sorosky and Scott-Conner 1998), corecut biopsy or excision biopsy. Imaging techniques such as mammography and ultrasound are often not useful in this group of patients. Physiologic changes in the breast make mammography more difficult to perform and to interpret during pregnancy. Max and Klamer (1984) found that the cancer could be detected mammographically in only a quarter of pregnant patients. Breast MRI in this population of patients is likely to be of little use as the breast shows widespread enhancement and there is low specificity for malignancy. There is some suggestion that MRI may cause foetal damage if performed during the first trimester. However it has been used to look for metastatic disease with good effect in pregnant women with other malignancies (M Hall-Craggs, 1999, personal communication).

Fine needle aspiration cytology (FNA) is useful in any trimester of pregnancy though the cytopathologist must be informed of the patient's obstetric condition as difficulties in diagnosis may arise leading to a false positive diagnosis of cancer (Finley et al. 1989). This is because the breast epithelium in pregnancy shows some of the features associated with carcinoma such as nuclear pleomorphism, prominent nucleoli and decrease in cell aggregation (Fig. 3.3). If FNA is inconclusive the next step is corecut biopsy. Infection rates after excision-biopsy are higher in these women and prophylactic antibiotics or suppression of lactation may be necessary if this is done.

Most staging investigations are not absolutely contraindicated in pregnancy. Bone scans should be performed only if warranted by symptoms or biochemical evidence of bony involvement (Shivvers and Miller 1997), and the patient should be adequately hydrated with a urinary catheter in situ throughout the procedure to allow prompt excretion of the radioisotope used.

Table 3.1. Differential diagnosis of breast lumps in pregnancy and lactation

Abscess
Galactocoele
Fibroadenoma (rapidly enlarging)
Infarct
Malignancy

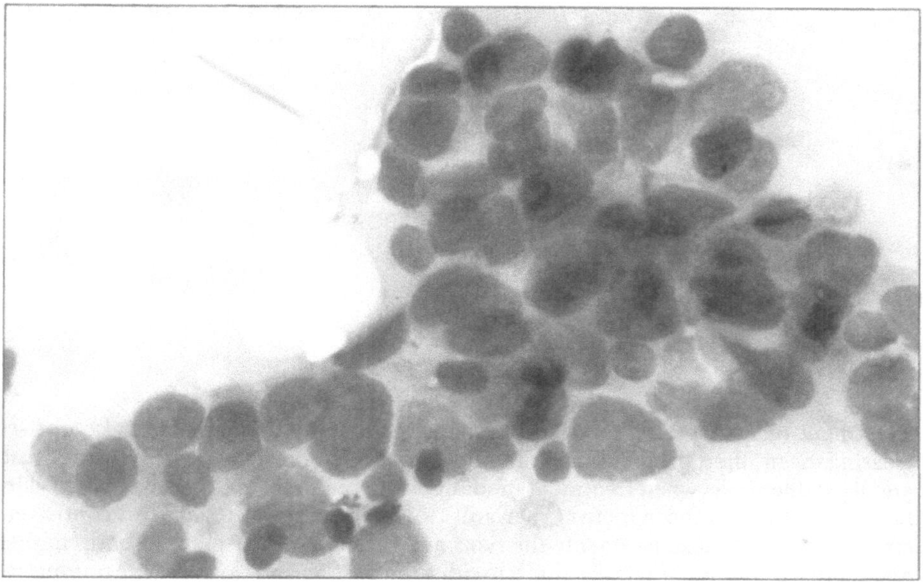

Figure 3.3. FNA of fibroadenoma in pregnancy. The breast epithelium shows nuclear pleomorphism. Mag x 600 (oil immersion). Cytology courtesy of Dr G Kocjan, University College London

Prognosis

Breast cancer survivors who decide to become pregnant may ultimately have a better outlook (Von Schoultz et al. 1995). Clark and Reid (1978) found that over half of those who became pregnant were alive at 15 years compared to only 35% of controls. They also found that the longer the time interval between diagnosis and pregnancy, the better the prognosis, and multiparous women did best of all.

Other studies seem to confirm these findings, i.e. that becoming pregnant does not lead to a worsened prognosis for breast cancer survivors (Velentgas et al. 1999). Kroman et al. (1997) identified 173 women from the Danish Cancer Registry who became pregnant after treatment for breast cancer, and found no evidence of a worse outcome. Furthermore they noted that those who had a full-term pregnancy had a reduced risk of death compared to those who had no full-term pregnancy, although this was not statistically significant (Kroman et al. 1997).

Usually a 2–3 year wait will be recommended after completion of treatment before trying for a pregnancy (Isaacs 1995) as this will allow identification of those with early recurrence and thus poor prognosis. However the decision to have a child is largely a social and personal decision and must involve full acknowledgement of the possibility of a shortened lifespan.

Contraception should take the form of barrier methods as there may be a small, albeit ill-defined, risk in taking the oral contraceptive pill.

Table 3.2. Reasons for low incidence of pregnancy following breast cancer

Under-reporting of cases
Poor survival rates in young women
Recurrence of cancer
Psycho-social reasons (Siegel 1997)
– fear of disease recurrence
– fear of offspring with genetic susceptibility
– personal stress

Treatment

Treatment of breast carcinoma in pregnancy is a complex matter as it comprises treating the mother, the foetus and the whole family. In addition, it gives rise to ethical and legal dilemmas when treatment modalities offered to the mother may potentially be harmful to the unborn foetus (Theriault 1992). The best way to face this controversial situation is to discuss openly the risks and benefits of treatment to both mother and foetus and strike a balance that provides the best options available. Appropriate psychological support for the patient and her partner is vital, as is the involvement of the obstetric team from the outset.

Treatment should begin as soon as possible after diagnosis. Termination of pregnancy does not confer a survival advantage to the mother (Sorosky and Scott-Conner 1998) and is therefore not routinely indicated. However if the patient is in the first trimester and requires chemotherapy, or if the diagnosis of pregnancy is made during radiotherapy, then abortion needs to be considered as the risk of teratogenesis is considerable (Doll et al. 1988). The ultimate decision in such a case, however, would rest with the patient and her partner.

Surgery

Surgery is usually first line treatment with mastectomy and axillary clearance being the treatment of choice as it circumvents the need for adjuvant radiotherapy. Anaesthesia can be carried out safely provided due allowance is made for the physiological changes of pregnancy, such as increase in circulatory volume, postural hypotension and delayed gastric emptying. Foetal monitoring may also be advisable (Peterson and Finster 1979). If breast reconstruction is to be done it should probably be performed at a later date i.e. after pregnancy and lactation, when the contralateral breast reverts to its former size.

Radiotherapy

Breast irradiation is contraindicated in pregnancy (Winchester and Cox 1992; Mayr et al. 1998). Substantial foetal exposure occurs in spite of abdominal shielding. This can therefore only be an option in women who are nearing the end of the third trimester, in whom it is possible to delay the radiotherapy until after delivery, or in women who decide to terminate their pregnancy on diagnosis.

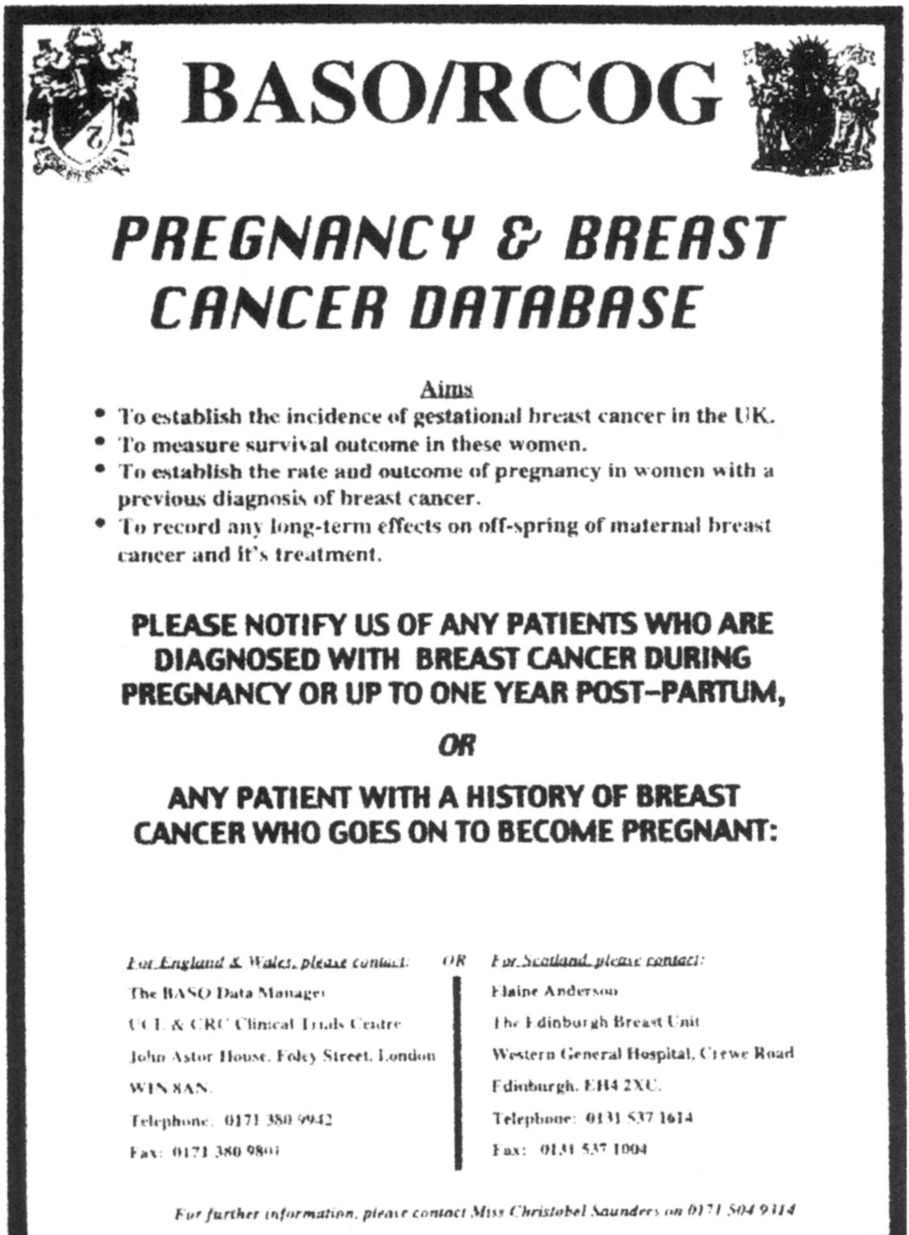

BASO/RCOG

PREGNANCY & BREAST CANCER DATABASE

Aims

- To establish the incidence of gestational breast cancer in the UK.
- To measure survival outcome in these women.
- To establish the rate and outcome of pregnancy in women with a previous diagnosis of breast cancer.
- To record any long-term effects on off-spring of maternal breast cancer and it's treatment.

PLEASE NOTIFY US OF ANY PATIENTS WHO ARE DIAGNOSED WITH BREAST CANCER DURING PREGNANCY OR UP TO ONE YEAR POST-PARTUM,

OR

ANY PATIENT WITH A HISTORY OF BREAST CANCER WHO GOES ON TO BECOME PREGNANT:

For England & Wales, please contact:	OR	For Scotland, please contact:
The BASO Data Manager		Elaine Anderson
UCL & CRC Clinical Trials Centre		The Edinburgh Breast Unit
John Astor House, Foley Street, London		Western General Hospital, Crewe Road
W1N 8AN.		Edinburgh, EH4 2XU.
Telephone: 0171 380 9942		Telephone: 0131 537 1614
Fax: 0171 380 9801		Fax: 0131 537 1004

For further information, please contact Miss Christobel Saunders on 0171 504 9314

Fig. 3.4. The UK pregnancy and breast cancer database circular.

The scatter dose to the foetus can be estimated, being dependent on the dose of radiation, field size and positioning of the field centre and on the trimester of pregnancy (van der Vange and van Dongen 1991). Thus in the first trimester, while the foetus is still lying within the true pelvis, with shielding in place, only 0.2 to 0.3% of the total radiation dose will reach the foetus (van der Vange and van Dongen 1991). However a foetus nearing full term will receive nearly 4%. On the other hand, the greatest risk to the foetus is during the first trimester when organogenesis is taking place (Petrek 1994).

Chemotherapy

Combination chemotherapy improves both disease-free survival and overall survival in premenopausal women (Bonadonna et al. 1995). Therefore it would be wrong to deny pregnant women this form of treatment for breast cancer. However this raises important questions regarding foetal teratogenesis and carcinogenesis. Doll's review of the literature (1988) showed that there was a high incidence of foetal malformations if chemotherapy was given in the first trimester, especially if folate antagonists like methotrexate were used. Conversely the risk of teratogenesis in the second and third trimesters is very low, and the use of chemotherapy should therefore be restricted to this period of pregnancy. There may however be growth restriction in a proportion of infants and increased rate of stillbirths in women treated with cytotoxics in the second and third trimesters (Zemlickis et al. 1992).

A recent study (Berry et al. 1999) has reported that pregnant women can be safely treated with combination chemotherapy during the second and third trimesters. The regimen used was cyclophosphamide, doxorubicin and fluorouracil, and they found that all infants were born with normal Apgar scores and normal birthweights.

Breastfeeding is contraindicated in women receiving chemotherapy as these drugs are excreted in breast milk (Theriault et al. 1992).

Long-term effects such as future sterility in offspring of these women remain undocumented so far, but it is hoped that such data will be forthcoming.

Neo-adjuvant chemotherapy is increasingly offered to young women with inoperable tumours. Again there is no absolute contraindication to this regimen in pregnant women in the second and third trimester.

Most oncologists using chemotherapy to treat these patients will liaise with the patient's obstetrician to plan a delivery, so that the timing of chemotherapy treatments can be arranged accordingly.

Hormonal Therapy

Most gestational breast cancers are ER negative so the patient will not benefit from hormonal therapy. At present there is insufficient data on the use of hormonal ablation therapy for breast cancer during pregnancy. Tamoxifen is potentially teratogenic and the effects of LHRH analogues on human pregnancy are not yet known.

LHRH analogue treatment, in the form of the drug Zoladex, is now advocated for the treatment of premenopausal women with ER positive early breast cancer. The results of a large multi-centre randomized controlled trial has shown definite benefit of Zoladex therapy over other forms of adjuvant therapy in terms of disease-free survival (Rutqvist 1999). In animal models, research carried out by the manufacturers showed that Zoladex did not display significant teratogenic effects although there was evidence of transfer across the placental barrier in both rats and rabbits. As its potential effect on human pregnancy is at present unknown it should not be used in such circumstances.

Treatment of Advanced Stage Disease

If diagnosed in early pregnancy termination is usually recommended, followed by palliative control of the patient's symptoms. However, diagnosis of advanced breast cancer in late pregnancy can present a complex problem, and delivery of the baby by Caesarian section should be carried out as soon as feasible. Close co-ordination is required between the obstetricians, breast care surgeon and oncologist and the nurse counsellors.

There have been no reports of metastases to the foetus but there have been documented cases of metastases to the placenta, although very rare (Eltorky et al. 1995).

Breastfeeding

Breastfeeding is contraindicated while a patient is receiving chemotherapy as the cytotoxic drugs can be excreted in the mother's milk (Theriault 1992), but it can be safely carried out in any pregnancies subsequent to prior treatment of breast cancer. Radiotherapy produces considerable changes in the breast epithelium and thus decreases the likelihood of successful lactation, while surgery for centrally placed lesions probably decreases the capacity to lactate more than surgery to the breast periphery (Varsos and Yahalom 1991, Higgins and Haffty 1994).

Pregnancy After Breast Cancer

Pregnancy subsequent to breast cancer is usually uneventful and thus may be overlooked or undocumented at follow-up (Clark and Reid 1978). This will lead to under-recording the rate of subsequent pregnancies in breast cancer survivors.

The available data suggest that only a very small minority of patients go on to produce offspring after treatment for breast cancer. The reasons for this are manifold. The decision to have children after breast cancer is not made lightly. Patients and their families are aware of the enormous social, psychological and economic implications involved that require a great deal of soul-searching before such a decision can be taken. This will lead to them either avoiding pregnancy or opting for termination. Moreover a significant proportion of women will be rendered infertile by their treatment.

Fertility After Breast Cancer

Adjuvant radiotherapy to the breast does not affect fertility in premenopausal patients. Tamoxifen can cause menstrual irregularities in young women and increase serum oestradiol levels, thus leading to sub-fertility. In older, perimenopausal women, it appears to hasten the onset of ovarian failure.

Chemotherapy, on the other hand, is far more likely to cause menstrual disturbances and infertility in the long term. Chemotherapy is used extensively in the treatment of premenopausal women with breast cancer (Rose and Davis 1977; Padmanabhan et al. 1986; Pagani et al. 1998) and has been shown to cause amenorrhoea in more than 60% of patients (Padmanabhan et al. 1986; Pagani et al. 1998). The incidence of amenorrhoea after CMF chemotherapy was higher in older patients with a reported incidence of 74% in patients above 40 years old and only 18% in women below 40 (Pagani et al. 1998).

Cytotoxic agents that attack rapidly dividing cells can destroy the proliferating granulosa and theca cells which are the main components of developing follicles. Secondly, alkylating agents that alter cellular DNA can also destroy non-proliferating primordial follicles. Since these cells cannot regenerate the resulting loss of ova is irreversible. This has been well illustrated by experiments showing that cyclophosphamide causes a reduction in the number of ovarian follicles in mature rats (Ataya et al. 1985). It has been proposed that this occurs in two phases, initially destruction of large follicles and, on prolonged treatment, loss of primordial follicles as well (Ataya et al. 1985).

It is not yet known for certain if chemotherapy can induce primordial follicles to undergo apoptosis in a manner similar to the processes seen in the ovary in foetal life (Brook and Marshall 1996) and adult life (Amsterdam et al. 1997).

There are a number of options available to young women who wish to preserve their fertility. Embryo cryopreservation, in vitro fertilisation (IVF) and oocyte donation are the main available options. Some studies have shown that concurrent LHRH analogue administration with chemotherapy may protect the ovary from damage and thus preserve fertility (Blumenfeld et al. 1996). The value of LHRH analogue therapy in preventing chemotherapy-induced ovarian failure has recently been explored in a group of premenopausal breast cancer patients (Shah 1999). However, the results are not conclusive at the present time, and the authors are collecting further data for analysis. The most recent development in this area is that of ovarian tissue autografting, which has been tried successfully in animal models (Gosden et al. 1994) and has now been reported in two human patients (unpublished data). Cancer patients can now be offered ovarian tissue banking prior to starting cytotoxic treatment with a view to re-implantation at a future date when their disease is in remission. This technique is still in its infancy and further results will be awaited with much interest.

Conclusion

Pregnancy-associated breast cancer is rare and thus the individual clinician's experience is likely to be sparse. Management of this condition requires a team approach involving obstetrician, oncologist, surgeon and nurse counsellors.

The relative lack of compiled data on this subject may soon be rectified by a United Kingdom database that is already up and running. This seeks to keep a record of all women presenting with breast cancer during pregnancy or lactation and also those breast cancer patients who go on to become pregnant (Fig. 3.4).

Current evidence suggests that breast cancer during pregnancy follows a similar pattern to breast cancer in non-pregnant premenopausal women and as such, should be treated along similar lines with a few exceptions (Saunders and Baum 1993). Termination of pregnancy is not routinely indicated unless there is a risk to the foetus from chemotherapy or radiotherapy in the first trimester, or the mother has advanced disease.

Treatment for breast cancer, especially chemotherapy, can affect future fertility and patients need to be forewarned about this and the various options open to them fully discussed and made available. If a woman does become pregnant after breast cancer, her prognosis will not change for the worse, and paradoxically, it may even improve.

References

Amsterdam A, Dantes A, Selvaraj N and Aharoni D (1997). Apoptosis in steroidogenic cells: structure-function analysis. Steroids 62, 207–11

Ataya KM. McKanna JA. Weintraub AM, Clark MR and LeMaire WJ. (1985). A luteinising hormone-releasing hormone agonist for the prevention of chemotherapy-induced ovarian follicular loss in rats. Cancer Res 45, 3651–6

Bani D, Masini E, Bello MG, Bigazzi M and Sacchi TB (1995). Relaxin activates the L-arginine-nitric oxide pathway in human breast cancer cells. Cancer Res 55(22):5272–5

Berry DL, Theriault RL, Holmes FA, et al. (1999). Management of breast cancer during pregnancy using a standardized protocol. J Clin Oncol 17(3):855–61

Blumenfeld Z, Avivi I, Linn S, Epelbaum R, Ben-Shahar M and Haim N (1996). Prevention of irreversible chemotherapy-induced ovarian damage in young women with lymphoma by a gonadotrophin-releasing hormone agonist in parallel to chemotherapy. Hum Reprod 11:1620–6

Bonadonna G, Valagussa P, Moliterni A, Zambetti M, Brambilla C (1995). Adjuvant cyclophosphamide, methotrexate, and fluorouracil in node-positive breast cancer: the results of 20 years of follow-up. N Engl J Med 332(14):901–6

Bonnier P, Romain S, Dilhhuydy JM, et al. (1997). Influence of pregnancy on the outcome of breast cancer: a case–control study. Int J Cancer 72:720–7

Botelho F and Clark DA (1998). How might pregnancy immunize against breast cancer? Am J Reprod Immunol 39(4):279–83

Brook CGD and Marshall NJ (1996). Reproductive endocrinology. In: Essential Endocrinology. Oxford: Blackwell Science

Bunker ML and Peters MV (1963). Breast cancer associated with pregnancy or lactation. Am J Obstet Gynecol 85:312–21

Byrd BF, Bayer DS, Robertson JC et al. (1962). Treatment of breast tumours associated with pregnancy and lactation. Ann Surg 155:940–7

Clark RM and Chua T (1989). Breast cancer and pregnancy: the ultimate challenge. Clin Oncol 1:11–18

Clark RM and Reid J (1978). Carcinoma of the breast in pregnancy and lactation. Int J Radiat Oncol Biol Phys 4:693–8

Doll D, Ringenberg Q, Yarbro J (1988). Management of cancer during pregnancy. Arch Intern Med 148:2058–64

Eltorky M, Khare UK, Osborne P, Shanklin DR (1995). Placental metastasis from maternal carcinoma. A report of three cases. J Reprod M 40(5):399–403

Finley JL, Silverman JF, Lannin DR (1989). Fine-needle cytology of breast masses in pregnant and lactating women. Diagn Cytopathol 5:255–60

Gallenberg MM and Loprinzi CL (1989). Breast cancer and pregnancy. Semin Oncol 16(5):369–76

Gosden RG, Baird DT, Wade JC and Webb R (1994). Restoration of fertility to oophorectomized sheep by ovarian autografts stored at −196°C. Hum Reprod 9:597–603

Hermon C, Beral V (1996). Breast cancer mortality rates are levelling off or beginning to decline in many western countries: analysis of time trends, age–cohort and age–period models of breast cancer mortality in 20 countries. Br J Cancer 73:955–60

Higgins S and Haffty BG (1994). Pregnancy and lactation after breast-conserving therapy for early stage breast cancer. Cancer 73(8):2175–80

Isaacs JH (1995). Cancer of the breast in pregnancy. Surg Clin North Am 75(1):47–51

Kroman N, Jensen M-B, Melbye M, Wohlfahrt J, Mouridsen HT (1997). Should women be advised against pregnancy after breast cancer treatment? Lancet 350:319–22

Max MH and Klamer TW (1984). Breast cancer in 120 women under 35 years old. Ann Surg 50:23–5

Mayr NA, Wen BC, Saw CB (1998). Radiation therapy during pregnancy. Obstet Gynecol Clin North Am 25(2):301–21

McManus MJ and Welsch CW. (1984). The effect of oestrogen, progesterone, thyroxine and human placental lactogen on DNA synthesis of human breast ductal epithelium maintained in athymic nude mice. Cancer 54:1920–7

Meduri G, Charnaux N, Loosfelt H, et al. (1997). Leutinizing hormone/human chorionic gonadotrophin receptors in breast cancer. Cancer Res 57:857–64

Merkel DE (1996). Pregnancy and breast cancer. Semin Surg Oncol 12(5):370–5
Moolgavkar SH, Day NE and Stevens RG (1980). Two-stage model for carcinogenesis: epidemiology of breast cancer in females. J Natl Cancer Inst 65(3):559–69
Nagasawe H. (1989). Prolactin and oestrogen in mammary tumorigenesis. Cancer Growth Prog 6:80–86
Nugent P and O'Connell TX (1985). Breast cancer and pregnancy. Arch Surg 120:1221–4
Padmanabhan N, Howell A and Rubens RD (1986). Mechanism of action of adjuvant chemotherapy in early breast cancer. Lancet ii, 411–4
Pagani O, O'Neill A, Castiglione M, et al. (1998). Prognostic impact of amenorrhoea after adjuvant chemotherapy in premenopausal breast cancer patients with axillary node involvement: results of the international breast cancer study group (IBCSG) trial VI. Eur J. Cancer 34, 632–40
Peterson H and Finster M (1979). Anesthetic risk in the pregnant surgical patient. Anesthesiology 51:430–51
Petrek JA (1994). Breast cancer during pregnancy. Cancer supplement 74(1):518–27
Prosperi Porta R, Montruccoli-Salmi D, Lalle M, et al. (1998). Pregnancy-associated breast cancer. Eur J Gynaecol Oncol 19(4):401–4
Purtillo DT, Hallgren HM, Yunis EJ (1972). Depressed maternal lymphocyte response to phytohaemagglutinin in human pregnancy. Lancet i:769
Ribeiro G, Jones DA, Jones M. (1986). Carcinoma of the breast associated with pregnancy. Br J Surg 73:607–9
Rose DP and Davis TE (1977). Ovarian function in patients receiving adjuvant chemotherapy for breast cancer. Lancet i: 1174–6
Rutqvist LE (1999). Zoladex and tamoxifen as adjuvant therapy in pre-menopausal breast cancer: a randomised trial by the Cancer Research Campaign (CRC) Breast Cancer Trials Group, the Stockholm Breast Cancer Study Group, the South-East Sweden Breast Cancer Group and Gruppo Interdisciplinare Valutazione Interventi in Oncologia (GIVIO). Proceedings of ASCO. 18, 67a
Saunders CM and Baum M. (1993) Breast cancer and pregnancy: a review. J Royal Soc Med 86:162–5
Shah EF (1999). The role of Goserelin in the prevention of ovarian damage during chemotherapy for primary breast cancer. MSc thesis, University of London
Shivvers, SA and Miller, DS (1997). Preinvasive and invasive breast and cervical cancer prior to or during pregnancy. Clin Perinatol 24:369–89
Siegel K, Gorey E, Gluhoski V (1997). Pregnancy decision making among women previously treated for breast cancer. J Psychosocial Oncol 15(1):27–42
Sorosky JI and Scott-Conner CE (1998). Breast disease complicating pregnancy. Obstet Gynecol Clin North Am 25(2): 353–63.
Theriault RL, Stallings CB, Buzdar AU. (1992). Pregnancy and breast cancer: Clinical and legal issues. Am J Clin Oncol 15(6):535–9
van der Vange N and van Dongen JA (1991). Breast cancer and pregnancy. Eur J Surg Oncol 17:1–8
Varsos G and Yahalom J (1991). Lactation following conservation surgery and radiotherapy for breast cancer. J Surg Oncol 46:141–4
Ventura SJ (1989). First births to older mothers 1970–1986. Am J Public Health 79:1675–84
Velentgas P, Daling JR, Malone KE, et al. (1999). Pregnancy after breast carcinoma: outcomes and influence on mortality. Cancer 85(11)2301–4.
Von Schoultz E, Johansson H, Wilking N, Rutqvist L-E (1995). Influence of prior and subsequent pregnancy on breast cancer prognosis. J Clin Oncol 13(2):430–4
White TT (1955). Carcinoma of the breast in the pregnant and nursing patient. Am J Obstet Gynecol 69:1277–86
Williams SF and Bitran JD (1985). Cancer and pregnancy. Clin Perinatol 12(3): 609–23.
Winchester DP and Cox JD (1992). Standards for breast-conservation treatment. CA Cancer J Clin 42(3):134–62
Zemlickis D, Lishner M, Degendorfer P, Panzarella T, Sutcliffe SB, Koren G (1992) Fetal outcome after in utero exposure to cancer chemotherapy. Arch Intern Med 152:573–6

4. Gynecologic Malignancies in Pregnancy

Matthew L. Anderson, Giancarlo Mari and Peter E. Schwartz

Cancers originating in the reproductive tract of pregnant women challenge physicians, patients and their families in many respects. Once diagnosed, these malignancies require effective and timely treatment. However, many of the treatments presently available either risk fetal wellbeing or necessitate early delivery. Attempts to simultaneously optimize maternal and fetal wellbeing are further complicated by the paucity of well-controlled clinical evidence to guide treatment decisions. As a result, difficult ethical and moral considerations are often required of both parents and the medical team.

This chapter will review the diagnosis and treatment of gynecologic malignancies in pregnant women. Screening for cervical cancer and the evaluation of adnexal masses will receive particular attention. Focused management algorithms for both scenarios will be presented.

Cervical Cancer

The uterine cervix is the most common site of malignancy observed in pregnant women.[1] Although estimates vary, more than 1 out of every 2,200 pregnancies are associated with invasive cervical cancer. Cervical dysplasia occurs even more commonly, complicating as many as 5% of all pregnancies.[2,3] Histologically, the majority of cervical cancers (93.1%) which occur in both pregnant and non-pregnant women are squamous cell carcinomas. Adenocarcinomas (3%), anaplastic carcinomas (2.6%), adenosquamous carcinomas (1.1%), adenoacanthoma (0.1%) and sarcoma (0.1%) also occur. This distribution does not appear to differ between gravid and non-gravid women.[4,5] Several case reports of a small cell neuroendocrine carcinoma of the cervix in pregnancy have also been published.[6]

Epidemiologically, women who develop cervical intraepithelial neoplasia or invasive cancer in pregnancy tend to marry at an earlier age, have a higher parity and be diagnosed at an earlier age than non-gravid controls. Similar to the non-pregnant woman, human papilloma virus (HPV) is strongly associated with both cervical dysplasia and invasive cervical cancer and is believed to play an important etiologic role in the sequential development of these lesions.[7] Because the squamocolumnar junction of the cervix migrates out along the ectocervix in response to the increased

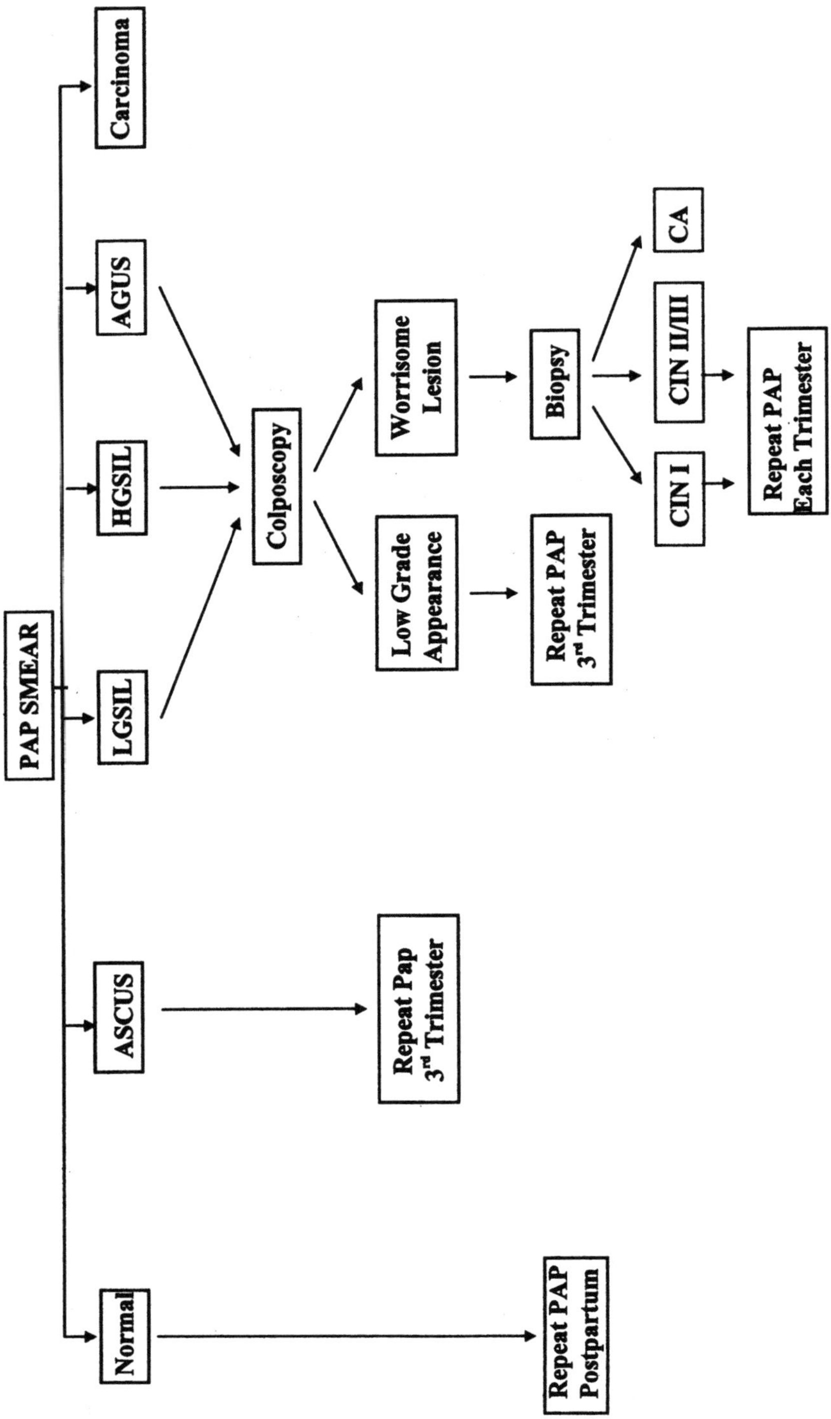

Fig. 4.1. Evaluation of cervical cytology in the gravid patient.

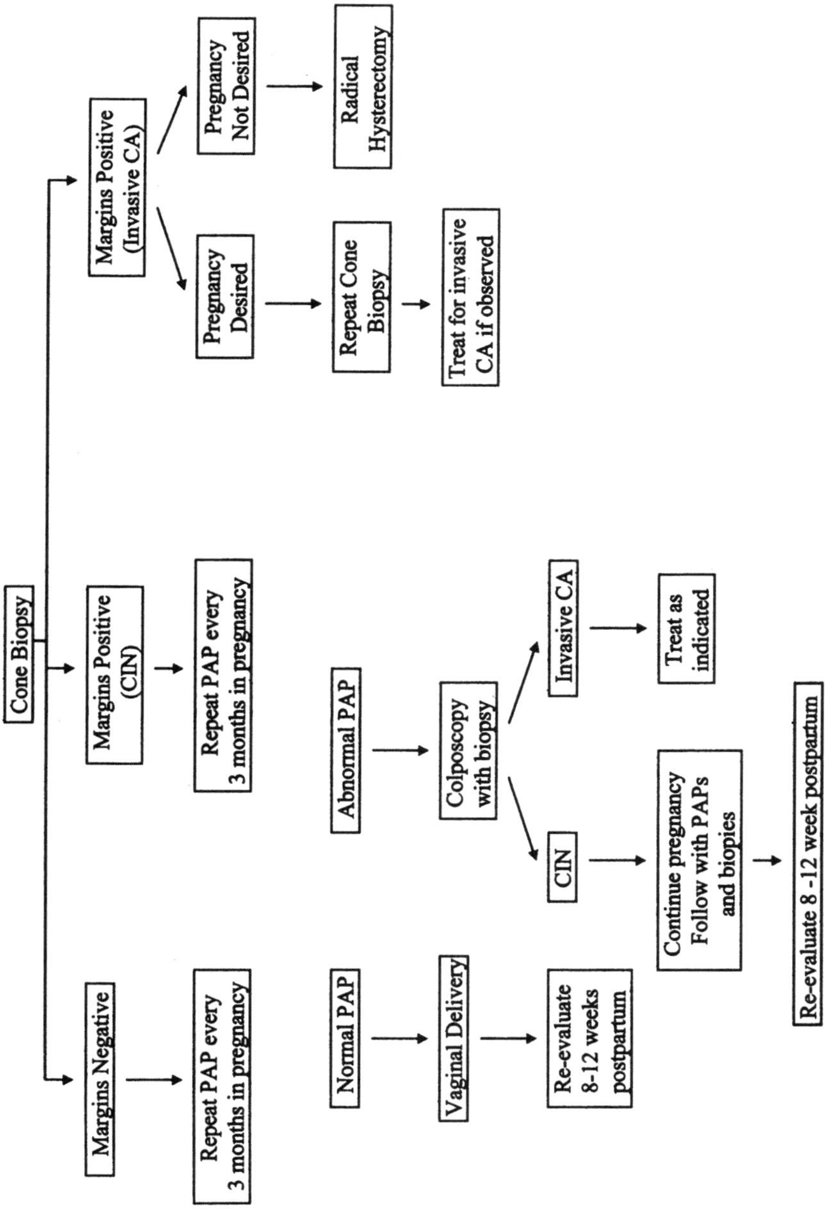

Fig. 4.2. Management of Stage Ia1 and Ia2 cervical cancer in pregnancy.

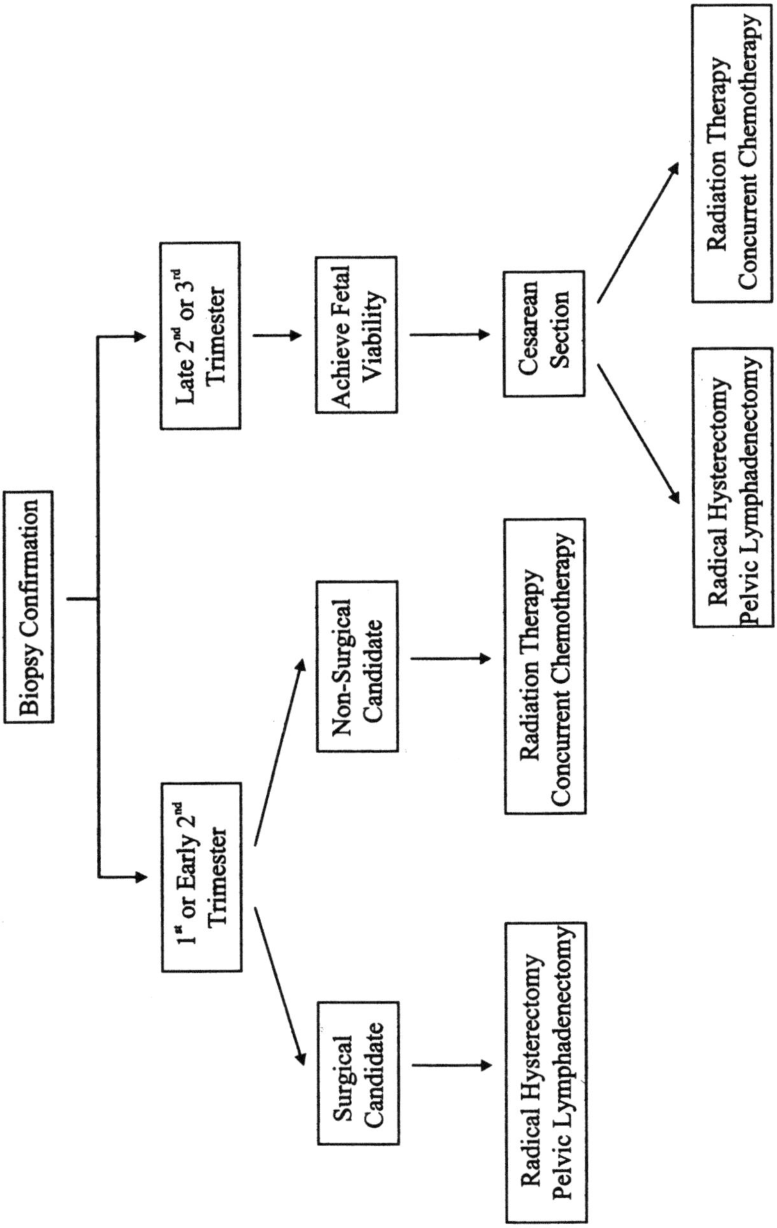

Fig. 4.3. Management of Stage Ib1 or IIa cervical cancer in pregnancy.

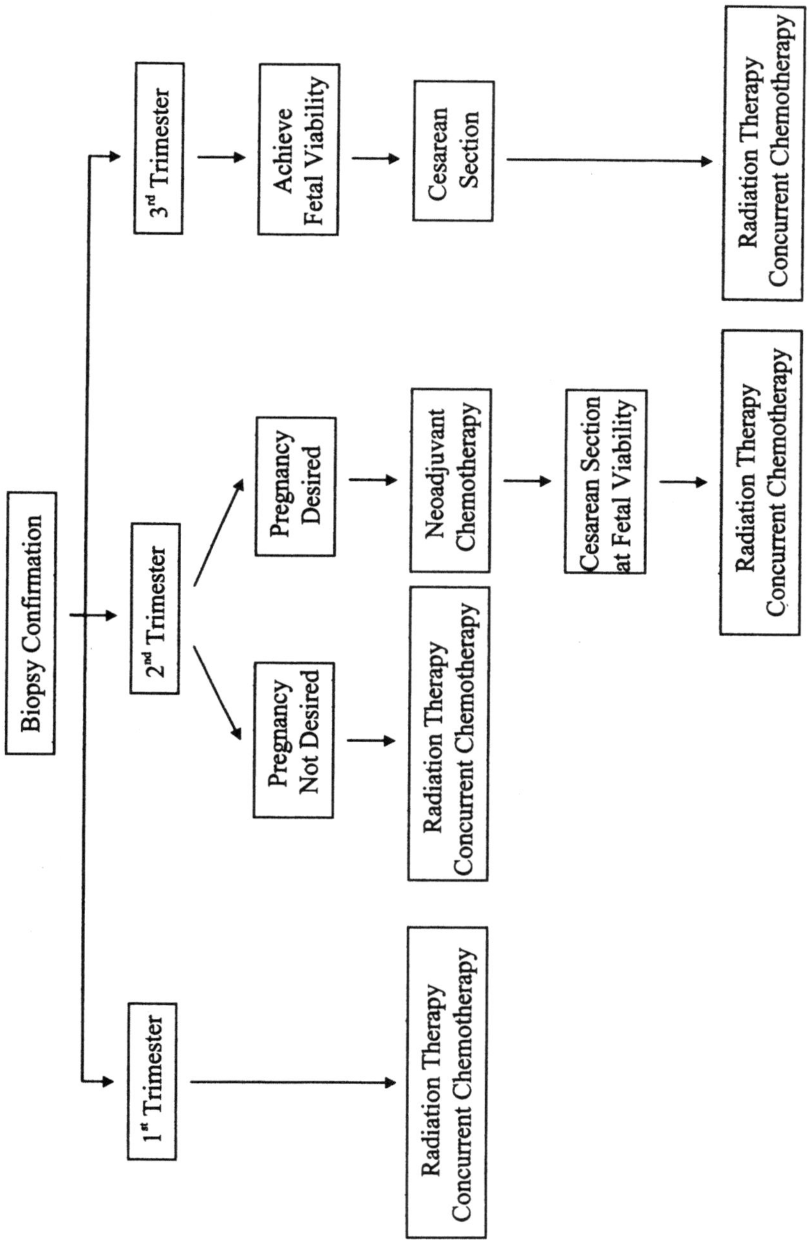

Fig. 4.4. Management of Stages Ib2, IIb–IV cervical cancer in pregnancy.

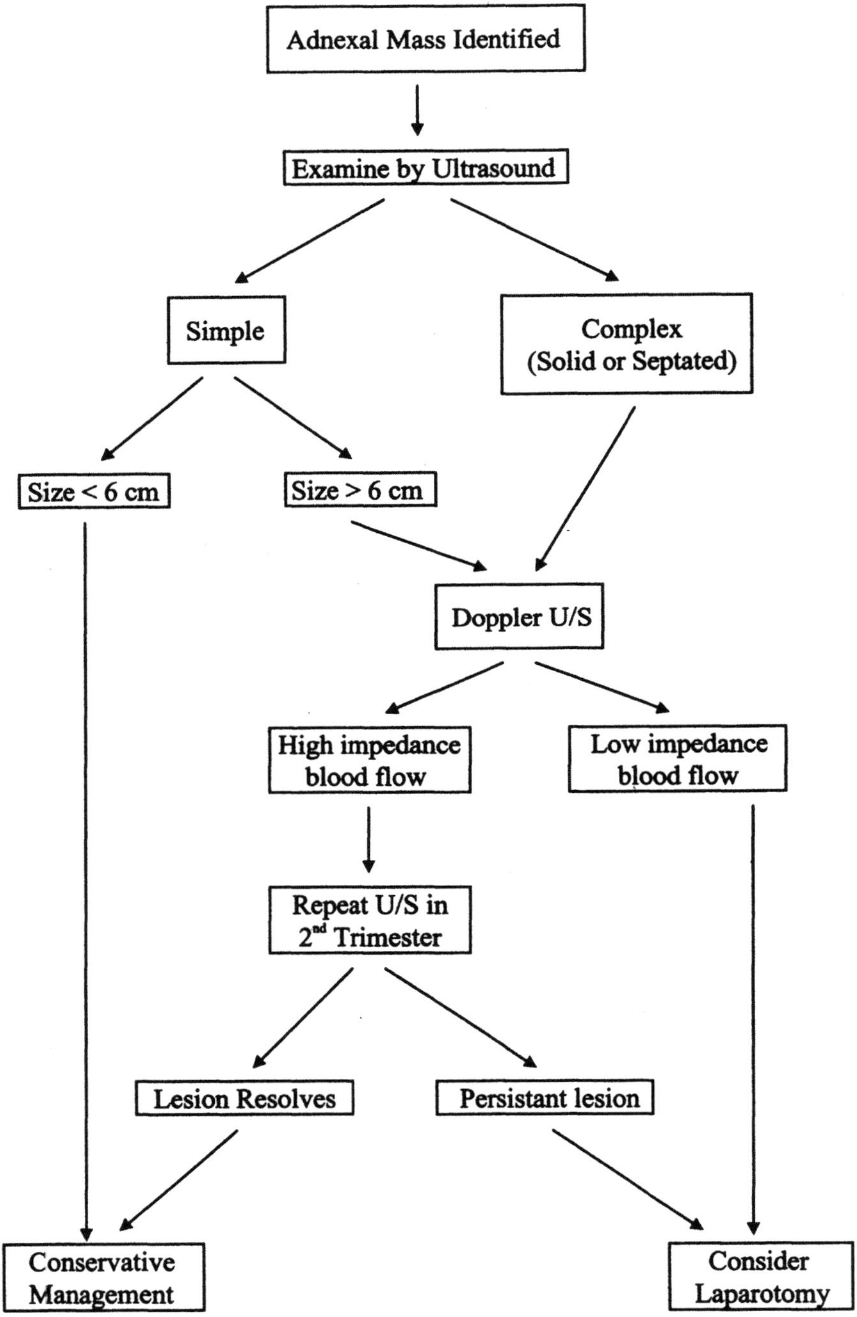

Fig. 4.5. Management of the adnexal mass in pregnancy.

levels of estrogen, pregnant women may be more vulnerable to infection with HPV than their non-gravid counterparts. Several investigators have measured a higher rate of clinical HPV infection in pregnant women using both PCR and serologic techniques to detect HPV DNA.[8,9] However, this observation has not been confirmed by other investigators.[10,11] Pregnancy appears to have little effect on the natural history of HPV infection or cervical dysplasia, once either are established.[12]

Screening Techniques for Pre-invasive and Invasive Cervical Lesions

The majority of women with cervical cancer are clinically asymptomatic.[13] If symptoms do occur, pain, vaginal bleeding and discharge are typical. However, these symptoms are non-specific and frequently masked by pregnancy, delaying appropriate evaluation of the pregnant woman with cervical cancer.[13] For this reason, all initial prenatal evaluations should include a thorough physical examination, including careful cervical inspection, bimanual examination and a smear for cytology. Suspicious cervical lesions should be biopsied. Techniques for performing cervical smears for pregnant women differ little from standard smears. The surface of the ectocervix should be sampled thoroughly and a specimen of endocervical cells collected. Use of the cytobrush and cervical brooms to collect endocervical cells has been controversial, given the potential risks of bleeding from the cervix and injury to the pregnancy. However, two randomized prospective trials have demonstrated that more abrasive techniques for collecting endocervical cells, such as the cytobrush, increase the yield of endocervical cells and decrease the frequency of inadequate smears without additional complications.[14,15]

Evaluation of Abnormal Cervical Cytology

Interpretation of cervical smears collected from gravid women is frequently complicated by the presence of atypical cells. For example, decidualized cells are frequently exfoliated from the endocervix of gravid women. Cytologically, these cells are small, have sharp cytoplasmic borders and hypochromatic nuclei and may appear similar to dysplastic cells. However, unlike dysplastic cells, decidualized cells contain regular chromatin and distinct nucleoli,[16,17] which allow proper identification with careful inspection of the PAP smear. Atypical cells may also be shed from portions of the endocervix undergoing the Arias-Stella reaction or from trophoblastic tissue within the uterus.[18] Cytologically, trophoblastic cells are large and are frequently multinucleated. In particular, they may be confused with similar noted cells shed from cervical epithelia infected by human papilloma virus, herpes simplex or, less commonly, mycobacterium tuberculosis.[19]

Despite these pitfalls, the Papanicolaou smear remains an excellent tool for screening gravid women for cervical dysplasia. Given the slow progression of cervical dysplasia to more advanced disease and the infrequency with which dysplasia conceals an invasive lesion, cervical smears with evidence of low grade squamous intraepithelial lesions (LGSIL) or atypical cells of undetermined significance (ASCUS) may be followed conservatively.[20] Repeat cytology should be performed in the third trimester and colposcopy performed if the lesion persists or progresses. More abnormal Papanicolaou smears, such as high-grade intraepithelial lesions (HGSIL) or atypical glandular cells (AGUS), require immediate colposcopic evaluation.

Over the past 30 years, the introduction of colposcopy has helped to reduce the need for cone biopsy with a minimal (<0.5%) rate of false negative results.[4] Several studies have concluded that colposcopy is a reliable tool for evaluating cervical dysplasia during pregnancy.[20,23] In some respects, colposcopy is facilitated by pregnancy-induced eversion of the normal cervical ectropion.[21,22] Serious morbidity, such as hemorrhage, preterm labor, abortion or infection, occurs only infrequently when directed biopsies are performed.[4] However, the atypical, papillary appearance of the normal columnar endocervical epithelium during pregnancy can complicate colposcopic interpretation of cervical findings. Pregnancy-induced increases in cervical vascularity also exaggerate the response of immature metaplastic epithelium to acetic acid and may produce a confusing distribution of blood vessels which mimics a severe lesion. For this reason, colposcopy should be performed by an experienced clinician, with directed biopsies performed for any lesion suggestive of severe dysplasia or invasive carcinoma. Random colposcopic biopsies should be avoided, due to a high rate of false negative results.[4]

At the Yale-New Haven Medical Center, pregnant women with HGSIL on Pap smears undergo colposcopy with directed biopsy of the site compatible with most advanced area of dysplastic change. Every effort is made to limit the number of biopsies to one in order to minimize bleeding. If bleeding does occur, it may be controlled with 3 or 4 silver nitrate sticks applied directly to the biopsy site. If the results of cervical biopsies are consistent with the recent Pap smear, patients with cervical dysplasia may be followed with smears repeated every third month.

For patients without evidence of progressive disease, repeat colposcopy and Pap smear should be performed 8 to 12 weeks postpartum. Appropriate follow-up is important, as one study indicates that the colposcopic impression of low grade lesions may underestimate disease severity and that more advanced lesions, such as carcinoma-in-situ (CIS) persists more frequently in pregnant women.[24] A more recent study, however, contradicts this conclusion and instead suggests that there is a high incidence of regression for severe cervical dysplasia, particularly among gravidas delivering vaginally.[25] Regardless, these patients should receive the close follow-up characteristic of any patient in whom cervical dysplasia has recently been evaluated or treated.

The immunodeficient patient diagnosed with cervical dysplasia should also register particular concern. Very limited data is presently available which directly addresses the natural history of cervical dysplasia specifically in HIV-positive pregnant women. One recent study suggests that HIV infection does increase the frequency or severity of cervical intraepithelial neoplasia (CIN) associated with atypical squamous cells of unknown significance (ASCUS) in pregnant women.[26] However, in non-pregnant women, cervical dysplasia occurs much more frequently in women infected with HIV.[27] Cervical dysplasia in HIV-positive women also persists longer, recurs more frequently after therapy and is more likely to progress to severe lesions or invasive carcinoma.[28,29,30] For these reasons, frequent evaluation of the HIV-infected, pregnant women should be performed. Aggressive antiretroviral therapy is associated with the regression of many cervical lesions.[31] However, appropriate follow-up of all immunodeficient patients affected with cervical dysplasia is critical.

Cone Biopsy

Cone biopsy is reserved for patients in whom microinvasive or invasive disease is suspected, as a result of either routine screening cytology or colposcopic biopsy. The decision to perform cone biopsy should be considered carefully, as several factors limit the usefulness of this procedure in pregnant women. First, cone biopsies are associated with first trimester pregnancy loss and preterm delivery.[32,33,34] Second, severe bleeding occurs with as many as 20% of cone biopsies performed in gravid patients.[4,35] Lastly, cone biopsy cannot be considered therapeutic in the gravid patient, as 30–57% of cone biopsies performed in pregnancy have margins positive for dysplasia or frank carcinoma.[36] In addition, cone biopsy does not appear to be effective in treating CIN in HIV-positive women.[37] Large loop excision of the transformation zone (LEETZ) or laser conization does not appear to confer any therapeutic or diagnostic advantage over cold-knife cone biopsy when evaluating cervical dysplasia.[36,38] Similar to cold-knife cone biopsy, LEETZ is also associated with a significant proportion of patients left with residual disease.[36]

To reduce the incidence of both hemorrhage and preterm labor following cone biopsy in the gravid patient, several authors have proposed combining cone biopsy with cervical cerclage. Despite initial promise, as many as 30% of patients experience preterm labor despite the presence of a cerclage.[39] Similar safety concerns also severely limit the use of other forms of therapy, such as cryoablation or LEETZ, in gravid women.[36]

Treatment for Invasive Cervical Cancer

Once identified, invasive cervical cancer requires prompt treatment. However, with early stage disease, therapy may be briefly delayed for patients in the late second or third trimester until fetal viability is established. This latter conclusion is supported by a number of small series which indicate that treatment delays for delivery by as much as 17 weeks do not significantly affect maternal outcome.[40-43]

For patients with microinvasive disease, either Stage Ia1 or Ia2, pregnancies more than 20 weeks of gestational age may be safely continued if surgical margins are histologically free of disease following cone biopsy and the patient is willing to be assessed with frequent Pap smears and colposcopy. However, if the patient no longer desires pregnancy, prompt therapy with a simple hysterectomy, leaving the ovaries in place, can be performed. Patients who desire definitive therapy following the conclusion of pregnancy may be delivered vaginally and have a subsequent hysterectomy (Stage Ia1) or be delivered by Cesarean section followed by an extrafascial or modified radical hysterectomy (Stage Ia2).

Patients with Stage Ib and IIa cervical cancer recognized in the first trimester of pregnancy are routinely recommended a type II radical hysterectomy and bilateral deep pelvic lymphadenectomies. This approach affords the patient the opportunity to preserve her ovaries with better postoperative function than that afforded by radiation therapy. At the Yale-New Haven Medical Center, this approach also appears to produces a five-year survival of 90%, regardless of tumor size. However, the primary treatment for more advanced cervical cancer, Stage IIb or higher, remains radiation therapy.[5] Women diagnosed with earlier stage malignancies may also be considered for radiation therapy if the risk for surgical morbidity or mortality is considered unacceptable. External beam radiation therapy has generally been employed first and, in most cases, will induce a spontaneous abortion. Intracavitary radiation follows completion of the external beam regimen. Pregnancy loss occurs at a threshold of 40cGy, which most commonly occurs between 30 and 60 days of therapy.[40,41] Although only limited data is available, one study indicates that the outcome of patients treated with radiation therapy does not appear to differ between gravid and non-gravid patients.[41] In that study, neither acute nor long-term complications in pregnant women were increased. More recent regimens for chemoradiation for the treatment of bulky cervical disease prior to hysterectomy have yet to be evaluated in gravid women, but should be considered, given their recently proven efficacy in the non-pregnant patient. These regimens include cisplatin (40mg/m^2) adminstered intravenously at weekly intervals while the patient is receiving radiation therapy or a combination of intravenous cisplatin (50 mg/m^2) and 5-fluoruracil (4g/m^2) adminstered on days 1 and 29.

From an obstetrical standpoint, there is little data to indicate which route of delivery is preferable for the pregnant woman diagnosed with cervical cancer. As mentioned earlier, vaginal deliveries have been considered acceptable for early stage cancers (Ia1) or more advanced cancers in patients experiencing pregnancy loss after radiation therapy. However, recent data appears to indicate that vaginal delivery worsens the prognosis for pregnant patients regardless of the clinical stage of disease.[44] In part, poor maternal outcomes following a vaginal delivery may result from recurrences at the prior site of episiotomy.[45,46] Cervical cancer can recur at the sites of perineal lacerations or episiotomies performed with vaginal delivery. These recurrences frequently occur in the first several years following delivery, progress rapidly and are usually fatal once discovered.[46] Thus, Cesarean section may be indicated even for those patients with early stage disease. Careful consideration should be made prior to performing hysterotomy for the evacuation of uterine contents during the second trimester prior to radiation therapy. The vertical uterine incision necessary for this procedure results in significant blood loss, which, in turn, decreases the effectiveness of radiation therapy administered shortly after delivery.

The role for neoadjuvant chemotherapy in the control and treatment of patients with cervical cancer in pregnancy has yet to be critically assessed. In part, this is due to the lack of long-term studies demonstrating the efficacy of such treatment and concern for potential injury to the fetus. However, several case reports have documented the successful use of regimens with cisplatin and vincristine in pregnant patients with a significant reduction in tumor volume.[47] In both cases, treatment appeared to render radical hysterectomy possible at the time of delivery in the third trimester with favorable neonatal outcomes. Thus, it may be appropriate to consider a role for neoadjuvant chemotherapy in the management of locally advanced cervical cancer, particularly when definitive treatment will be delayed for the fetus to reach viability.

Postpartum Evaluation

Although many of the atypical findings on Papanicolaou smear resolve following delivery, changes may persist as long as 6 months postpartum and require adequate follow-up. Some investigators have documented that the number of inadequate Pap smears due to a lack of endocervical cells decreases after delivery and that the rate of cervical dysplasia is actually higher at this time.[3] In contrast, more recent data suggests there is a high rate of regression for patients diagnosed with severe dysplasia who deliver vaginally.[25] Regardless, all patients, particularly immunosuppressed individuals, should be followed closely similarly to any patient recently diagnosed with cervical dysplasia. Postpartum therapy for cervical dysplasia should be considered in all cases, as appropriate.

Ovarian Cancer

The incidence of ovarian cancer is slowly increasing in the United States. Ovarian cancer in pregnancy remains a rare occurrence, complicating only 1 in 9000 to 1 in 25,000 pregnancies.[48] However, adnexal masses are frequently observed in gravid women, complicating as many as 1 in 190 pregnancies.[49] This observation can be partly attributed to the widespread use of ultrasound. At least one third of adnexal masses discovered during pregnancy are found during routine obstetrical ultrasonography.[50]

Both benign and malignant ovarian masses tend to be asymptomatic when discovered in the pregnant woman.[51] Careful evaluation is therefore necessary to differentiate benign from malignant processes. In this regard, the sonographic appearance of the mass in question may be helpful. Simple structures are most consistent with physiologic cysts. Most physiologic cysts resolve by the end of the first trimester. Failure of a simple cyst to resolve spontaneously by this time may be considered an indication for surgery. Other potential indications for laparotomy include tumor size greater six centimeters, a solid or complex ultrasonographic appearance and the presence of bilateral abnormalities. Magnetic resonance imaging may be helpful in situations where ultrasound findings are equivocal or the lesion cannot be distinguished from a uterine neoplasm. However, Doppler ultrasound is potentially useful for differentiating high and low risk adnexal masses. Regardless of size, adnexal masses with blood flow characterized by a high resistive index appear to carry little risk, even when these masses fail to resolve by the second trimester.

Histologically, most ovarian cancers complicating pregnancy are either epithelial cancers of borderline malignant potential or germ cell tumors.[52] This latter observation reflects the younger age of gravid women when compared to the typical ovarian cancer patient. Dysgerminomas are the most common ovarian germ cell tumors that occur during pregnancy, followed by endodermal sinus tumors.[53] Sex cord or stromal ovarian tumors, such as granulosa cell or Sertoli-Leydig cell tumors also occur. Great care must be taken to differentiate sex cord-stromal tumors from ovarian decidualization, luteoma of pregnancy or benign granulosa cell proliferations observed with pregnancy.[54] Although elevated levels of tumor markers may be helpful in non-pregnant women for differentiating benign from malignant masses, elevations of these markers during pregnancy for reasons unrelated to malignancy further reduces their diagnostic value. For example, elevations of serum alpha-fetoprotein (AFP) and human chorionic gonadotropin (ß-hCG) can be effective circulating tumor markers for the diagnosis and follow-up of endodermal sinus tumors and non-gestational trophoblastic tumors, respectively.[55] Likewise, the combination of elevated AFP and ß-hCG levels may be an excellent means to diagnose and follow embryonal carcinomas. However, titers of each of these markers, including CA-125, are routinely elevated in pregnancy for reasons unrelated to malignancy. Their levels may be misleading even when normalized as a multiple of the mean for prenatal patients.[56]

Only 3% to 5% of adnexal masses detected in pregnancy will ultimately prove to be malignant.[57] Thus, most may be managed conservatively, provided that the patient's symptoms and the characteristics of the identified mass are consistent with a benign etiology. Because adnexal masses are more likely to undergo torsion during pregnancy, exploratory laparotomy is not infrequently required when torsion is suspected in the patient with severe or intermittant abdominal pain, nausea and vomiting. If possible, surgical intervention should be delayed until the second trimester to reduce the risk of pregnancy loss. However, when first trimester exploration and ovarian resection is necessary, supplemental progesterone has been administered to decrease the likelihood of pregnancy loss.[58] The efficacy of this intervention, however, remains unproved.

Surgical Staging of Ovarian Malignancies

Complete surgical staging should be performed for ovarian malignancies in a manner similar to the non-pregnant woman. Although the gravid uterus makes assessment of the retroperitoneum more difficult, every effort should be made to remove the tumor intact. The remaining ovary should be carefully inspected and biopsied, if suspicious. Because germ cell malignancies are almost invariably unilateral, it is inappropriate to remove both ovaries when a germ cell tumor is diagnosed by frozen section. More recent evidence suggests that occult dysgerminomas may also be present in a grossly normal contralateral ovary.[59] In this situation, it is not absolutely necessary to remove the entire contralateral ovary. However, if both ovaries are involved by malignancy and the gestation has reached second trimester, both ovaries should be removed as the pregnancy no longer requires hormonal support from the corpus luteum. Because dysgerminomas are more likely to spread to para-aortic nodes, every effort should also be made to sample these lymph nodes at the time of laparotomy. An omentectomy and peritoneal sampling along with cytologic assessment of the peritoneal cavity should be routinely performed as part of the staging process.

Therapy of Ovarian Malignancies in Pregnancy

Patients with either Stage Ia or Ib invasive epithelial ovarian cancer, grades 1 and 2, may be managed conservatively with surgery alone and the pregnancy allowed to continue to term. Subsequent therapy is dictated by the histologic type and stage of malignancy identified. Epithelial tumors of borderline malignant potential appear to be adequately treated by surgery alone.[60] In these circumstances, chemotherapy is reserved for patients with invasive metastases associated with borderline primary tumors. However, a recent study has suggested that many features suggestive of aggressive biologic behavior in borderline tumors regress following delivery, potentially obviating the need for further therapy.[61] Although cytotoxic chemotherapy should be avoided during the first trimester, case studies suggest that platinum-based chemotherapy may be successfully administered for epithelial ovarian carcinomas in the second and third trimester with little apparent injury to the fetus.[62,63,64] For this reason, pregnant women with Stage Ic or greater invasive epithelial ovarian cancer or any grade 3 cancer diagnosed in the second and third trimesters should be offered the opportunity to receive platinum-based chemotherapy without terminating their pregnancy. Following delivery, a total abdominal hysterectomy, bilateral salpingo-oophorectomy, omentectomy and paraaortic and pelvic lymph node sampling with resection of all gross tumor is recommended. In all instances, extra-ovarian tumor should be debulked as best possible, both at the time of initial laparotomy and following re-exploration if indicated.

Management of ovarian germ cell malignancies depends upon the histologic identity of the tumor. Stage Ia dysgerminomas may be effectively treated with surgery, but advanced staged tumors should be treated with chemotherapy.[55] Dysgerminomas are exquisitely sensitive to both radiation and chemotherapy and chemotherapy can and should be administered in the second or third trimester with the intent to cure. A regimen of vincristine, actinomycin-D and cyclophosphamide (VAC) has been used in a limited number of pregnant patients with few adverse neonatal sequelae apparent either at delivery or following limited follow-up.[55,65-67] Cesarean section is used to deliver the fetus at the time of viability. Other germ cell tumors include endodermal sinus tumors, embryonal carcinomas, immature teratomas, choriocarcinomas and mixed germ cell tumors. The management of each is based on both the stage of disease and the presence or absence of circulating oncofetal proteins that can be used as markers for response to therapy. Endodermal sinus tumors, although virulent, are exquisitely sensitive to chemotherapy and advanced stage tumors with this histology can be treated with regimens of vincristine, adriamycin and cisplatin (VAC) or cisplatin, etoposide and bleomycin (BEP). Three case reports have appeared in the literature in which the patient delivered a normal, healthy child with no evidence of maternal disease at completion of combination chemotherapy.[65,66,68]

Sex cord-stromal tumors may be managed similarly to germ cell malignancies. In general, most of these malignancies are found at an early stage at the time of diagnosis and may be managed with surgery alone, resecting all visible tumor.[69] For more advanced disease, surgery should be followed by intense combination chemotherapy. However, experience with treating these latter tumors in pregnancy is limited by their rarity.

Vulvar Cancer

As many as 5% of vulvar malignancies are diagnosed during the puerperum.[70] Histologically, squamous carcinomas comprise the majority of vulvar lesions. Sarcomas, melanomas and even adenocarcinomas of the Bartholin's gland have also been reported.[70] Similar to cervical and ovarian cancers, there is no evidence that the natural history of invasive squamous carcinoma of the vulva is affected by pregnancy. Human papilloma virus is believed to play an important etiologic role and smoking is a strong risk factor for the progression of vulvar dysplasia to invasive disease. Often the slow rate of disease progression allows definitive therapy to be delayed until completion of the pregnancy, unless associated with an immune deficiency.

Radical surgical excision remains the mainstay of curative therapy. More recently, less extensive surgery has been effective for superficially invasive carcinomas.[71] Bilateral inguinal lymphadenectomies have also been reduced to ipsilateral lymphadenectomies for unilaterally invasive lesions, provided frozen section analysis reveals no evidence of lymph node metastases. Furthermore, lymph node sampling, rather than a complete lymphadenctomy, may be performed when frozen histology indicates microinvasive disease. Regardless of the procedure ultimately chosen, the perioperative management of the gravid woman with vulvar carcinoma should be handled appropriately for the gestational age of the pregnancy. Extensive vulvectomies may be performed, with the knowledge that the risk of spontaneous abortion or premature labor increases substantially with more radical procedures. Chemotherapy, usually based on a regimen including cis-platinum, may be administered for metastatic disease once organogenesis has concluded.[72] Adjuvant radiotherapy should be postponed until after delivery of the fetus.

For the obstetrician, vulvar malignancy presents less of a conflict in the managment of the gravid or laboring patient than its cervical or ovarian counterparts. Vaginal delivery appears permissible, provided that groin healing is complete and an adequate vaginal introitus remains.

Endometrial Cancer

Approximately 20 cases of endometrial adenocarcinoma have been reported in pregnancy.[73-78] Most of these malignancies were discovered incidentally at the time of curettage for pregnancy termination or retained products of conception. Histologically, most are well-differentiated endometrial adenocarcinomas or adenoacanthomas and are clinically associated with vaginal bleeding.[76] One case of mixed mesodermal tumor of the uterus has also been reported.[79] In part, the infrequent occurrence of endometrial malignancies in pregnant women may reflect the association of infertility with endometrial adenocarcinoma. Standard therapy for patients with adenocarcinoma of the endometrium is a total abdominal hysterectomy and bilateral salpingo-oophorectomy. However a recent case report has described the use of progesterone therapy following uterine dilation and curettage to preserve fertility.[80] This patient subsequently conceived triplets and delivered at 30 weeks gestational age. Definitive surgical therapy performed four weeks following delivery revealed no evidence of residual disease. This latter approach cannot, however, be encouraged as standard therapy.

References

1. Haas JF. Pregnancy in association with a newly diagnosed cancer: a population-based epidemiologic assessment. Int J Cancer 1984;34:229–35.
2. Pairwuti S. Pap smear examinations in women with near-term pregnancy. J Med Assoc Thailand. 1991;74:156–8.
3. Londo R BT, Girod C, Glasser M. Prenatal and postpartum Pap smears: do we need both? Fam Pract Res J 1984;14:359–67.
4. Hacker NF, Berek JS, LaGasse LD, Charles EH, Savage EW, Moore JG. Carcinoma of the cervix associated with pregnancy. Obstet Gynecol 1982;59:735–46.
5. Sood AK Soroksky J, Krogman S, Anderson B, Benda J, Buller RE. Surgical management of cervical cancer complicating pregnancy: a case–control study. Gynecol Oncol 1996;64:294–8.
6. Chang DH, Hsueh S, Soong YK. Small cell carcinoma of the uterine cervix with neurosecretory granules associated with pregnancy. A case report. J Reprod Med 1994;39:537–40.
7. Wright JR Richart R. Role of human papilloma virus in the pathogenesis of genital tract warts and cancer. Gynecol Oncol 1990;37:151.
8. Anderson JR. Cancer-associated human papillomavirus types are selectively increased in the cervix of women in the first trimester of pregnancy. J Women's Health 1997;6:162–5.
9. Schneider A, Hutz M, Gissman L. Increased prevalence of human papilloma viruses in the lower genital tract of pregnant women. Int J Cancer 1987;40:198–201.
10. Smith EM, Johnson SR, Jiang D, Jiang D, Zaleski S, Lynch CF, Brundage S. The association between pregnancy and human papilloma virus prevalence. Canc Detect Prevent 1991;15:397–402.
11. Kemp E, Hakenewerth AM, Laurent SL, Gravitt PE, Stoerker J. Human papillomavirus prevalence in pregnancy. Obstet Gynecol 1992;79:649–56.
12. Chang-Claude J, Schneider A, Smith E, Blettner M, Wahrendorf, J, Turek L. Longitudinal study of the effects of pregnancy and other factors on detection of HPV. Gynecol Oncol 1996;60:355–62.
13. Mikuta JJ. Invasive carcinoma of the cervix in pregnancy. South Med J 967;60:843–7.
14. Orr JW, Barrett J, Orr PF, Holloway RW, Holimon JL. Efficacy and safety of the cytobrush during pregnancy. Gynecol Oncol 1992;44:260–2.
15. McCord ML, Stovall TG, Meric JL, Summitt RL, Coleman SA. Cervical cytology: a randomizd comparison of four sampling methods. Am J Obstet Gynecol 1992;166:1772–7.
16. Murad TM, Terhas TK, Flint A. Atypical cells in pregnancy and postpartum smears. Acta Cytol 1981;25:623–30.
17. Schneider V, Barnes L. Ectopic decidual reaction of the cervix: frequency and cytologic presentation. Acta Cytol 1981;25:616–22.

18. Rhatigan RM. Endocervical gland atypia secondary to Arias-Stella change. Arch Pathol Lab Med 1992;116:943–6.
19. Pisharodi L, Jovanoska S. Spectrum of cytologic changes in pregnancy. A review of 100 abnormal cervicovaginal smears with emphasis on diagnostic pitfalls. Acta Cytol 1995;39:905–8.
20. LaPolla JP, O'Neill C, Wetrich D. Colposcopic management of abnormal cervical cytology in pregnancy. J Reprod Med 1988;33:301–6.
21. Jones EG, Schwinn CP, Bullock WK, Varga A, Dunn JE, Friedman H, Weir J. Cancer detection during pregnancy. Am J Obstet Gynecol 1968;101:298–307.
22. Campion MJ, Sedlacek T. Colposcopy in pregnancy. Obstet Gynecol Clinics North America 1993;20:153–63.
23. McDonnell JM, Mylotte MJ, Gustafson RC, Jordan JA. Colposcopy in pregnancy: a twelve year review. Br J Obstet Gynecol 1981;88:414–20.
24. Coppola A, Soroksky J, Casper R, Anderson B, Buller RE. The clinical course of cervical carcinoma-in-situ diagnosed during pregnancy. Gynecol Oncol 1997;67:162–5.
25. Aikens JK, Sehdev H, Warshal DP, Rocereto TF. Recurrent cervical dysplasia following spontaneous regression after delivery. Gynecol Oncol 1999;72:460.
26. Holcomb KM, Mathews RP, Abulafia O, Chapman J, Lee YC, Buhl A. The significance of ASCUS in HIV-positive women. Gynecol Oncol 1999;72:458.
27. Spinillo A, Tenti P, Baltaro F, Piazzi G, Iasci A, DeSantolo A. Cervical intraepithelial neoplasia in pregnant intravenous drug users infected with human immunodeficiency virus type 1. Eur J Obstet Gynecol Reprod Biol 1996;68:175–8
28. Heard I, Bergeron C, Jeannel D, Henrion R, Kazatchkine MD. Papanicolaou smears in human immunodeficiency virus-seropositive women during follow-up. Obstet Gynecol 1995;86:749–53.
29. Maiman M. Management of cervical neoplasia in human immunodeficiency virus-infected women. J Nat Canc Inst 1998;23:43–9.
30. Maiman M, Fruchter R, Sedlis A, Feldman J, Chen P, Burk RD, Minkoff H. Prevalence, risk factors and accuracy of cytoloig screening for cervical intraepithelial neoplasia in women with the human immunodeficiency virus. Gynecol Oncol 1998;68:233–9.
31. Heard I, Schmitz V, Costagliola D, Orth G, Kazatchkine MD. Early regression of cervical lesions in HIV-seropositive women receiving highly active antiretroviral therapy. AIDS 1998;12:1459–64.
32. Kristensen J, Langhoff-Roos J, Kristensen FB. Increased risk of preterm birth in women with cervical conization. Obstet Gynecol 1993;81:1005–8.
33. Leiman G, Harrison NA, Rubin A. Pregnancy following conization of the cervix: complications related to cone size. Am J Obstet Gynecol 1980;136:14–18.
34. Jones JM, Sweetnam P, Hibbard BM. The outcome of pregnancy after cone biopsy of the cervix: A case–control study. Br J Obstet Gynecol 1979;86:913–6.
35. Hannigan EV, Whitehouse HH, Atkinson WD, Becker SD. Cone biopsy during pregnancy. Obstet Gynecol 1982;60:450–5.
36. Robinson WR, Webb S, Tirpack J, Degefu S, O'Quinn AG. Management of cervical intraepithelial neoplasia during pregnancy with LOOP excision. Gynecol Oncol 1997;64:153–5.
37. Holcomb KM, Mathews RP, Abulafia O, Chapman J, Lee YC, Buhl A. The efficacy of cervical conization in the treatment of cervical intraepithelial neoplasia in HIV-positive women. Gynecol Oncol 1999;72:456.
38. Raio L, Ghezzi F, Di Naro E, Gomez R, Luscher KP. Duration of pregnancy after carbon dioxide laser conization of the cervix: Influence of cone height. Obstet Gynecol 1997;90:978–82.
39. Goldberg G, Altaras M, Bloch B. Cone cerclage in pregnancy. Am J Obstet Gynecol 1991;77:315–7.
40. Prem KA, Makowski EL, McKelvey JL. Carcinoma of the cervix associated with pregnancy. Am J Obstet Gynecol 1966;95:99–108.
41. Sood AK, Sorokshy JI, Mayr N, Krogman S, Anderson B, Buller RE, Hussey DH. Radiotherapeutic management of cervical cancer complicating pregnancy. Cancer 1997;80:1073–8.
42. Monk BJ, Montz FJ. Invasive cervical cancer complicating intrauterine pregnancy: treatment with radical hysterectomy. Obstet Gynecol 1992;80:199–203.
43. Duggan B, Muderspach L, Roman LD, Curtin JP, d'Ablaing G, Morrow CP. Cervical cancer in pregnancy: Reporting on planned delay in therapy. Obstet Gynecol 1993;82:598–602.
44. Sood AK, Sorokshy JI, Mayr NA, Anderson B, Buller RE, Niebyl JR. Cervical cancer after recent pregnancy: does route of delivery influence survival? Gynecol Oncol 1999;72:460.
45. Gordon AN, Jensen R, Jones HW. Squamous carcinoma of the cervix complicating pregnancy: Recurrence in episiotomy after vaginal delivery. Obstet Gynecol 1989;73:850–2.
46. Cliby WA, Dodson M, Podratz KC. Cervical cancer complicated by pregnancy: Episiotomy site recurrences following vaginal delivery. Obstet Gynecol 1994;84:179–82.

47. Tewari K, Cappuccini F, Gambino A, Kohler MF, Pecorelli S, Disaia PJ. Neoadjuvant chemotherapy in the treatment of locally advanced cervical carcinoma in pregnancy. Cancer 1998;82:1529–34.
48. Chung A, Birnbaum SJ. Ovarian cancer associated with pregnancy. Obstet Gynecol 1973;41:211–4.
49. Hogston P, Lilford RJ. Ultrasound study of ovarian cysts in pregnancy: prevalence and significance. Br J Obstet Gynecol 1986;93:625–8.
50. Buttery BW, Beischer NA, Fortune DW, Macafee CA. Ovarian tumors in pregnancy. Med J Aust 1973;1:345–9.
51. Jubb ED. Primary ovarian carcinoma in pregnancy. Am J Obstet Gynecol 1963;85:345.
52. Degani R, Shohan Z, Atar E. Ovarian carcinoma during pregnancy: a study of 23 cases in Israel between the years of 1960 and 1984. Gynecol Oncol 1989;33:326.
53. Karlen JR, Akbari A, Cook WA. Dysgerminoma associated with pregnancy. Obstet Gynecol 1979;53:330–5.
54. Clement PB. Tumor-like lesions of the ovary associated with pregnancy. Int J Gynecol Pathol 1993;12:108.
55. Schwartz PE. Combination chemotherapy in the management of ovarian germ cell malignancies. Obstet Gynecol 1984;64:564–72.
56. Schwartz PE, Chambers SK, Chambers JT, Gutmann J, Katopodis N, Foemmel R. Circulating tumor markers in the monitoring of ovarian germ cell malignancies. Cancer 1987;60:353–61.
57. Creasman WT, Rutledge F, Smith JP. Carcinoma of the ovary associated with pregnancy. Obstet Gynecol 1971;38:111–6.
58. Hopkins MP, Duchon MA. Adnexal surgery in pregnancy. J Reprod Med 1986;31:1035–7.
59. Bianchi UA, Sarteri E, Favall G. New trends in treatment of ovarian dysgerminoma. Gynecol Oncol 1986;23:246.
60. Julian CG, Woodruff, JD. The biologic behavior of low-grade papillary serous carcinoma of the ovary. Obstet Gynecol 1972;40:860–7.
61. Mooney J, Silva E, Tornos C, Gershenson D. Unusual features of serous neoplasms of low malignant potential during pregnancy. Gynecol Oncol 1997;65:30–5.
62. King LA, Nevin PC, Williams PP, Carson LF. Treatment of advanced epithelial ovarian carcinoma in pregnancy with cisplatin-based chemotherapy. Gynecol Oncol 1991;41:78–80.
63. Koc ON, McFee M, Reed E, Gerson SL. Detection of platinum-DNA adducts in cord blood lymphocytes following in utero platinum exposure. Eur J Cancer 1994;30A:716–7.
64. Henderson CE, Elia G, Garfinkel D, Poirier MC, Shamkhani H, Runowicz CD. Platinum chemotherapy during pregnancy for serous cystadenocarcinoma of the ovary. Gynecol Oncol 1993;49:92–4.
65. Metz SA, Day TG, Pursell SH. Adjuvant chemotherapy in a pregnant patient with endodermal sinus tumor of the ovary. Gynecol Oncol 1989;32:371–4.
66. Kim DS, Park MI. Maternal and fetal survival following surgery and chemotherapy of endodermal sinus tumor of the ovary during pregnancy: a case report. Obstet Gynecol 1989;73:503–7.
67. Montz FJ, Horenstein J, Platt LD, d'Ablaing G, Schlaerth JB, Cunningham G. The diagnosis of immature teratoma by maternal serum alpha-fetoprotein screening. Obstet Gynecol 1989;73:522–5.
68. Malone JM, Gershenson D, Creasy RK, Kavanagh JJ, Silva GE, Stringer CA. Endodermal sinus tumor of the ovary associated with pregnancy. Obstet Gynecol 1986;68:86S–89S.
69. Young RH, Dudley AG, Scully RF. Granulosa cell, Sertoli-Leydig cell and unclassified sex cord-stromal tumors associated with pregnancy. Gynecol Oncol 1984;18:181–205.
70. Lutz M, Underwood P, Rozier JC, Putney FW. Genital malignancy in pregnancy. Am J Obstet Gynecol 1977;129:536–42.
71. Gitsch G, Van Eijkeren M, Hacker NF. Surgical therapy of vulvar cancer in pregnancy. Gynecol Oncol 1995;56:312–5.
72. Moore DH, Fowler WJ, Currie JL, Walton LA. Squamous cell carcinoma of the vulva in pregnancy. Gynecol Oncol 1991;41:74–7.
73. Sandstrom R, Welch W, Green TH. Adenocarcinoma of the endometrium in pregnancy. Obstet Gynecol 1979;53:73S–76S.
74. Schammel DP, Mittal KR, Kaplan K, Deligdisch L, Tavassoli FA. Endometrial adenocarcinoma associated with intrauterine pregnancy. A report of five cases and a review of the literature. Int J Gynecol Pathol 1998;17:327–35.
75. Suzuki A, Konishi I, Okamura H, Nakashima N. Adenocarcinoma of the endometrium associated with intrauterine pregnancy. Gynecol Oncol 1984;18:261–9.
76. Schneller J, Nicastri A. Intrauterine pregnancy conincident with endometrial carcinoma: A case study and review of the literature. Gynecol Oncol 1994;54:87–90.
77. Hoffman MS, Cavanagh D, Walter TS, Ionata F, Ruffolo EH. Adencarcinoma of the endometrium and endometroid carcinoma of the ovary associated with pregnancy. Gynecol Oncol 1989;32:82–5.

78. Zirkin HJ, Krugliak L, Katz M. Endometrial andeocarcinoma coincident with intrauterine pregnancy. A case report. J Reprod Med 1983;28:624–6.
79. Scocsia A, Merino MJ, Haas M, Copel JA, Schwartz PE. Malignant mixed mesodermal tumor of the uterus arising in association with a viable gestation. Obstet Gynecol 1988;71:1047–50.
80. Kimmig R, Strowitzki T, Muller-Hocker J, Kurzl R, Korell M, Hepp H. Conservative treatment of endometrial cancer permitting subsequent triplet pregnancy. Gynecol Oncol 1995;58:255–7.

5. Hematologic Malignancies in Pregnancy

Tanja Pejovic, Peter E. Schwartz and Giancarlo Mari

Hematologic malignancies are among the most commonly diagnosed neoplasms that occur during pregnancy.[1] Their incidence seems to be independent of pregnancy. Pregnant women with hematologic neoplasms present several diagnostic and therapeutic challenges to the clinician. Their rare occurrence and their nonspecific symptoms often delay the diagnosis. Hematologic malignancies are second only to melanoma in their ability to metastasize to the placenta. The chemotherapeutic agents used to treat hematologic malignancies have teratogenic potential, although human studies have not confirmed this theoretic risk.[2]

Hodgkin's Lymphoma

Hodgkin's lymphoma generally occurs during the reproductive years, with a mean age at diagnosis of 32 years. It comprises 40% of all lymphomas. One-third of women with Hodgkin's lymphoma are pregnant or have delivered a child within one year of diagnosis.[3]

The most common presenting symptom is peripheral lymphadenopathy, with 60–80% of the patients having enlarged cervical lymph nodes. In addition, patients have nonspecific symptoms of weight loss, malaise, pruritus, and night sweats.

The diagnosis of Hodgkin's lymphoma is based on presence of pathognomonic Reed–Sternberg giant cells. The disease is subclassified into four histologic subtypes. The lymphocyte-predominant subtype has the most favorable prognosis and is associated with early stage disease. The nodular sclerosis subtype has a relatively favorable prognosis, usually occurring in young women with positive supraclavicular and mediastinal lymph nodes. The mixed cellularity subtype occurs more frequently in middle-aged patients. The lymphocyte depletion subtype is the least favorable and is often associated with advanced disease.[3]

Lymphomas do not affect the course of pregnancy. A similar survival rate of 70% was found in pregnant and non-pregnant patients with Hodgkin's lymphoma.[4] The incidence of first-trimester miscarriages, prematurity and stillbirth in pregnant patients with Hodgkin's lymphoma is no higher than in age-matched pregnant women in control groups.[2] Similarly, pregnancy does not appear significantly to alter the clinical behavior of Hodgkin's lymphoma. A recent review of 17 cases of Hodgkin's lymphoma in pregnancy from Stanford University Medical Center confirmed that the clinical course of the disease was not changed in pregnancy.[5] Most of the patients deferred therapy until after delivery and had no evidence of disease on the last follow-up.[5]

Lymphoma staging is based on the physical examination, hematologic and biochemical tests, bone-marrow evaluation and radiographic imaging. The diagnosis is usually confirmed by a biopsy of an enlarged lymph node. When a chest X-ray is performed for detection of mediastinal disease in pregnancy, abdominal shielding must be used. However, magnetic resonance imaging is the preferred diagnostic technique because it has a high sensitivity and eliminates exposure of the fetus to ionizing radiation. If lymphography is believed to be needed, it should be limited to a single X-ray exposure 24 hours after the injection of dye.

The treatment of patients with Stage I and Stage II disease is radiotherapy. The reported 5-year survival is 89% and 67% respectively.[6] Radiation is also the treatment of choice for the Stage IIIa lymphocyte-predominant or nodular sclerozing subtypes. Other histologic subtypes presenting as stage IIIa are treated with radiation combined with chemotherapy. More advanced disease is treated with combination chemotherapy. Patients with Hodgkin's disease diagnosed in the first trimester should undergo therapeutic abortion prior to radiation. Internal radiation scatter from the standard mantle field cannot be shielded and would lead to an exposure rate to the fetus of more than 10 rads (0.1 Gy) which is allowed in the first trimester. Similar disease diagnosed in the third trimester is treated with early delivery of the infant once fetal maturity is achieved, followed by radiation.

Stages III and IV Hodgkin's disease has been successfully treated with nitrogen mustard (Mustagen), vincristine (Oncovin), procarbazine, and prednisone (MOPP regimen). Ward and Weiss[4] recommend that the patients who must receive chemotherapy in the first trimester receive vinblastine during the first trimester as it has been associated with a minimal risk to the fetus. When a patient enters the second trimester a modified mantle field of radiation and combined chemotherapy should be considered. Most clinicians recommend avoidance of pregnancy for two years after therapy for Hodgkin's disease because recurrence within this period denotes poor prognosis. It is at present unclear if prior radiation or chemotherapy for Hodgkin's disease has any adverse effect on subsequent pregnancies.[2]

Non-Hodgkin's Lymphoma

The mean age of the patients with a diagnosis of non-Hodgkin's lymphoma is 42 years, suggesting that most of the patients are past their reproductive age. Only seventy-five cases of non-Hodgkin's lymphoma in pregnancy have been described to date. The National Cancer Institute's Working Formulation is the most widely accepted classification of non-Hodgkin's lymphoma which established three main categories of the disease (low-, intermediate- and high-risk) according to histologic type and clinical performance.[7] Treatment choice depends on grade and extent of the disease. Low-grade non-Hodgkin's lymphoma can be observed throughout the gestation. Chemotherapy, most often as a single agent, can be given postpartum.

Because of the very aggressive nature of diffuse intermediate- and high-grade non-Hodgkin's lymphomas, therapy should not be delayed. Although therapeutic abortion followed by combination chemotherapy was recommended in the past, several reports demonstrated successful treatment of pregnant women who subsequently gave birth to healthy infants. Aviles et al.[7] reported on the largest series of patients with non-Hodgkin's lymphomas treated in pregnancy. Three of 19 patients died during induction treatment, while the remaining 16 gave birth to healthy children who were at normal levels of development 3–11 years after birth. Eight of the 16 women are alive and without evidence of disease 4–9 years after delivery. This series offers support for the administration of combined treatment to women with non-Hodgkin's lymphoma who wish to maintain their pregnancies.

Acute Leukemia

Since Virchow's first description of acute leukemia in pregnancy, more than 400 cases have been reported.[8] Acute leukemia is subdivided into acute myeloid leukemia (AML) and acute lymphoblastic leukemia (ALL). Histologic staining is used to classify leukemias according to French-American-British system.

Pregnancy does not influence the course of acute leukemia; however, spontaneous remissions after pregnancy termination have been described.[8] Almost all women treated with chemotherapy in pregnancy survive to delivery and 87% of fetuses survive.[8] The literature suggests a higher incidence of prematurity and low-birth weight in infants born to mothers with leukemia in pregnancy, but this may be due to the administration of chemotherapy and not to the disease. Placental involvement and metastases to the fetus are very rare, with only few documented cases.[9-11] Still, hematologic malignancies are second only to malignant melanoma in their ability to metastasize to the products of conception. Therefore, detailed histopathological examination of the placenta should always be performed in patients with leukemia.

When the diagnosis of acute leukemia is confirmed, treatment should be started immediately. Patients should be aware of potential teratogenic effects of treatment in the first trimester. Most authors consider treatment in the second and third trimester safe.[12,13] Supportive care should be instituted to minimize maternal morbidity. Maintenance goals of chemotherapy include a platelet count of 20,000/mm^3 and 50, 000/mm^3. Intensive chemotherapy allows complete remission rates of 72% and 76% in pregnant women with AML and ALL respectively.[8] Unfortunately, the disease usually relapses within one year.

Chronic Leukemia

Chronic myelocytic leukemia (CML) constitutes 90% of the chronic leukemias in pregnancy.[3] CML can be subdivided into three clinical phases: chronic, accelerated, and an acute blastic phase. Patients usually present with fatigue, low-grade fever, and night sweats. The diagnosis is based on leukocytosis of up to 700, 000 leukocytes/mm^3 with basophilia. Bone marrow examination reveals hypercellularity with a left-shift in myelopoiesis. Therapy of CML in pregnancy is supportive and specific therapy is delayed in early pregnancy to avoid potential risks to the developing fetus. Traditional chemotherapy with single agent busulfan has been palliative, and although it improves the patient's sense of wellbeing it does not change the course of the disease. Plasmapheresis and leukophoresis have been reported to decrease platelet and leukocyte counts. Because plasmapheresis has been successfully used in management of Rh-sensitized pregnancies, it is preferred over chemotherapy in the control of chronic phase of CML in pregnancy. Allogenic and autologous bone marrow transplants have been shown to be effective treatment, producing long-term disease-free survival in more than 60% of patients if performed in the chronic phase.[114] These treatment modalities are not applicable in treatment of CML in pregnancy. About 96% of pregnant women with CML survive to delivery. Fetal survival throughout gestation is 84%, however the disease inevitably progresses to the blastic phase with a median survival of 2 months after the onset of blastic crises.[14]

Chrisomalis et al[15] reported the only case of chronic lymphocytic leukemia (CLL) in pregnancy. A young pregnant woman did not require any chemotherapy and had a normal pregnancy outcome. The placenta showed an increased number of mature lymphocytes in the intervillous space, consistent with the diagnosis of CLL.[15]

References

1. National Cancer Institute. 1998 Annual Cancer Statistics Review. Washington, DC: US Department of Health and Human Service
2. Sadural E, Smith LG. Hematologic malignancies during pregnancy. Clin Obstet Gynecol 1995; 38:535–46
3. Schwartz PE, Marchant D. Cancer in pregnancy. In: E. Albert Reece, J. Hobbins (eds). Medicine of the Fetus and Mother. Philadelphia: Lippincott-Raven Publishers, 1999
4. Ward FT, Weiss RB. Lymphoma and pregnancy. Semin Oncol 1989; 16:397–409
5. Gelb AB, van de Rijn M, Warnke RA, Kamel OW. Pregnancy associated lymphomas. A cliniopathological study. Cancer 1996; 78:304–10
6. Mitchell MS, Capizzi RL. Neoplastic disease. In: Burrow GN, Merris TF, (eds). Medical complications during pregnancy. Philadelphia: WB Sauders, 1982
7. Aviles A, Diaz-Maqueo JC, Torra-Garcia EL, Guzman R. Non-Hodgkin's lymphoma and pregnancy: presentation of 16 cases. Gynecol Oncol 1990; 37:335–42
8. Caligiuri MA. Leukemia and pregnancy: effects of treatment on mother and child. Advan Oncol 1992; 8:10–17
9. Sheikh SS, Khalifa MA, Marley EF, Bagg A, Lage JM. Acute monocytic leukemia (FAB M5) involving the placenta associated with delivery of a healthy infant: case report and discussion. Int J Gyn Pathol 1996; 15:363–6
10. Honore LH, Brown LB. Intervillous metastases with maternal myeloid leukemia. Arch Pathol Lab Med 1990; 114:450
11. Dildy III GA, Moise Jr KJ, Karpenter Jr R. Maternal malignancy metastatic to the products of conception: A review. Obstet Gynecol Surv 1989; 44:535–40
12. Claahsen HL, Semmekrot BA, van Dongen PM, Mattijssen V. Successful fetal outcome after exposure to doxorubicin and cytosine-arabinoside during the second trimester of pregnancy – a case report. Am J Perinatol 1998; 15:295–7
13. Baer MR. Management of unusual presentations of acute leukemia. Hematol Oncol Clin North Am 1993; 7:286–92
14. Weibel KS, Tallman MS. Chronic leukemia. In: Gleicher N, (ed.). Principles and Practice of Medical Therapy in Pregnancy. New York: Appleton & Lange, 1992:1068–72
15. Chrisomalis L, Baxi LV, Heller D. Chronic lymphocytic leukemia in pregnancy. Am J Obstet Gynecol 1996; 175:1381–2

6. Melanoma in Pregnancy

Seth P. Harlow

Introduction

Over the past two decades in the United States, the incidence of melanoma has been rising at an alarming rate. It is estimated there will be approximately 44,000 new cases of melanoma in the United States in 1999.[1] This disease occurs in an age range such that 35% of women patients will be of childbearing age (16–45 years) when they develop this disease. It is therefore of no surprise that the diagnosis of melanoma may coincide with pregnancy in a substantial number of patients in this age group. The estimated incidence of melanoma occurring during pregnancy is 2.8 cases per 1,000 live births,[2] making this one of the most commonly diagnosed cancers during pregnancy. Since the first reports of melanoma occurring in pregnancy, there has been controversy as to the influence that pregnancy has on the development, rate of growth and prognosis of this disease. While no clear consensus exists on all of these issues, there have been several studies that have helped to clarify our understanding of the interactions that occur between these two conditions. This information should aid the treating physician in counseling pregnant patients with this disease and in helping to make treatment decisions.

Epidemiology

Risk Factors

Cutaneous melanoma is known to occur in greater frequency in people with fair skin, blonde or red hair and in those who tend to sunburn easily. Individuals who have a history of frequent sunburns, especially if there was blistering, are at higher risk for developing melanoma. There is a definite racial predisposition toward Caucasians, with melanoma being very uncommon in blacks or persons of Asian descent.[3] Genetic factors are also important. There are well-described familial syndromes with an inherited predisposition to developing melanoma. The best example is the Dysplastic Nevus Syndrome or Atypical Mole Syndrome, where affected individuals are at very high risk for developing melanoma, with some forms of this syndrome having lifetime risks exceeding 50%.[4] The search for the cause of melanoma has implicated sun exposure as the likely carcinogenic agent in most cases of this disease. More specifically ultraviolet B irradiation has been implicated as the specific wavelength of light that has the greatest potential for causing melanoma. This wavelength is known to induce the DNA damage that is thought to initiate the malignant process in melanocytes.[5]

Physical Findings and Diagnosis

Most cutaneous melanomas will present as an enlarging, darkly pigmented skin lesion; however, they may also be red or pale in color (amelanotic). In addition to the characteristic colors of these lesions, melanomas may present as skin lesions which itch or cause pain and some will have ulceration or bleeding. In women the most common site of melanoma is on the lower extremities. Any skin lesion which has shown an increase in size, change in coloration, variegation in color, recent bleeding, pain or itching should be promptly biopsied. There is minimal morbidity associated with a skin biopsy and potentially great harm if a diagnosis of melanoma is delayed.

Appropriate biopsies include either a full thickness excisional biopsy with a 1–2mm margin around the lesion, if the lesion is small, or a full thickness punch biopsy in the most raised portion of the lesion if it is large. Biopsies should be performed with local anesthesia and can be readily done as an office procedure. It is important not to perform shave biopsies of lesions suspected of being melanoma, as this may not allow an accurate determination of the maximum tumor depth, which may influence the appropriate margin of surgical excision required.

When a diagnosis of melanoma is made, a complete physical examination is required to assess the clinical stage of the disease. Careful evaluation for additional suspicious pigmented skin lesions should be performed, as there may be synchronous melanomas. Evaluation for satellite lesions near the primary tumor site, for in-transit lesions between the primary tumor and the regional nodal basins, and the regional nodal basins for metastatic disease should be performed. Any tumor found outside of the region of the primary tumor or regional nodal basins would be considered a distant or systemic metastasis. Appropriate initial staging studies should include a complete blood count, liver function tests and a chest X-ray. Extensive body scanning is not required for asymptomatic patients with clinical Stage I or II (localized) disease.

Pathology

Growth Patterns

There are four commonly described growth patterns of cutaneous melanoma, which differ in their locations and propensity to metastasize.

a) Lentigo Maligna Melanoma – These lesions typically appear as darkly pigmented patches of skin on the facial region of elderly patients. These lesions tend to be thin and rarely metastasize. Lentigo Maligna melanomas are associated with the best overall prognosis of the four melanoma subtypes.

b) Superficial Spreading Melanoma – These lesions are characterized by a radial (lateral) growth phase that later in its course becomes more vertical. Superficial spreading melanoma is the most common growth pattern seen in melanoma, accounting for 70–80% of cases. These lesions may appear anywhere on the body but are most

common in sun exposed areas and are often found to arise from pre-existing benign nevi. Superficial spreading melanomas tend to be thin lesions and hence are commonly associated with a good prognosis, however if left intact they may develop a vertical growth phase and have deeper invasion and a subsequent worse prognosis.
c) Nodular Melanoma – These lesions are characterized by a dominant vertical growth phase, creating a skin nodule or papule. These lesions usually arise de-novo without an associated benign pigmented nevus near by and can occur anywhere on the body. Nodular melanomas more frequently bleed or ulcerate than other sub-types and are more frequently found to be amelanotic. Nodular melanomas are typically deep at presentation and are therefore associated with the worst prognosis of the four melanoma subtypes.
d) Acral-Lentiginous Melanoma - These lesions occur on the soles of the feet, palms of the hands or under the nails. They typically have an early onset of a vertical growth phase hence are frequently quite deep on presentation. They present as a slightly raised irregular pigmented area of skin that is usually greater than 2cm in diameter. These lesions, like nodular melanoma, may be amelanotic. Prognosis for Acral Lentiginous melanoma is generally better than Nodular melanoma but is significantly worse than the other two subtypes.

Staging of Primary Tumor

Tumor thickness or depth of invasion has been found to be the primary tumor characteristic that has the greatest prognostic significance. Two separate micro-staging systems have been developed for staging the primary melanoma site. Each of these systems has been found to supply independent prognostic information, therefore both are routinely reported.

Clark's Classification

This system[6] determines the deepest level of invasion of the primary melanoma based on the anatomic layer of the skin to which the tumor extends. There are five levels of invasion reported.

Table 6.1 Clark's Classification

Level I	Tumor confined to the epidermis (melanoma in-situ).
Level II	Tumor extending into the papillary dermis.
Level III	Tumor extending to the junction of the papillary and reticular dermis.
Level IV	Tumor extending into the reticular dermis.
Level V	Tumor extending into the subcutaneous fat.

Breslow's Classification

This system[7] involves the measurement of the thickest portion of the primary tumor using an ocular micrometer. Measurements proceed from the most external surface of the tumor to its deepest location along a straight line perpendicular to the skin at the tumor's thickest location. The numerical measurement in millimeters is recorded. Breslow's depth has been correlated to patient prognosis with a near linear relationship between depth of invasion and risk of disease recurrence.

AJCC Staging

The American Joint Commission on Cancer has developed the following system for the staging of cutaneous melanoma.[8] This system incorporates both the Clark's and Breslow's microstaging systems for the primary tumor sites (T stage) along with the Nodal stage (N stage) and Metastasis stage (M stage) making up the TNM system.

Table 6.2 AJCC Staging

Stage	
0	In-situ melanoma (Clark's Level I)
1a	Localized melanoma, < 0.75mm thick or Clark's Level II (T1, N0, M0)
1b	Localized melanoma, 0.76mm–1.5mm thick or Clark's Level III (T2, N0, M0)
2a	Localized melanoma, 1.51mm–4.0mm thick or Clark's level IV (T3, N0, M0)
2b	Localized melanoma, > 4.0mm thick or Clark's level V (T4, N0, M0)
3	Limited nodal metastases, involving one regional nodal basin or fewer than five in-transit metastases without nodal disease. (any T, N1, M0)
4	Advanced regional metastases or distant metastases (any T, N2 or M1)

Melanoma in Pregnancy

Surgeons treating patients with melanoma in the 1940s and 1950s began making observations that led many to believe that an interaction could exist between the hormonal stimulation of pregnancy and the development or progression of melanoma. The first was the observation that melanoma was rarely seen in women before the onset of puberty and that a peak in the incidence curves of this disease occurred during the childbearing years. A second observation was that women in general had a better outcome from melanoma treatment when compared to men. This survival advantage, however, was lost when women became post-menopausal. A third observation was that there were well-known skin pigmentation changes that occurred in women during pregnancy. These skin changes included increased pigmentation of the face, nipples and labia as well as darkening of pre-existing nevi and other pigmented skin lesions. These pigmentary changes were thought to be due to the increased levels of circulating hormones that occur during pregnancy. In fact it is now known that levels of estrogens, progesterone, androgens and beta-melanocytic stimulating hormone (beta-MSH) amongst others increase in pregnancy and may be potential candidates as mediators of these clinical findings.

Supporting the theory of a hormonal effect is laboratory evidence demonstrating the binding of estrogen and progesterone to melanoma cell lines.[9] This, coupled with clinical trials that demonstrated the possibility of a small beneficial effect of tamoxifen (an anti-estrogen) in the treatment of melanoma,[10] raised the suspicion that there may be a significant hormonal influence in this disease. More recent studies, however, using immuno-histochemical techniques, have shown in fact that classic estrogen or progesterone receptors are not present in melanoma cells.[11] These findings however do not exclude the possibility that other hormones may stimulate melanoma proliferation or that there may be other avenues by which estrogen or progesterone affect these tumor cells outside of their classic receptor pathways.

In trying to assess the impact that pregnancy may have on the patient with melanoma, several important questions needed to be answered. First, was there evidence that pregnancy influenced the frequency in which melanoma occurred in the female patient? Second, was there a difference in the histologic subtype or the primary tumor location in the pregnant patient as compared to non-pregnant women? Third, was the stage of disease at diagnosis different in the pregnant patient as compared to non-pregnant women? Fourth, were the rates of disease recurrence and patient survival different in the pregnant patient as compared to non-pregnant women?

Some additional important clinical questions to be answered included: Were the risks of disease recurrence influenced by subsequent pregnancies after a diagnosis of melanoma has been made? Was there any evidence of a survival benefit for pregnant patients with melanoma to terminate their pregnancies? Were there differences in the recommended treatment for the pregnant patient as compared to the non-pregnant patient? In an attempt to answer these questions several studies over the past four decades have been performed assessing the effect that pregnancy has on melanoma. A review of the existing data will be discussed.

Effect of Pregnancy on the Incidence of Melanoma

The true effect that pregnancy has on the incidence of melanoma has proven to be a difficult question to answer. The difficulty arises because obtaining true incidence levels during pregnancy may be altered by delay in diagnosis, or by patients terminating their pregnancy before a tissue diagnosis is made. The best available data assessing this has come from large state registries such as the Connecticut Tumor Registry. Houghton et al[12] analyzed data from this registry and demonstrated that the observed rate of melanoma occurring during pregnancy was slightly less than that predicted based on the incidence of this disease in non-pregnant women of similar age (observed cases = 12, expected cases = 13.3) The authors noted, however, that even large databases such as this may underestimate the true incidence of melanoma occurring during pregnancy, as some patients may have terminated their pregnancy prior to diagnosis or treatment. The best available data, however, suggests that there is no significant increase in the incidence of melanoma during pregnancy when compared to non-pregnant women of childbearing age.

Several studies have evaluated the effect that previous pregnancies may have on the risk of developing melanoma. At least three studies have demonstrated an actual decrease in the risk of melanoma in parous women (in two studies the risk was least in women with three or more children) as compared to nulliparous women.[13,14,15] The reasons for this decreased risk are not known, but it is speculated that pregnancy leads to repeat exposure to fetal antigens which may be similar to those present on melanoma cells. This exposure may lead to an increased maternal immune surveillance in future years that helps to eliminate cells that express those antigens (melanoma cells).

While the overall incidence of melanoma may not be significantly different during pregnancy there is evidence that certain precursor lesions may become more active during pregnancy. As was stated, it is generally accepted that pigmented skin lesions will frequently change during pregnancy and it has been reported that 10–33% of women report changes of pre-existing nevi during pregnancy.[16,17] However when these changes were further studied, many actually occurred in non-melanocytic skin lesions that have no potential for developing into melanoma. There is however evidence linking pregnancy with increased activation of nevi in patients with documented Dysplastic Nevus Syndrome (DNS), a syndrome with a known increased risk of cutaneous melanoma. A prospective study by Ellis in 1991[18] found that patients with DNS had a 3.9-fold increased incidence of enlarging nevi during pregnancy as compared to when the same patients were not pregnant. The incidence of enlarging nevi was greater in those patients who fit the criteria for the familial form of the syndrome and higher yet in those patients with a family history of melanoma.

A second prospective study, by Pennoyer et al[19] (this in patients without a known history of DNS), followed women during the course of their pregnancies to document the incidence of melanocytic nevi being activated, either by a change in size or an increase in pigmentation. This study demonstrated that there was essentially no change in benign appearing nevi during pregnancy and that in those patients where there were changes, the nevi were as likely to decrease in size as increase. An unique aspect of this study was that it limited its observations to the nevi on the backs of patients, theorizing that nevi at other anatomic locations, such as the abdomen or breasts, would change in size as the skin in those areas stretched with the pregnancy. It was an assumption of this study that any effect pregnancy may have on benign nevi would affect lesions located on the back at the same rate as lesions located elsewhere on the body.

It is unclear from the Ellis study where the changing nevi were located anatomically. It is possible that some or most of the activated lesions were present in the regions noted above and that the change in lesion size was due more to the stretching of skin during pregnancy than to a true activation of the lesions. It is also possible that there is a true difference between the nevi of patients with DNS compared to those without the disorder, one that predisposes DNS patients to activation of their nevi during pregnancy and which may potentially increase their risk of developing melanoma in the future.

Histologic Subtypes and Tumor Location

Retrospective reviews of patients with melanoma detected during pregnancy have shown that there is essentially no difference in the relative ratio of different histologic subtypes of melanoma in pregnant women as compared to non-pregnant women. Superficial spreading melanoma remains the most common subtype, accounting for approximately 70–75% of cases in both pregnant and non-pregnant controls. Nodular melanoma is the second most common subtype accounting for 15–20% of cases in both groups. Acral Lentiginous and Lentigo Maligna Melanoma subtypes are both quite uncommon in both pregnant women and non-pregnant women of childbearing age.[20,21] The location of the primary tumor is a known prognostic factor as well. Melanomas arising on the head, neck or trunk are associated with a worse prognosis than lesions arising on the extremities. Controlled studies have demonstrated mixed results when comparing the tumor locations in pregnant versus non-pregnant women. Early reports of melanoma occurring in pregnancy suggested a higher rate of head, neck and trunk primaries in pregnant women, whereas more recent studies have shown similar distributions or a decrease in high-risk sites in the pregnant patient population.[20,21,22] When this data is taken as a whole, there appears to be no significant difference in the incidence of high-risk primary tumor locations in the pregnant patient as compared to age matched non-pregnant controls.

Stage of Disease

The current staging system for melanoma is dependent on characteristics of the primary tumor (depth of invasion) and the presence of lymphatic or distant metastases. The current AJCC system, however, was not used before the early 1980s, instead a three-stage system was used. In that system, Stage I tumors were localized (any thickness), Stage II tumors had lymphatic metastases and Stage III tumors had distant metastatic disease. Studies prior to this time, therefore, did not routinely evaluate tumor thickness or depth of invasion, which are known prognostic factors in the clinical Stage I patient. More recent studies have micro-staged the primary tumors on a routine basis and allow a comparison of disease in a more precise fashion based on Clark's and Breslow's levels. A review of recent studies in which these measurements were made in comparison to age-matched controls shows a relatively consistent finding of increased primary tumor thickness in melanomas diagnosed during pregnancy (Table 6.3). The reasons for this increased tumor depth are not immediately clear. It has been postulated that pregnancy may stimulate growth of the primary tumor, similar to that seen in patients with dysplastic nevi, leading to an increase in tumor depth. Another possibility is that pigmented skin lesions in pregnant patients are not biopsied as early as they should be, given the prevailing clinical teaching that benign nevi frequently enlarge during pregnancy. A delay in diagnosis caused by prolonged observation of a suspicious lesion may allow additional tumor growth and subsequently a thicker lesion at time of tissue diagnosis. Whatever the reason, there is good evidence from several controlled retrospective trials that primary tumor depth is significantly greater in pregnant patients with melanoma than non-pregnant age-matched women.

Another important factor in the staging of patients with melanoma is the presence or absence of lymphatic or distant metastases (N and M stage). Distant metastases (Stage IV) are associated with a very poor prognosis, with 5-year survival rates of 10–20%. Patients with lymphatic metastases (lymph nodes or in-transit metastases: Stage III) have a significantly worse prognosis when compared to patients with localized

Table 6.3. Relationship of primary tumor depth to pregnany.

Author	Patients	Breslow depth (mean)	Clark Level(% patients)			
			I/II	III	IV/V	Unknown
Wong[20]	Pregnant	1.24mm	35	32	24	9
	Non-pregnant	1.28mm	29	36	23	12
Slingluff[22]	Pregnant	2.17mm	11	49	33	7
	Non-pregnant	1.52mm	11	50	31	8
MacKie[29]	Pregnant	2.38mm	not available			
	Non-Pregnant (3 groups)	1.49, 1.96, 1.48mm	not available			
Travers[21]	Pregnant	2.28mm	not available			
	Non-pregnant	1.22mm	not available			

disease, with 5-year survival rates of 35–50%. As mentioned earlier, studies prior to the 1980s utilized a 3-stage system with lymphatic metastases signifying Stage 2 and systemic metastases Stage 3. Patients were generally staged based on their clinical presentation. However the ability of a clinical examination to assess the regional lymph nodes for the presence of metastatic disease is often inaccurate. Therefore, studies which relied on the clinical assessment of nodes rather than a pathologic evaluation would inherently under-stage a significant number of those patients. This is a matter of importance, as elective lymph node dissections (ELND) have never been universally performed in melanoma due to the associated morbidity and a lack of conclusive evidence showing a survival benefit to these procedures. Therefore these procedures have often been omitted in pregnant patients because of a perceived increased risk to the fetus caused by a more prolonged operation. While there may be debate as to the impact that ELND has on patient survival, it is clear that disease staging is more accurate in the groups undergoing these procedures. Comparisons of groups based on pathologic staging will therefore give a more accurate assessment of the influence that pregnancy has on disease outcome on a stage for stage basis.

In a report by Wong et al. in 1989,[20] pregnant patients with clinical Stage I melanoma were compared to age-matched controls. In this report, the authors performed routine elective node dissections in all patients with primary tumors >0.65 mm thick or Clark's Level III or higher. By using such stringent criteria it is unlikely that any lymph node metastases were missed, as the expected nodal involvement rate in the patients not undergoing ELND would be 1% or less. In this study 47% of pregnant patients had elective node dissections compared to 45% of age-matched non-pregnant controls. The incidence of node positivity in the pregnant patients was 14%. Unfortunately, the incidence of positive nodes in the control group was not disclosed. This rate however falls in the range of what would be expected in a cohort of clinically node negative melanoma patients in the general population. This study compares to that of Slingluff et al,[22] where elective node dissections were performed in 16% of pregnant patients and 17% of controls. In this study patients had similar presenting clinical stages but subsequent lymph node recurrences occurred in 39% of pregnant patients as compared to 26% of controls, suggesting a higher rate of lymph node involvement in the pregnant patients. The increased incidence of lymphatic recurrences in this study is not completely unexpected, however, as the pregnant patient group had significantly thicker primary tumors than the control group (mean thickness 2.17 mm vs 1.52 mm). Additional studies have suggested a higher incidence of lymphatic or distant metastases in pregnant patients at presentation. Houghton et al[12] found 33% of pregnant patients in their series presented with clinically palpable nodal disease or distant metastases as compared to 12% of non-pregnant women. A similar increase in presenting stage was reported by George et al[23] and Shiu et al[24] Trapeznikov et al,[25] however, reported similar stages at presentation in pregnant women when compared to age- and site-matched non-pregnant controls.

In summary, it appears that pregnant patients do present with thicker primary tumors compared to age-matched non-pregnant controls and hence may have an increased risk of lymphatic metastases because of these thicker lesions. The incidence of distant metastases, however, in most series does not appear to be significantly different in the pregnant population despite the tendency for thicker primary lesions.

Recurrence Rates and Survival

Older Studies

Interest in the possible effects of pregnancy on the outcome of melanoma was spurred on by early reports of impaired survival in pregnant patients with this disease. In 1951 Pack and Scharnagel[26] reviewed 1,050 cases of melanoma and found 10 cases diagnosed during pregnancy. Five of those patients died of their disease within 30 months of diagnosis. The authors found an additional eleven patients who reported a growth or change in a nevus during a previous pregnancy who subsequently were diagnosed with melanoma. Three of those eleven patients died of disease in short follow-up of less than three years while follow-up of the other patients was of very limited duration. The authors suggested that malignant transformation of benign nevi could occur as a result of pregnancy and that pregnancy caused "dynamic growth propensities" to occur in melanoma that could not be slowed down once started, even with termination of the pregnancy. This report, however, had no age-matched non-pregnant controls with which to compare survival rates and therefore these conclusions are debatable. This study did initiate further investigation, however, into the effect of pregnancy on melanoma. A follow-up study from this institution in 1960 by George and Fortner[23] added an additional 67 patients to those reported by Pack and Scharnagel. These patients were compared to 141 age-matched patients who were not pregnant during the course of their disease. The pregnant patients had a higher incidence of lymphatic metastases at presentation and a greater frequency of lesions on the head, neck and trunk. Tumor thickness was not yet considered at this time as a prognostic factor and therefore was not analyzed. Despite the seemingly higher risk lesions in the pregnant group there was no difference in five or ten year survival between the groups.

In 1976 Shiu et al[24] reviewed the course of women with melanoma categorized into four groups:

1 Nulliparous women (n = 47)

2 Parous women who observed no changes in nevi during previous pregnancies (n = 134)

3 Parous women who noted growth, irritation or other change in nevi during a previous pregnancy (n = 36)

4 Women treated for melanoma during pregnancy (n = 34)

The authors found no difference in survival in clinical Stage I (localized) disease between the four groups; there was however an increased incidence of Stage II (lymphatic metastases) disease in groups 3 and 4 (tumor thickness was not reported). Survival rates in Stage II patients were significantly lower in patients from groups 3 and 4; however as this combined both pregnant and non-pregnant patients at diagnosis, it is difficult to determine the effect of pregnancy alone in these patients.

In 1981, Houghton et al[12] reviewed cases of twelve patients diagnosed with melanoma during pregnancy. The authors compared this group to two control groups; the first, a group of 24 non-pregnant women with melanoma who were matched for age, stage and primary tumor site with the study group, the second being a group of 175 non-pregnant women of childbearing age who were otherwise not matched for tumor characteristics. Survival rates at 3 and 5 years were considerably lower in the pregnant patients when compared to the unmatched control group but there was no significant difference in survival when compared to the matched controls.

In 1983, Sutherland et.al.[27] identified 18 patients with melanoma either diagnosed during pregnancy, noted to have arisen in pregnancy or clearly documented to have been stimulated during pregnancy. Fifteen patients presented with stage I (localized) disease and of those 13 had sufficient follow-up for analysis. Tumor thickness was not documented. Of these thirteen patients, only 4 were alive at 5 years of follow-up. Although a control group was not used the investigators concluded that patients with melanoma diagnosed, initiated or stimulated during pregnancy had a disproportionately high mortality rate.

In 1989 Colbourn et al[28] reviewed outcomes of three groups of women with melanoma:

1 Women with melanoma diagnosed before or during a pregnancy (n = 13)

2 Women whose melanoma was diagnosed after their last pregnancy (n = 43)

3 Women who were nulliparous for the time of the study (n = 16)

Information on patient age, tumor location and tumor thickness were not available on all patients. Almost all patients had clinical Stage I (localized) disease. The authors found a 15% increased 5-year survival rate in the control group (group 3) when compared to group 1 patients. Unfortunately enough significant information was lacking from this study, such as the proportion of women in group 1 who were actually diagnosed during pregnancy, as well as the location and thickness of the primary tumors, to make any strong conclusions possible.

Matched Control Studies

A recent group of five retrospective studies have been reported that incorporate information on the known prognostic factors of tumor thickness and stage of the tumors as well as making use of age- and stage-matched control groups in their analyses. These studies avoided possible inconsistencies by allowing only women diagnosed with melanoma during pregnancy into their study groups. These studies at present offer the best available data set for analyzing the effect pregnancy may exert on the outcome of patients with melanoma. A synopsis of these studies follows.

Slingluff et al[22] made a study in which the authors review the results of 100 patients diagnosed with melanoma during pregnancy as compared to 86 non-pregnant age-matched controls. Pregnant patients had thicker primary tumors (mean 2.17 mm vs 1.52 mm) but had similar clinical stages at presentation Stage I: 88% of pregnant, 92% non-pregnant). All patients with clinical Stage I disease were analyzed for disease free and overall survival. Patients diagnosed during pregnancy did have significantly shorter disease free intervals ($p = 0.039$); however, this was largely due to lymphatic and local recurrences that did not translate into significantly different overall survival rates between the two groups. The incidence of lymphatic recurrences in the pregnant group may well have been lower if more frequent elective lymph node dissections had been performed on the pregnant patients (only 16% had ELND). This possibly may have equalized the disease free interval rates seen in this study by eliminating the occult nodal disease that was the source of most of the disease recurrences seen.

The study by Wong et al[20] reviewed the results of 77 women with melanoma diagnosed during pregnancy. Of these patients, 66 had clinical Stage I (localized) disease. These patients were compared to 619 non-pregnant age-matched controls with Stage I disease. In this study there was a much more liberal use of ELND (47% of pregnant and 45% of non-pregnant patients had ELND) which made pathologic staging more accurate. In this study there was no difference in the tumor thickness of melanomas diagnosed during pregnancy compared to controls (mean tumor thickness 1.24mm in pregnant women vs 1.28 mm in controls). The overall and disease free survival rates were equivalent in the two patient groups at three and five year follow-up.

MacKie et al[29] reviewed 92 patients diagnosed with clinical Stage I (localized) melanoma diagnosed during pregnancy. The study group was compared to three other groups:

1 women who had their first pregnancy after the diagnosis of melanoma (n = 85)

2 women who completed all pregnancies before the diagnosis of melanoma (n = 143)

3 women who were treated for melanoma between pregnancies.

The latter two groups served as controls for this study. Patients diagnosed with melanoma during pregnancy presented with thicker primary tumors and a higher incidence of lesions on the head, neck, or trunk as compared to controls. Overall survival rates however were equivalent when adjusted for depth of primary tumor invasion by log rank adjustment. This finding was suggestive that pregnancy itself did not alter patient outcome from melanoma.

McManamny et al[30] reviewed 23 patients diagnosed with Stage I (localized) melanoma during pregnancy. The control groups were women between the ages of 15 and 40 who were not pregnant at the time of, nor became pregnant after the diagnosis of, their clinical Stage I melanoma. There was no significant difference in tumor thickness or location of the primary tumors between the two groups. Survival analysis demonstrated no significant difference in disease free or overall survival between the two groups.

Trapeznikov et al[25] is a study from the Russian literature and is reviewed in the English literature in 1993 by Kjems and Krag.[31] In this study 102 patients were diagnosed with melanoma during pregnancy. This group was compared to 599 non-pregnant women matched for age, primary site, tumor thickness and clinical stage. Overall survival rates were less in the pregnant group at 5 years of follow-up (44.4% vs 53.6%), but this difference did not reach statistical significance. However at 10 years of follow-up this survival difference continued and did reach statistical significance (26.0% vs 43.0%). Survival rates were also evaluated for women who had full term pregnancies or an abortion before the twentieth week. For clinical Stage I patients the survival rates were higher in the group completing their pregnancy (66.5% vs 33.5% at 5 years), but for clinical Stage II patients survival was better in the group receiving an abortion (27% vs 53.6% at 5 years). This study is the only recent study using matched controls that has demonstrated a difference in survival in patients diagnosed with melanoma during pregnancy. It is unclear why these differences were noted. However as the survival rates in this study are quite low compared to similar stage patients treated in the west, this data should be evaluated cautiously.

In summary, review of the existing literature, which at its best is limited to matched retrospective comparisons, suggests that pregnancy does not significantly influence patient survival rates with melanoma. There may be a tendency towards more frequent lymphatic recurrences, but this finding is inconsistent and may be an artifact caused by inadequate pathologic staging at the time of initial diagnosis. There is a consistent association of increased tumor thickness in melanomas diagnosed during pregnancy, however, it is unclear as to whether this increased thickness is due to a "stimulatory" effect on the tumor caused by the pregnancy itself or is due to delays in the diagnosis of melanoma caused by clinicians ascribing changes seen in skin lesions as being a normal consequence of pregnancy.

Treatment of Melanoma

The primary treatment for melanoma today remains complete surgical excision of all known disease. The extent of surgery is dependent on the stage of disease at presentation. A careful history and physical examination to identify potential sites of satellite lesions, in-transit lesions and lymph node metastases should be made before a surgical plan is made. Evaluation for systemic metastases should include liver function tests, complete blood count and a chest X-ray. Further studies for metastatic disease are not cost effective in the asymptomatic patient presenting with clinical Stage I or II (localized) disease.

The surgical treatment of the primary tumor site involves a wide excision to include the full thickness of skin and subcutaneous fat tissue around the tumor site. The recommended width of the wide excision will be dependent on the tumor thickness found on biopsy but may need to be tailored depending on the anatomic location of the tumor to allow better functional results in areas such as the face, hands, feet or bony prominences. Current recommendations for wide excision margins are 1cm for primary tumors <1.0 mm in thickness and 2 cm for lesions 1.0 to 4.0 mm in thickness. Lesions which are deeper than 4.0 mm thick, should be excised with a 3 cm margin if possible. In most cases primary closure of the wide excision site is feasible and is recommended. This requires the use of elliptical incisions and the frequent use of local undermining or rotation flaps. If primary closure is not feasible then use of split thickness skin grafts will suffice in most cases for wound closure. The above recommendations for margin width were based on results of two prospective randomized clinical trials: The World Health Organization (WHO)[32] published results of a prospective randomized trial comparing wide excision margins of 1 cm vs 3 cm around primary tumor sites. In this study there were no local recurrences noted in patients with lesions less than 1mm in depth in either treatment group. Survival rates in this subset of patients were the same in either group as well. Because of the decreased morbidity associated with the 1cm margins, this became the recommended surgical treatment for lesions <1 mm in depth. The Intergroup Melanoma Committee[33] subsequently performed a prospective randomized study comparing wide excision margins of 2 cm vs 4 cm for patients with primary melanomas between 1.0 and 4.0 mm in depth. Results of this study showed identical rates of local recurrence with either margin width; however, this rate increased equally in both groups with increasing tumor thickness. In patients with lesions greater than 4.0 mm in depth the local recurrence rates have been reported as high as 10–20% which has led many surgeons to advocate wider margins (3 cm or more) despite the fact there is no prospective randomized data comparing this to 2 cm margins.

The management of regional lymph nodes in the setting of clinically negative nodes has been an issue of debate in past. Routine elective lymph node dissection has been advocated by many surgeons for intermediate thickness melanomas (1.0 to 4.0 mm deep) based on retrospective studies showing a survival advantage in those groups. However more recently reported prospective randomized trials[34,35] have failed to confirm this survival advantage except in certain small subgroups of patients. The debate over elective node dissections fortunately has largely been put to rest with the introduction of Sentinel lymph node mapping techniques. These techniques utilize a vital blue dye (isosulfan blue), a radiolabeled colloid (Technetium-99m-Sulfur colloid), or both, which are injected into the dermis around the primary melanoma site. The agents then travel to the first draining lymph node or nodes and label those nodes, which can then be selectively removed by the surgeon. Using these methods, sentinel node biopsies can identify the presence of metastatic disease in a regional node basin with great accuracy (98% accuracy at identifying nodal metastases), while subjecting the patient to a much less morbid procedure than an elective lymph node dissection.[36,37] The sentinel node techniques have now become widely practiced and are considered the standard of care in many institutions performing large volumes of melanoma surgery.

The surgical treatment of melanoma in many cases can be performed safely and comfortably for the patient under local anesthesia. This should allow minimal risk to the mother and her fetus. The surgical treatment of the primary tumor should not be delayed unduly because of the pregnancy. Management of the regional lymph nodes can be delayed until after delivery, or with sentinel node techniques can be done at the time of the primary tumor wide excision. If a sentinel node procedure is indicated, use of the blue dye is most appropriate; however, the dose of radiation used if the radiolabeled method is chosen is minimal and should be of no consequence to the fetus.

Until recently the only treatment modality of proven benefit for melanoma was surgical resection. Recent data reported from the Eastern Cooperative Oncology Group (ECOG) [38] however has shown for the first time that an adjuvant treatment in high-risk patients can improve survival in melanoma. The agent used was Interferon-alfa-2b. This treatment is given as a high dose intravenous treatment for 1 month followed by lower dose subcutaneous injections for an additional 11 more months. With this regimen, high-risk patients (node positive disease or primary tumors > 4.0 mm deep) had an 11% reduction in mortality rate compared to controls (no adjuvant treatment). This treatment however came at the expense of significant toxicity. A subsequent study from ECOG comparing the same dose of interferon-alfa-2b to a low dose interferon arm and an untreated arm have not yet shown the same improvement in overall survival as seen in the initial study.[39] Based on this data it would therefore be recommended that any adjuvant treatment of the pregnant patient be delayed until after delivery. Additional trials are investigating the use of immunomodulators and tumor vaccines as adjuvant therapies for melanoma but would need to be considered investigational at this time.

Treatment of the pregnant patient with distant metastases is a difficult problem with very few good options. In the select group of patients with isolated single or a limited number of metastases, surgical resection should be strongly considered and done without delay. The chance for long-term survival in the patient with resectable lesions is in the range of 10–20%.[40] If the patient is not a candidate for surgical resection, the chance for long-term survival is near 0%. A discussion should be made of the patient's desires to complete the pregnancy knowing the prognosis. There is no evidence that terminating the pregnancy will affect the patient's prognosis, however. In rare cases chemotherapy has been given for metastatic melanoma during the second trimester with successful delivery of a healthy child,[41] but given the small number of such cases treated this way, this cannot be considered as standard procedure.

Melanoma is known as the malignancy with the greatest propensity to metastasize to the products of conception; this remains an extremely rare event, however, with less than 60 cases reported in the literature. Despite this very rare finding the placenta should be checked carefully for evidence of metastases in any patient with a history of melanoma, as there is a 40–50% risk of fetal involvement if this is found.[42]

Subsequent pregnancies to date have not been found to increase a patient's risk for melanoma recurrence.[29,43] Some authors have made recommendations, however, that patients should avoid pregnancy for 2 to 3 years following treatment of melanoma, as this corresponds to the time interval where most recurrences will occur. In the patient with a thin Stage I melanoma, who is at minimal risk for recurrence, this waiting period is probably excessive and earlier pregnancy should pose no risk to the patient.

Summary

With the increasing incidence of melanoma in the United States and the frequent occurrence of this disease during the childbearing years in women, the number of cases of melanoma occurring during pregnancy is likely to increase in the future. Prompt diagnosis is crucial to maximize patient survival, therefore any skin lesion which has enlarged, changed color, bled or otherwise changed should be biopsied to rule out the possibility of melanoma. If melanoma is diagnosed, prompt surgical treatment of the primary tumor site with consideration of a sentinel lymph node biopsy should be undertaken. In many cases general anesthesia can be avoided for these procedures. To date there is no clear consensus on the effect that pregnancy may have on the outcome of melanoma, but there is a tendency for pregnant patients to present with thicker lesions and perhaps a higher incidence of lymph node metastases. The bulk of data in controlled studies indicates that on a stage for stage basis, pregnant patients fare the same as non-pregnant patients with melanoma. This fact suggests that pregnancy itself probably has little effect on the outcome of this disease and that earlier diagnosis is needed for these patients. There is no data to suggest that termination of the pregnancy is needed or is of benefit in these patients and there is no evidence that subsequent pregnancies will affect disease recurrence. Adjuvant biologic or chemotherapy is of uncertain benefit to the pregnant patient and has potential serious toxicity and therefore would not be recommended as a standard treatment during pregnancy.

References

1. Landis SH, Murray T, Bolden S, Wingo PA. Cancer Statistics 1999. CA-A Cancer Journal for Clinicians1999; 49:8–31
2. Wong DJ, Strassner HT. Melanoma in pregnancy. Clinical Obstetrics Gynecology 1990; 33:782–91
3. Balch CM, Reintgen DS, Kirkwood JM, Houghton A, Peters L, Ang KK. Cutaneous melanoma. In: Devita VT Jr., Hellman S, Rosenberg SA (eds). Cancer: Principles and Practice of Oncology, 5th Edn. Philadelphia: Lippincott-Raven Press, 1997
4. Elder DE, Green MH, Guerry D, et al. The dysplastic nevus syndrome: our definition. AM J Dermatopathol 1982; 4:455–60
5. Ananthaswamy HN, Pierceall WE. Molecular mechanisms of ultraviolet radiation carcinogenesis. Photochem Photobiol 1990; 52:1119–36
6. Clark WH Jr. The histogenesis and biological behavior of primary malignant melanoma of the skin. Cancer Research 1969; 29:705–27
7. Breslow A. Thickness, cross sectional areas and depth of invasion in the prognosis of cutaneous melanoma. Ann Surg 1970: 902–8
8. Beahrs OH, Henson DE, Hutter RVP, Kennedy BJ. (eds) Handbook for Staging of Cancer: From the Manual for Staging of Cancer, 4th edn. Philadelphia: JB Lippincott Co, 1993:155–60.
9. Neifeld JP, Lippman ME. Steroid Hormone Receptors and Melanoma. J Invest Dermatol 1980; 74:379–81
10. Nesbet RA, Woods RL, Tattersall MHN et al. Tamoxifen in malignant melanoma. New England J Med 1979; 301:1241–2
11. Duncan LM, Travers RL, Koerner FC, Mihm MC Jr., Sober AJ. Estrogen and progesterone receptor analysis in pregnancy-associated melanoma: absence of immunohistochemically detectable hormone receptors. Human Pathology 1994; 25(1):36–41
12. Houghton AN, Flannery J, Viola MV. Malignant melanoma of the skin occurring during pregnancy. Cancer 1981; 48:407–10
13. Zanetti R, Franceschi S, Rosso S, Bidoli E, Colonna S. Cutaneous malignant melanoma in females: the role of hormonal and reproductive factors. Int J Epidemiol 1990; 19:522–6

14. Gallagher RP, Elmood JM, Hill GB, Coldman AJ, Threllfall WJ, Spinelli JJ. Reproductive factors, oral contraceptives and risk of malignant melanoma: western Canada melanoma study. Br J Cancer 1985; 52:901–7
15. Wyshak G, Frisch RE, Albright NL, Albright TE, Schiff I. Reproductive factors and melanoma of the skin among women. 1989: 28:527–30
16. Foucar E, Bentley TJ, Laube DW, et al. A histopathologic evaluation of nevocellular nevi in pregnancy. Arch Dermatol 1985; 121:350–4
17. Sanchez JL, Figueroa LD, Rodriguez E. Behavior of melanocytic nevi during pregnancy. Am J Dermatopathol 19984; 6(suppl 1):89–91
18. Ellis DL. Pregnancy and sex steroid hormone effects on nevi of patients with the dysplastic nevus syndrome. J Am Acad Dermatol 1991; 25:467–82
19. Pennoyer JW, Grin CM, Driscoll MS, et al. Changes in size of melanocytic nevi during pregnancy. J Am Acad Dermatol 1997; 36:378–82
20. Wong JH, Sterns EE, Kopald KH, et al. Prognostic significance of pregnancy in Stage I melanoma. Arch Surg 1989; 124:1227–31
21. Travers RL, Sober AJ, Berwick M, et al. Increased thickness of pregnancy associated melanoma. Br J Dermatol 1995; 132:876–83
22. Slingluff CL Jr., Reintgen DS, Vollmer RT et al. Malignant melanoma arising during pregnancy: a study of 100 patients. Ann Surgery 1990; 211:552–9
23. George PA, Fortner IG. Melanoma with pregnancy: a report of 115 cases. Cancer 1960; 13:854–9
24. Shiu MH, Schottenfeld D, Maclean B, et al. Adverse effects of pegnancy on melanoma: a reappraisal. Cancer 1976; 37:181–7
25. Trapeznikov NN, Khasanov SR, Yavovsky VV. Skin melanoma and pregnancy. Voproxy Onkologii 1987; 33:40–6
26. Pack GT, Scharnagel IM. The prognosis for malignant melanoma in the pregnant woman. Cancer 1951; 4:324–34
27. Sutherland CM, Loutfi A, Mather FJ, et al. Effect of pregnancy upon malignant melanoma. Surg Gynec Obstet 1983; 157:443–6
28. Colbourn DS, Nathanson L, Belilos E. Pregnancy and malignant melanoma. Seminars in Oncology 1989; 16:377–87
29. MacKie RM, Bufalino R, Morabito A, Sutherland C, Cascinelli N. Lack of effect of pregnancy on outcome of melanoma. Lancet 1991; 337:653–5.
30. McManamny DS, Moss AL, Pocock PV, Briggs JC. Melanoma and pregnancy: a long-term follow-up. Br J Obstet Gyn 1989; 96:1419–23
31. Kjems E, Krag C. Melanoma and pregnancy, a review. Acta Oncolog 1993; 32:371–8
32. Veronesi U, Cascinelli N, Adamus J, et al. Thin Stage I primary cutaneous melanoma. Comparison of excision margins of 1 or 3cm. NEJM 1988; 318:1159–62
33. Karakousis C, Balch C, Urist M, et al. Local recurrence in malignant melanoma: long term results of the multi-institutional randomized surgical trial. Ann Surg Oncol 1996; 3:446–52
34. Veronesi U, Adamus J, Bandieva DC, et al. Delayed regional lymph node dissection in Stage 1 melanoma of the skin of the lower extremities. Cancer 1982; 49:2420–30
35. Balch CM, Soong S-J, Bartolucci AA, et al. Efficacy of an elective regional lymph node dissection of 1 to 4mm thick melanomas for patients 60 years of age and younger. Ann Surg 1996; 224:255–66
36. Morton DC, Wen DR, Wong JH, et al. Technical details of intra-operative lymphatic mapping for early stage melanoma. Arch Surg 1992; 127:392–9
37. Krag DN, Meijer SJ, Weaver DC, et al. Minimal access surgery for staging malignant melanoma. Arch Surg 1995; 130:654–8
38. Kirkwood JM, Strawderman MH, Ernstoff MS, et al. Adjuvant therapy of high risk resected cutaneous melanoma: The Eastern Cooperative Oncology Group trial EST 1684. J Clin Oncol 1996; 14:7–17
39. Mastrangelo M. Conference report Third International Conference Adjuvant Therapy of Malignant Melanoma. Melanoma Research 1999; 9:306–8
40. Feun LG, Gutterman J, Burgess MA, et al. The natural history of resectable metastatic melanoma (Stage IVa melanoma). Cancer 1982; 50:1656–63
41. Dipaola RS, Goodin S, Ratzall M, et al. Chemotherapy for metastatic melanoma during pregnancy. Gyn Oncol 1997; 66:526–30
42. Dildy GA, Moise KJ, Carpenter RJ, et al. Maternal malignancy metastatic to the products of conception: a review. Obst Gyn Surv 1989; 44:535–40
43. Reintgen DS, McCarty KS, Vollmer R, et al. Malignant melanoma and pregnancy. Cancer 1985; 55:1340–4

7. Rare Tumors in Pregnancy

Tanja Pejovic, Giancarlo Mari and Peter E. Schwartz

Cancer is among the leading causes of non-accidental death in the United States in women aged 15–35, accounting for 19% of mortality in this age group, and it is the leading cause of death in women age 35–54, accounting for 41% of deaths in this group.[1] About 1 in 1000 women will be affected by cancer while pregnant. As the tendency for delaying pregnancy until the late reproductive years continue, more cases of cancer complicating pregnancy are expected.

Gastrointestinal Cancer

Colorectal Cancer

Colorectal cancer is rarely seen in pregnancy. The incidence of colon cancer during pregnancy in the United States in the period 1981–1989 was 1 per 13, 000 live births.[2] To date over 200 cases of colon cancer in pregnancy have been reported, most of them being reported before 1985.[3] The subject is discussed in detail in Ch. 8.

Pancreatic Cancer

Only 3 cases of pancreatic cancer have been reported to be associated with pregnancy.[4] Supportive care with biliary drainage and hyperalimentation may be necessary to maintain the mother through pregnancy. Eight cases of insulinoma in pregnancy have been described, all recognized in the first trimester as a result of hypoglycemic crises.[5]

Gastric Cancer

Only 0.4–0.5 % of gastric carcinomas occur in women under 30 years of age. Given the high pregnancy rate in this group about 9 cases of gastric cancer complicating pregnancy per year may be expected in the United States. The literature on gastric cancer in pregnancy consists of isolated case reports[6,7] and a Japanese study on a larger group of patients.[8]

The symptoms of gastric cancer are similar to those frequently seen in normal pregnancies. They include gastrointestinal discomfort, nausea, vomiting and exacerbation of pre-existing ulcer disease. The diagnosis is frequently delayed. During the first trimester, emesis affects 50–70% of women. Gastroscopy is an effective means of diagnosing gastric carcinoma. However, it would not be cost-effective to perform gastroscopy on all pregnant patients presenting with emesis. However, since hyperemesis gravidarum usually improves after 16 week of gestation, vomiting beyond the sixteenth week requires a careful work up including ruling out of gastric carcinoma.

As in the general population, half of the patients with gastric cancer present with resectable disease, the remaining cases are fatal. In a series by Maeta et al[9] a significant proportion of gastric cancer in pregnancy were Borrmann Type 4 cancers and poorly differentiated adenocarcinoma with a scirrhous type of growth and peritoneal metastases. The prognosis is dismal.

Liver Cancer

Hepatocellular carcinomas are very rare in women and usually occur in postmenopausal women. Until 1995, only 28 cases of hepatocellular carcinoma were described in women.[10,11] An isolated case of hepatocellular carcinoma in pregnancy resulted in a maternal death. A single case of extrahepatic biliary tract carcinoma in pregnancy has been reported.[12] Routine management of choledochal cysts with excision and a Roux-en-Y reconstruction should be deferred until after delivery because of the risk of maternal morbidity and fetal mortality associated with the procedure.

Endocrine Tumors

Thyroid Cancer

Although thyroid disorders and thyroid nodules are frequently diagnosed in pregnancy, thyroid cancer is infrequent in pregnancy. Pregnancy does not promote or increase the frequency of thyroid neoplasm.[13] To date there is no convincing evidence that pregnancy has an adverse effect on maternal prognosis or fetal outcome.

The most common histologic types of thyroid cancer are the papillary, follicular, and anaplastic carcinoma, whereas medullary carcinomas account for less than 5% of all thyroid cancers.[14] The most common histologic type in pregnancy is papillary carcinoma. The prognosis is very good with 15-year survival rate of 90–95%. Prognosis is not affected by sub-clinical metastases to regional lymph nodes, which are present in 50–70% of the patients. As papillary carcinomas occur most frequently in women 30–34 years of age, with the current tendency toward delaying childbearing, it is possible that more papillary carcinoma of the thyroid will be diagnosed in the future. Follicular carcinoma occurs most frequently in women over 40 years of age and it has a slightly worse prognosis than the papillary variant. Anaplastic carcinoma is very aggressive. It is rare in pregnancy as it is most frequently found in women over 50 years of age. Medullary carcinomas are rare; they occur as a part of MEN II syndrome, are bilateral and have been reported only once in pregnancy.[15]

Pregnancy should not delay the diagnosis of thyroid cancer. Fine needle aspiration is considered safe in pregnancy.[16] It is associated with false negative rate of only 6%.[17]

Radionucleotide scanning is contraindicated in pregnancy because of the risk of destroying the fetal thyroid.

The majority of thyroid cancers in pregnancy are well differentiated. Pregnancy does not change the course of these tumors and there is no reason to terminate pregnancy or avoid subsequent pregnancies.[17,18] Thyroid suppression may be administered until delivery, regardless of the trimester in which diagnosis has been established.[19] Patients should undergo surgery if metastases develop during suppression therapy or if the tumor is fixed to surrounding tissue. Usually, subtotal thyroidectomy is performed. Radioactive iodine therapy is never used in pregnancy because iodine-131 can cross the placenta and cause fetal hypothyroidism and cretinism.[13] Extensive surgery should be avoided in pregnancy as miscarriage can occur as a result of it.

Patients diagnosed with medullary thyroid carcinoma in the first two trimesters of pregnancy should undergo prompt total thyroidectomy and a prophylactic neck dissection, while those diagnosed in the third trimester can await fetal maturity. One must be aware of the risks of concurrent additional tumors that are part of MEN II (pheochromocytoma, parotid and parathyroid cancers). Standard therapy for anaplastic carcinoma is a total thyroidectomy and radiation therapy. Patients undergoing thyroidectomy in pregnancy should be substituted with levothyroxine postoperatively in doses sufficient to keep their thyroid-stimulating hormone levels low.[20]

Pheochromocytoma

Pheochromocytoma during pregnancy is rare, occurring in 1 of 54, 000 term pregnancies.[21] Over 200 cases have been reported in the literature to date.[22] Malignant pheochromocytomas accounted for only four of these cases.[22,24] Although rare, the association between pregnancy and pheochromocytoma deserves special consideration since its clinical picture is easily mistaken for pregnancy-induced hypertension, eclampsia, or essential hypertension. Delay in diagnosing pheochromocytoma in pregnancy may have catastrophic consequence.[25]

In the past pheochromocytoma has been associated with a high maternal mortality (58%) and fetal mortality (55%). However, when diagnosis is made in pregnancy the maternal mortality was 0 and fetal loss was 15%.[22] Because of its rarity, there are no studies comparing mortality and morbidity of pheochromocytoma in the pregnant and non-pregnant population. Characteristic symptoms associated with even benign pheochromocytoma include hypertension, headache, palpitations, anxiety, and congestive heart failure. During pregnancy complicated by pheochromocytoma there are many precipitants of a potentially catastrophic hypertensive episode, such as anesthesia, vaginal delivery, uterine contractions, vigorous fetal movements and anti-emetics such as metoclopramide.[26]

MRI may be used to confirm the presence and the location of the tumor. Provocative tests should not be used, because this may lead to maternal death.[24] A 24-hour urine collection for levels of cathecholamines, vanilmandelic acid, and metanephrines may confirm the diagnosis.

The management of pheochromocytoma in the first two trimesters has been surgical removal of the tumor, while medical management with alpha- and beta-blocking agents has been reserved for tumors diagnosed later in pregnancy.[27] Specific risks are associated with pheochromocytoma surgery included elevated blood pressure and tachycardia. Technical advances in surgery however have allowed safe removal of the tumors with minor intra- and postoperative complications. Recently, Janetschek et al. have reported a series of 19 patients who successfully underwent laparoscopic surgery for pheochromocytoma.[28] Two of these patients were pregnant and had tumors removed at 16 and 20 gestational weeks respectively.[28] Most authors consider vaginal delivery to be contraindicated and in cases treated medically without surgical removal of the tumor, delivery was by Cesarean section.[29]

Controversy exists concerning medical management of pheochromocytoma in pregnancy. Arguments against it include unknown long-term effects of alpha- and beta-blockers, teratogenic potential of phenoxybenzamine (alpha-blocker of choice), and the risk of delaying removal of a malignant pheochromocytoma.[30,31] However, several authors have reported successful medical management of pheochromocytoma with phenoxybenzamine to lower blood pressure and propranolol to prevent arrhythmias.[31,32,33]

Parathyroid Carcinoma

One case of parathyroid carcinoma in pregnancy has been reported. The patient presented with a clinical picture of acute pancreatitis at 31 weeks of gestation, underwent a partial parathyroidectomy and subsequently delivered a viable child.[34]

Parotid Gland Carcinoma

The only case of mucoepidermoid carcinoma of the parotid gland in pregnancy was described in 19 year old woman who was treated with radioactive iodine for thyroid cancer 3 years prior to diagnosis of parotid gland cancer.[35]

Central Nervous System Tumors

Central nervous system tumors rarely complicate pregnancy, as they tend to occur in women beyond childbearing age.[36] The types of brain tumors in pregnant women are similar to those in non-pregnant population of the same age group.[37] Thirty-two percent of brain tumors in pregnancy are gliomas, 29% meningiomas, 15% acoustic neuromas, and other types each account for 6% or less. Spinal tumors are very rare and account for only 12% of central nervous tumors in pregnancy; 61% of these tumors are vertebral hemangiomas and 18% are meningiomas.[37]

Patients usually present with nonspecific symptoms such as headache and nausea, which can be mistaken as associated with a normal pregnancy and thereby delaying diagnosis. MRI is the modality of choice for diagnosing central nervous system tumors, and it also has the benefit of avoiding the risk of radiation exposure.

Pregnancy may have dramatic effects on some tumors including meningiomas, pituitary adenomas, acoustic neuromas and vertebral hemangiomas.[36] The rapid enlargement of tumors may be brought about by the hormonal stimulation of responsive tumors. About 90% of meningiomas have high affinity progesterone receptors and about 30% have estrogen receptors, suggesting that there may be hormonal influence on growth of these tumors in pregnancy.[36] Similarly, 30% of pituitary macroadenomas are known to enlarge in pregnancy to the extent that they require medical or surgical treatment.

DeAngelis[36] recommended that labor should be as pain-free as possible in patients with central nervous system tumors, because any maternal effort may cause increase in intracranial pressure.[37] For the same reasons, forceps delivery is recommended to shorten the second stage of labor. There is continued need for data concerning the influence of anesthetic management on the outcome of labor and delivery of patients with these tumors.[38]

Low-grade glial tumors such as astrocytomas and oligodendrogliomas almost never require urgent treatment.[23] By contrast, high-grade glial tumors (anaplastic astrocytoma, anaplastic oligodendroglioma and glioblastoma multiforme) require prompt treatment. Therapeutic abortions have been recommended for patients diagnosed in the first trimester because of the rapid course of these tumors and to avoid adverse effects of radiation therapy to the fetus.[39] In the second and third trimester decisions should be made on an individual basis. Corticosteroids are used to reduce symptoms of increased intracranial pressure. Prednisone is preferred in pregnancy because it is metabolized before crossing the placenta.

There are several reports on good fetal outcomes with surgical treatment of central nervous system tumors at different stages of pregnancy.[40-44]

Bone Tumors

Benign and malignant bone tumors rarely complicate pregnancy. The diagnosis can be suspected from the characteristic radiographic appearance. When diagnosis is not certain, a biopsy must be done.

Two benign bone tumors, which can affect pregnancy and delivery, are endochondromas and benign exostosis, both of which may occur at the pelvic brim. These tumors may interfere with progression of labor by causing mechanical obstruction at the pelvic inlet, thus necessitating Cesarean section.

The most common primary malignant tumors seen in those of childbearing age are Ewing's sarcoma, osteogenic sarcoma, and osteocytoma. They usually involve the clavicle, sternum, spine, humerus or femur and are associated with local pain, mass, and disability.[45]

Primary bone tumors are aggressive and frequently metastasize hematogenously already at the time of diagnosis. The prognosis of these tumors was uniformly poor with most patients dying of disease within 24 months. Pregnancy does not change the natural course of the disease.[46]

Within the last 20 years the treatment of osteogenic sarcoma with limited surgery followed by aggressive chemotherapy has brought about significant improvement in survival rates. Therefore, it is appropriate to recommend termination of pregnancy for patients diagnosed in the first or early second trimester.[46] If the diagnosis is made later in pregnancy, early delivery of the infant followed by aggressive chemotherapy is advised. Alternatively, because the risk of fetal malformations induced by chemotherapy during the second half of pregnancy is low, continuation of pregnancy despite chemotherapy may be considered. As most recurrences from bone malignancy occur within first 3 years of treatment, future pregnancy should be deferred until that interval has passed.

Bladder Cancer

Bladder cancer is very rare in pregnancy and may be mistaken for other more common conditions such as urinary tract infection, pyelitis, and miscarriage. Waser et al (1927) reported the first patient with bladder cancer during pregnancy and a further 12 cases have been reported since then.[47-49] Ten of these 12 patients presented with hematuria, although in 4 patients this was initially thought to be vaginal bleeding. Therefore it is essential that if the source of bleeding in pregnancy cannot be proven to originate from the cervix, serious consideration be given to urethral catheterization and urine cytology.

The most common histologic type of bladder cancer in pregnancy is transitional cell carcinoma, followed by squamous cell carcinoma and adenocarcinoma, the distribution being similar to that in non-pregnant patients. Treatment of bladder cancer in pregnancy is similar to that in non-pregnant patient. The standard treatment for a superficial, well-differentiated bladder cancer is fulguration. Treatment of invasive carcinoma includes radiation therapy followed by partial or complete cystectomy. Bladder cancer in early pregnancy requires a therapeutic abortion if radiation is needed. In late pregnancy, treatment may be delayed until fetal maturity is achieved.[50]

Three-year survival of early stage bladder cancer (Stages 0, A, B1) is estimated to be 54%, whereas deep-invasion stages (Stages B2 and C) are associated with 42% 3-year survival.[50]

References

1. Wingo PA, Tong T, Bolden S. Cancer statistics. CA Cancer J Clin 1995; 45:8–30
2. Woods JB, Martin JN, Jr, Ingram FH, Odom CD, Scott-Conner CE, Rhodes RS. Pregnancy complicated by carcinoma of the colon above the rectum. Am J Perinatol 1992; 9:102–10
3. Bernstein MA, Madoff RD, Caushaj PF. Colon and rectal cancer in pregnancy. Dis Colon Rectum 1993; 36:172–8
4. Schwartz PE, Marchant D. Cancer in pregnancy. In: E Albert Reece and JC Hobbins (eds). Medicine of the Fetus and Mother, 2nd edn. Philadelphia: Lippincott-Raven Publishers, 1999
5. Garner PR, Tsang R. Insulinoma associated with pregnancy. Obstet Gynecol 1989; 73:847–9
6. Davis JL, Chen MD. Gastric carcinoma presenting as an exacerbation of ulcers during pregnancy: a case report. J Reprod Med 1991; 36:450–2
7. Scharl A, Huber P, Lorenzen J, U-J Gohring. Gastric cancer during early pregnancy. Two case reports. Arch Gynecol Obstet 1996; 258:151–4
8. Ueo H, Matsuoka H, Tamura S, Sato K, Tsunematsu Y, Kato T. Prognosis of gastric cancer associated with pregnancy. World J Surg 1991; 15:293–7
9. Maeta M, Yamashiro H, Oka A, Tsujitani S, Ikeguchi M, Kaibara N. Gastric cancer in the young, with special reference to 14 pregnancy associated cases: analysis based on 2325 consecutive cases of gastric cancer. J Surg Oncol 1995; 58:191–5
10. Entezami M, Becker R, Ebert A, Pritze W, Weitzel TT. Hepatocellular carcinoma as a rare cause of an excessive increase in alpha-fetoprotein during pregnancy. Gynecol Oncol 1996; 62:405–7
11. Hsich TT, Hou HC, Hsu JJ, Hsieh CC, Jeng LB. Term delivery after hepatocellular carcinoma resection in previous pregnancy. Acta Obstet Gynecol Scand 1996; 75:77–8
12. Binstock D, Moosa AR, Levin B. Pregnancy complicated by extrabiliary tract carcinoma. J Reprod Med 1983; 28:153
13. Ringenberg QS, Doll DC. Endocrine tumors and miscellaneous cancers in pregnancy. Semin Oncol 1989; 16:445–55
14. Chodander CM, Abhyankar SC, Deodhar KP. Sipple's syndrome (multiple endocrine neoplasia) in pregnancy (case report). Aust NZ J Obstet Gynecol 1982; 22:243–44
15. Goldman MH, Tisch B, Chattock AG. Fine needle biopsy of a solitary nodule arising during pregnancy. J Med Soc NJ 1983; 80:525–6
16. Tan GH, Gharib H, Goellner JR, van Heerden JA, Bahn RS. Management of thyroid nodules in pregnancy. Arch Intern Med 1996; 156:2317–23
17. Herzon FS, Morris DM, Segal MN, Rauch G, Parnell T. Coexisting thyroid cancer and pregnancy. Arch Otorhinolaringol Head Neck Surg 1994; 120:1191–4

18. Hill CS, Clark RL, Wolf M et al. The effect of subsequent pregnancy in patients with thyroid carcinoma. Surg Gynecol Obstet 1996; 122:1219–21
19. Mestman JH. Thyroid disease in pregnancy. Clin Perinatol 1985; 12:651–67
20. Choe W, McDougall IR. Thyroid cancer in pregnant women: diagnostic and therapeutic management. Thyroid 1994; 4:433–40
21. Harper MA, Murnaghan GA, Kennedy L. Pheochromocytoma in pregnancy. Five cases and review of literature. Br J Obstet Gynaecol 1989; 96:594–606
22. Antonelli NM, Dotters DJ, Katz VL, Kuller JA. Cancer in pregnancy: a review of the literature. Part I. Obstet Gynecol Surv 1996; 51:125–35
23. Ellison GT, Mansberger JA, Mansberger Jr AR. Malignant recurrent pheochromocytoma during pregnancy: case report and review of the literature. Surgery 1988; 103:484–9
24. Easterling TR, Carlson K, Benedetti TJ, Manusco JJ. Hemodynamics associated with the diagnosis and treatment of pheochromocytoma in pregnancy. Am J Perinatol 1992; 9:464–6
25. Takai Y, Seki H, Kinoshita K. Pheochromocytoma in pregnancy manifesting as hypertensive crisis induced by metoclopramide. Int J Gynaecol Obstet 1997; 59:133–7
26. Freier DT, Thompson NW. Pheochromocytoma and pregnancy: The epitome of high risk. 1993; 114:1148–52
27. Janetschek G, Finkenstedt G, Gasser R et al. Laparoscopic surgery for pheochromocytoma: adrenelectomy, partial resection, excision of paragangliomas. J Urol 1998; 160:330–4
28. Takahashi K, Sai Y, Nosaka S. Anaesthetic management for Cesarean section combined with removal of pheochromocytoma. Eur J Anaest 1998; 15:364–6
29. Oliver MD, Brownjohn AM, Vinall PS. Medical management of pheochromocytoma in pregnancy. Aust NZ J Obstet Gynaecol 1990; 30:268–71
30. Santeiro ML, Stromquist C, Wyble L. Phenoxybenzamine placental transfer during the third trimester. Ann Pharm 1996; 30:1249–51
31. Stenstrom G, Swolin K. Pheochromocytoma in pregnancy. Experience of treatment with phenoxybenzamine in three patients. Acta Obstet Gynecol Scand 1985; 64:357–62
32. Armaroli R, Simoni S, Artuso S, Mattioli G. Pheochromocytoma during pregnancy. Ital J Surg Sci 1989; 19:75–8
33. Hess HM, Dickson J, Foh HE. Hyperfunctioning parathyroid carcinoma presenting as acute pancreatitis in pregnancy. J Reprod Med 1980; 25:83–5
34. Rodrique-Chevas S, Ocampo LB. A case report of mucoepidermoid carcinoma of the parotid gland developing after radioiodine therapy for thyroid carcinoma. Eur J Surg Oncol 1995; 21:692–5
35. DeAngelis LM. Central nervous system neoplasms in pregnancy. Adv Neurol 1994; 64:139–52
36. Roelvink NCA, Kamphorst W, August H, van Alphen M, Rao BR. Pregnancy-related primary brain and spinal tumors. Arch Neurol 1987; 44:209–15.
37. Finfer SR. Management of labor and delivery in patients with intracranial neoplasms. Br J Anaesth 1991; 67:784–7
38. Lunardi P, Rizzo A, Missori P, Braioli B. Pituitary apoplexy in an acromegalic woman operated on during pregnancy by transphenoid approach. Int J Gynecol Obstet 1990; 34:71–4
39. Coyne TJ, Atkinson RL, Prins JB. Adrenocorticotropic hormone-secreting pituitary tumor associated with pregnancy: case report. Neurosurgery 1992; 31:953–5
40. Johnson RJ Jr, Voorhies RM, Witkin M, Robichaux AG 3rd, Braussard WAJr. Fertility following excision of a symptomatic craniopharyngeoma during pregnancy: Case report. Surg Neurol 1993; 39:257–62
41. Tokuda Y, Hatayama T, Sakoda K. Metastasis of malignant struma ovarii to the cranial vault during pregnancy. Neurosurgery 1993; 33:515–18
42. Doyle KJ, Luxford WM. Acoustic neuroma in pregnancy. Am J Oto 1994; 15:111–13
43. Simon MA, Phillips WA, Bonfiglio. Pregnancy and aggressive or malignant bone tumors. Cancer 1984; 53:2563–4
44. Cruikshank SH, McNellis TM. Carcinoma of the bladder in pregnancy. Am J Obstet Gynecol 1983; 145:768–71
45. Keegan GT, Forkowitz MJ. Transitional cell carcinoma of the bladder during pregnancy. A case report. Texas Med 1982; 8:44–5
46. Loughlin KR, Ng B. Bladder cancer in pregnancy. Case report. Br J Urol 1995; 75:421–2
47. Hendry WF. Management of urological tumours in pregnancy. Br J Urol 1997; 80 Suppl 1:24–8

8. Colorectal Cancer in Pregnancy

Shlomo M. Stemmer

Colorectal cancer in pregnancy is uncommon. Colorectal cancer is the second most prevalent cancer in women in the United States.[1] In general this is a disease of the middle-aged and the elderly. It is estimated that only 10% of colorectal cancers develop in women under the age of 40, or about 1 in 2000. In women under 30 only about 2% of colorectal cancers occur in this age group.[2,3] A review by Bernstein et al[4] of 42 cases of colorectal cancer in pregnancy showed that the mean age of the patients at time of diagnosis was 31 years. Recent estimates of the incidence of colorectal cancer in pregnancy are 1 in 10,000.[5] This incidence might continue to rise as women tend to delay pregnancy to the mid–late thirties and early forties.

Many reported cases of colorectal carcinoma during pregnancy have presented with advanced disease. The difficulty in making early diagnosis of colorectal cancer in pregnancy is attributed to the similarity in the presenting signs and symptoms of colorectal cancer and gastrointestinal complaints often experienced by pregnant patients. Adding to the delay in diagnosis is that standard tests used to diagnose and evaluate the extent of the disease, such as colonoscopy and abdominal CT scan, are either not proven to be safe or contraindicated in pregnancy. Therefore, complications from colorectal cancer such as bowel obstructions, perforation and metastasis are more common in pregnancy.[6]

Since colorectal cancer is relatively uncommon in young patients, there is a proportionally higher rate of hereditary syndromes in young patients with colorectal cancer including pregnant patients.[7,8] Hereditary syndromes and strong risk factors for colorectal cancer are familial polyposis, hereditary nonpolyposis colorectal cancer (Lynch syndromes) and chronic inflammatory bowel syndrome. In a review by Girard et al. out of 19 pregnant patients with colon cancer, four gave a history of predisposing factors.[9]

The distribution of the tumor within the colon and rectum in pregnancy is different from non-pregnancy. The American Cancer Society reported in 1981 that in non-pregnant patients under the age of 40 about 70% of the tumors were located in the colon and about 30% in the rectum.[10] In contrast, Bernstien et al reported after reviewing 205 published cases of colorectal cancer in pregnancy, 86% were rectal tumors. It is speculated that a diagnosis bias occurs in pregnant patients with colorectal cancer as pelvic and rectal exams are more common during the prenatal period accounting for a higher detection rate of rectal cancer.

Diagnosis

Diagnosis of colorectal cancer during pregnancy is generally difficult and often made late when advanced disease is present. Many of the symptoms and signs of colorectal cancer may be attributed to pregnancy. However, an alert medical provider may note several differences between the clinical presentation of pregnancy alone and that of colorectal cancer complicating pregnancy (Table 8.1). Symptoms of colorectal cancer depend on the size and location of the tumor, and the presence of complications such as partial or complete bowel obstruction, perforation or hemorrhage. The most common presenting symptoms of colorectal cancer are abdominal pain, changes in bowel habits, rectal bleeding and weight loss.[11] Nausea or vomiting occurs in about 10% to 15% of the patients.[12]. Similarly in pregnant patients with colorectal cancer, the most common presenting symptoms are abdominal pain, constipation, nausea, vomiting and rectal bleeding.[6] These symptoms might start at any gestational age. In normal pregnancy, nausea and vomiting, or "morning sickness", usually starts between 4 to 8 weeks gestation and ends at about 14 weeks. Rarely a pregnancy is complicated by hyperemesis gravidarum which causes persistent nausea, vomiting, weight loss, dehydration and electrolyte imbalance. In these patients an underlying cause such as pancreatitis, liver or gallbladder disease, pyelonephritis and colorectal cancer should be considered. Persistent abdominal or pelvic pain in a normal pregnancy might be due to heartburn, ligament pain or placental abruption. In pregnancy complicated by colorectal cancer the pain might be referred to the upper abdomen

Table 8.1. Differences in the clinical presentation between normal pregnancy and colorectal cancer complicating pregnancy.

Clinical presentation	Normal pregnancy	Pregnancy complicated by colorectal cancer
Nausea and vomiting	Uncommon after first trimester	Might start at any gestational age and may be present throughout the pregnancy
Weight	Gain after first trimester	Inadequate weight gain or loss during the pregnancy
Bowel functions	Diarrhea is rare	Constipation and diarrhea may occur
Rectal bleeding	Uncommon, usually due to hemorrhoids	Common, hemorrhoids might not be present
Persistent abdominal pain and/or tenderness	Uncommon	Common, might be referred to upper abdomen
Abdominal mass	Enlarging uterus or attached lieomyoma	Separate from the uterus
Abdominal distension	Usually not until second half of the pregnancy	At any gestational age, may indicate perforation
Anemia	Mild to moderate	Moderate to severe
Peripheral lymphadenopathy and hepatomegaly	None	May be present with metastatic disease

and would not be relieved with anti-acid therapy. The average weight gain during pregnancy is 25 to 35 lbs., most of this weight gain occuring after the first trimester when the nausea and vomiting subsides. By contrast in pregnancy complicated by colorectal cancer, weight gain may be small to none or there might be weight loss. Constipation is common in pregnancy due mainly to decrease in the motility of the colon, and mechanical obstruction by the uterus. Colon cancer, especially if located in the left side, may cause constipation due to partial or complete obstruction. As stool moves past the obstruction, diarrhea usually occurs. Rectal bleeding during pregnancy is usually due to bleeding from hemorrhoidal veins. The development or aggravation of hemorrhoids during pregnancy is due to the obstruction of venous return and from constipation. In the absence of bleeding hemorrhoids, the presence of rectal bleeding should be evaluated as it might be due to colorectal cancer. Since most colorectal tumors are located in the rectum, digital rectal examination is very important as many rectal tumors are palpable. Many of the reported cases of colorectal cancer during pregnancy have presented with advanced disease mainly due to delayed diagnosis. Persistent abdominal pain, tenderness, abdominal distention or a palpable abdominal mass are usually secondary to advanced colorectal cancer. Complications from colorectal cancer such as an obstruction produce hypoactive or high-pitched bowel sounds. Bowel perforation from colorectal cancer is rare, though more common in pregnancy.[6] Abdominal cramping, rebound tenderness and distension along with fever and hypoactive or absent bowel sounds is highly suspicious for bowel perforation. Anemia of pregnancy is usually mild and caused mainly by the relatively greater increase in plasma volume compared to the increase in hemoglobin mass and red cell volume. In healthy iron-sufficient pregnant women only 1% will have a hemoglobin count of less that 10.[13] Rectal bleeding due to colorectal cancer may worsen the anemia of pregnancy as significant amounts of blood loss may occur over time. Advanced metastatic colorectal cancer may present with hepatomegaly and peripheral lymphadenopathy. Peripheral lymphadenopathy may include metastases to the left supraclavicular space (Virchow's node). Depending on the location of the tumor, final diagnosis is usually made by rectal examination, proctoscopy, flexible sigmoidoscopy or colonoscopy.

Evaluation

The clinical evaluation of the pregnant patient with colorectal cancer is similar to the non-pregnant patient except that barium enema and abdominal CT scan are contraindicated in pregnancy because of radiation teratogenicity. Colonoscopy, although not yet proven safe in pregnancy, is essential in obtaining preoperative tissue diagnosis and should be offered to all patients following perinatal counseling. Rectal ultrasound is indicated for staging rectal tumors and metastatic disease to the liver can be evaluated with abdominal ultrasonography. Serum carcinoembryonic antigen (CEA) levels are unchanged in normal pregnancy and therefore can be used the same way as in non-pregnant patients with colorectal cancer.[14] CEA levels are useful in determining cancer prognosis, incomplete resection of the tumor if the levels fail to normalize after surgery, or recurrence if the levels rise after a period of normalization following surgery. Patients in the third trimester of pregnancy with rectal tumors need to be evaluated for the feasibility of a vaginal delivery, specifically that there is no obstruction to the birth canal from the tumor.

Treatment

The treatment of colorectal cancer during pregnancy depends mainly on the size, location, extent of the tumor and gestational age of the fetus. Colorectal tumors diagnosed in the first half of the pregnancy should be resected as soon as possible. The size of the uterus at this gestational age rarely preclude a complete tumor resection. Several reports have described successful tumor resection followed by the birth of a healthy infant.[15] Laparoscopic tumor resection if indicated is at times possible at this gestational age. Tumor resection of colorectal cancer diagnosed after the second half of pregnancy should be delayed until delivery. The infant should be delivered as soon as fetal lung maturity is achieved. Definitive surgery should be performed after several weeks allowing for resolution of the vascular congestion of pregnancy and involution of the uterus. There are reports that delay of definitive therapy resulted in increase in tumor size and metastases,[16] therefore consideration should be given to the administration of steroids to accelerate fetal lung maturity. In case that a Cesarean delivery is indicated for obstetrical reasons, concomitant tumor excision may be considered. Complications from colorectal cancer such as obstruction, perforation or metastases warrant immediate surgical intervention regardless of gestational age. In cases in which the tumor is inoperable, the pregnancy should be allowed to continue until viability and surgery performed only as a palliative measure. Adjuvant chemotherapy with Levamisole and 5-fluorouracil (5-FU) has a limited role in the pregnant patient with colorectal cancer. Treatment with levamisole and 5-FU reduced the risk of cancer recurrence by 41% and the overall mortality by 31% in patients with Duke's C tumors.[17] Pregnant patients with colorectal cancer Duke Stage C may be offered adjuvant chemotherapy with levamisole and 5-FU after the first trimester. There are reports that these chemotherapeutic agents are safe after the first trimester,[18,19] however, the patient should be counseled regarding the limited data and the increase in the rates of intrauterine growth restriction and prematurity[20] with the use of these agents. The treatment of colorectal cancer in pregnancy is further complicated by the relatively high rate of ovarian metastases. The incidence of ovarian metastases in patients under 40 years old with colorectal cancer is 24%.[21] Similarly, pregnant patients with colorectal carcinoma have a 25% incidence of ovarian metastases.[22]. Because of the relatively high incidence of ovarian metastases in pregnant patients with colorectal cancer, bilateral ovarian biopsies with frozen section are recommended,[19] and bilateral salpingo-oophorectomy is performed if the ovaries are involved.

Conclusion

The prognosis for pregnant patients with colorectal cancer is similar to non-pregnant patients of the same age. Patients less than 40 years old and especially pregnant patients have poor prognosis due to delay in diagnosis. A high index of suspicion should be kept on all pregnant patients presenting with rectal bleeding or persistent gastrointestinal complaints (Table 8.1). A gastrointestinal evaluation should be obtained which may include a rectal examination, sigmoidoscopy, colonoscopy and ultrasonography. Tumor resection should be performed without delay during the first half of the pregnancy and following delivery if the diagnosis is made late in the pregnancy. A team approach consisting of an obstetrician, gastroentrologist, oncologist, general surgeon and perinatologist is recommended to optimize outcome for mother and infant.

References

1. Parker SL, Tong T, Bolden S, et al. Cancer statistics, 1996. Cancer J Clin 1996; 46:5–27
2. Coffey RJ, Cardenas F. Cancer of the bowel in the young adult. Dis Colon Rectum 1964; 7:491–2
3. Falterman KW, Hill CB, Markey JC, et al. Cancer of the colon, rectum and anus. A review of 2313 cases. Cancer 1974; 84:951–9.
4. Bernstein MA, Madoff RD, Caushaj PF. Colon and rectal cancer in pregnancy. Dis Colon and Rectum 1993; 36:172–8
5. Woods JB, Martin JN Jr, Ingram FH, et al. Pregnancy complicated by carcinoma of the colon above the rectum. Am J Perinatology 1992; 9:102–10
6. Shushan A, Stemmer SM, Reubinoff BE, et al. Carcinoma of the colon during pregnancy. Obstet Gynecol Surv 1992; 47:222–5
7. Isbister WH, Frasier J. Large-bowel cancer in the young: A national survival study. Dis Colon Rectum 1990; 33:363–6
8. Ransohoff DF, Lang CA. Screening for colorectal cancer. N Engl J Med 1991; 325:37–41
9. Girard RM, Lamarche J, Baillot R. Carcinoma of the colon associated with pregnancy: Report of a case. Dis Colon Rectum 1981; 24:472–5
10. Silverberg E. Cancer Statistics. New York: American Cancer Society, 1981
11. Falterman KW, Hill CB, Markey JC, et al. Cancer of the colon, rectum, and anus: A review of 2313 cases. Cancer 1974; 34:951–9
12. Cappell MS, Goldberg ES. The relationship between the clinical presentation and spread of colon cancer in 315 consecutive patients: A significant trend of earlier cancer detection from 1982 through 1988 at a university hospital. J Clin Gastroenterol 1992; 14:227–35
13. Scott DE, Prichart JA. Iron deficiency in healthy young college women. JAMA 1967; 199:147
14. Lamerz R, Reuder H. Significance of CEA determination in patients with cancer of the colon-rectum and the mammary gland in comparison to physiological states in connection with pregnancy. Bull Cancer 1976; 63:575–86
15. Walsh C, Fazio V. Cancer of the colon, rectum, and anus during pregnancy. Gastroenterol Clin of North America, 1998; 27:257–67
16. Heres P, Witltink J, Cuest MA, Burger CW, van Groeningen CJ, Meijers S. Colon Carcinoma during pregnancy: A lethal coincidence. Eur J Obstet Gynecol Reprod Biol 1993; 48:149–52
17. Moertel CG, Fleming TR, MacDonald JS, et al. Levamisole and fluorouracil for adjuvant therapy of resected colon carcinoma. N Engl J Med 1990; 322:352–8
18. Aviles A, Diaz-Maqueo JC, Talavara A, et al. Growth and development of children of mothers treated with chemotherapy during pregnancy: Current status of 43 children. Am J Hematol 1991; 36:243–8
19. Nesbitt JC, Moise KJ, Sawyers JL. Colorectal carcinoma in pregnancy. Arch Surg 1985; 120:636–40
20. Sommers GM, Kao MS. Using chemotherapeutic agents during pregnancy. Contemp Obstet Gynecol 1987; 30:45–8
21. Pitluk H, Poticha SM. Carcinoma of the colon and rectum in patients less than 40 years of age. Surg Gynecol Obstet 1983; 157:335–7
22. Matsuyama T, Tsukamoto N, Matsukuma K, et al. Malignant ovarian tumors associated with pregnancy. Report of six cases. Int J Gynecol Obstet 1989; 28:61–6

9. Radiologic Diagnosis of Cancer in Pregnancy

Kunle Odunsi, Peter E. Schwartz and Giancarlo Mari

Introduction

Cancer and pregnancy often result in two opposing emotional reactions in young women. One leads to dismay and horror, while the other usually to joyous elation. The patient is inevitably distraught and terrified, whilst the obstetrician and medical advisers are faced with a therapeutic dilemma involving diagnostic, obstetric, perinatal, surgical, physiological and moral issues. The situation is further complicated by the fact that pregnancy may limit adequate physical examination, and make clinical evaluation of the extent of malignant disease difficult. Yet an estimated 1 in 1000 women will be affected by cancer in some form while pregnant.[1] The most common malignancies in women aged 15 to 34 years are of the breast, cervix and central nervous system, as well as leukemia, and non-Hodgkin's lymphoma. In the 35 to 54 age group, cervical, lung, colorectal and ovarian cancer also become more common[2] and it is likely that more cases of cancer during pregnancy will be seen as the trend for delaying pregnancy into later reproductive years continues.

Although recent advances in diagnostic imaging have resulted in an increased ability to evaluate specific organs and anatomic regions with precision, there is generally no agreement about which test is superior in its diagnostic accuracy and in which sequence the various tests should be used. Four basic principles must be adhered to in order to reach a coherent plan of imaging in pregnancy. First, the information being sought should be clearly defined. Is the examination being used for screening, staging or surveillance? Second, the availability and quality of the imaging technology to be used for the study should be known. Third, the diagnostic radiologist should be familiar and adept with the imaging modality. Finally, the possible effects of the imaging modality on the developing fetus should be known. This chapter reviews the evidence of the effect of radiation on the developing fetus, provides the general physical principles of how images are generated by the various technologies, and the imaging strategies used for the most common malignancies occurring in pregnant women.

Effects of Diagnostic Imaging on the Developing Fetus

Proliferating cells are radiosensitive, and this makes the pre-implantation stage of the developing embryo most vulnerable to ionizing radiation, followed by the period from 2 to 15 weeks.[3] Radiation doses of 10 to 90cGy in the 8–15 week postconceptional period have been associated with an increased risk of mental retardation, while exposure greater than 1 Gy almost always result in fetal death.[4,5] The United Nations Scientific Committee on the Effects of Anatomic Radiation and the International Commission of Radiologic Protection currently recommend the limit of cumulative fetal radiation exposure to less than 500 mrem and suggest that doses above 100 mrem be avoided from 8 to 15 weeks post-conception. Fetal exposure to ionizing radiation has been estimated during CT pelvimetry to be 8.2 to 13 cGy (820 to 1300mrem) at the center of the CT slice.[6]

Several groups have examined the effect of ionizing radiation on the risk of childhood cancers. The principal results of a meta-analysis carried out by Bithell are summarized in Table 9.1.[7] The largest of these studies, the Oxford Survey of Childhood Cancers (OSCC) covered all children dying from malignant disease in Britain under 16 years of age and included 15, 276 case–control pairs.[8] Approximately three-quarters of the total amount of information worldwide comes from the OSCC, so that the quantitative conclusions about the risk of childhood cancers from irradiation in utero essentially depend on the validity of these data. Nevertheless, whether attention is restricted to the OSCC, to all other studies, or to the grand total, a highly significant relative risk of 1.4 is seen. The excess relative risk coefficient is 0.038 per cGy of radiation (95% confidence interval 0.007–0.079) from which an absolute risk coefficient of 6% per cGy (95% confidence interval 1.0–12.6) may be derived.[6]

In spite of theoretical concerns about cellular damage from tissue heating and cavitation at high-power outputs, there are no documented adverse effects of ultrasound on the developing fetus. There is no increased risk of childhood cancers in the individ-

Table 9.1. Relative risk of cancer in childhood associated with irradiation in utero found in different studies (after Bithel 1993)

Study (period covered)	Relative risk (unadjusted)	95% Confidence interval
OSCC (1953–1981)	1.39	1.30–1.49
NE United States (1947–1967)	1.47	1.22–1.77
Inter-regional study, UK (1980–1982)	1.23	0.90–1.68
Los Angeles (1950–1957)	1.34	0.90–2.00
Louisiana (1951–1955)	1.70	1.08–2.69
Helsinki (1959–1968)	1.18	0.74–1.87
California (1955–1956)	1.68	1.06–2.67
Tri-state (US) (1959–1962)	1.40	0.87–2.27
Swedish twins (1952–1983)	1.38	0.78–2.46
Minnesota (1953–1957)	1.28	0.69–2.37
All except OSCC	1.37	1.22–1.53
All	1.38	1.31–1.47

uals born to women who undergo ultrasonography during pregnancy.[9] In addition, there is no dose response relationship between the number of ultrasound examinations and the occurrence of cancer.

In the case of Magnetic Resonance Imaging (MRI), the biologic effects of electromagnetic radiation, the static magnetic field gradients, and radiofrequency electromagnetic energy involved in MR imaging is not yet known. Alterations in the gradient of magnetic fields may induce electric current. This may lead to power deposition (thermal effects) as well as producing direct electrical effects. However, in a study in which frog embryos were exposed to 4.5T (clinical imaging 1.5T), there was no teratogenic effect.[10] Further, when pregnant mice were exposed to MRI (1.5T) with and without the administration of contrast agent, there were no differences in the incidence of early miscarriage, fetal death, low birthweight, abnormal morphology or litter size.[11] Despite theoretical concerns, in humans there are no reported adverse fetal effects of MRI during pregnancy.

Basic Principles

Since the introduction of computed tomography (CT) into clinical service in the late 1970s, it has become the mainstay of diagnostic imaging in cancer patients. CT offers non-invasive, easily reproducible results with high sensitivity and specificity for a wide range of organ sites, while being both widely available and relatively low in cost. Standard CT is able to acquire data as single slices every 5 to 10 seconds. More recently, with spiral CT, it is possible to acquire a volume of data over a 24–40-second period, which enables rapid, optimal timing of data acquisition and contrast injection.

Recent improvements in transducer technology and the development of color Doppler imaging have significantly enhanced the role of ultrasound in cancer diagnosis. In general, no patient preparation is required, and no contrast material is administered. High-frequency transducers (7–10 MHz) are used for near field imaging of superficial anatomic structures, while lower-frequency transducers (3–5 MHz) are used for most routine abdominal imaging. For evaluation of the female pelvis, dedicated endovaginal probes (5 to 7MHz) are routinely utilized.

Color Doppler sonography enables real time visualization of blood flow without use of contrast agents. Based on the Doppler equation, the frequency of the reflected signal is proportional to both the velocity of the blood flow and the cosine of the angle of the interrogating ultrasound beam. Because the cosine of 90 degrees is zero, Doppler signals are unobtainable when examining vessels perpendicular to the plane of insonation. Doppler information may be displayed graphically by the use of spectral Doppler analysis. The combination of real-time images and spectral Doppler analysis is referred to as duplex scanning.

Magnetic resonance imaging (MRI) is a cross-sectional imaging technique utilizing strong magnetic fields and multiple radiofrequency pulses to generate an image with outstanding spatial resolution and tissue contrast. MRI is based on the principles of nuclear magnetic resonance (NMR), a non-destructive technique used in physical chemistry to analyze the composition of substances. Nuclei are composed of an odd number of protons and neutrons and have magnetic moments. When placed in a magnetic field, the nuclei attempt to align with the field and rotate about the axis of the magnetic field. The frequency of rotation (Lamour frequency) is dependent upon the specific nuclei and the strength of the magnet. This relationship, the Lamour equation is expressed as

$$f = yB_0$$

where f = Lamour frequency, y = gyromagnetic ratio, a constant for each type of nucleus, and B_0= the external magnetic field strength. Hydrogen (^1H) is the most commonly imaged nucleus in the body because of its relative abundance and high gyromagnetic ratio compared with other nuclei with a magnetic moment such as phosphorous (^{31}P), sodium (^{23}Na), and carbon (^{13}C).

The longitudinal or T1 relaxation is a measure of the time for the processing nuclei to return to their baseline state (i.e. oriented parallel to the magnetic field) after the radiofrequency pulse has been turned off. It is also the time for the MR signal to rise to 63% of its maximum equilibrium value and varies between 200 and 800 ms for most tissues. Tissues with a short T1 will appear bright on T1-weighted images (Table 9.2). By contrast, the transverse (T2) relaxation is the time taken for the MR signal to decrease to 63% of its original value and varies between 50 and 200ms for most tissues. Tissues with a long T2 will appear bright on a T2-weighted image (Table 9.2).

Nuclear medicine uses radioisotopes as tracers to assess normal and abnormal physiology of living tissues. "Hot spots" are detected when the process concentrates radioactivity, as with tumors concentrating gallium-67, thallium-201, [F-18]deoxyglucose (FDG) or radiolabeled monoclonal antibodies. "Cold spots" occur when tumors displace normal structures and tissues such as space-occupying liver lesions on Tc-99m sulfur colloid liver scans. Single photon emission computed tomography (SPECT) creates tomographic or cross-sectional images of radioactivity distribution, while positron emission tomography (PET) provides quantitative

Table 9.2. Relative signal intensities of tissues

Tissue	T1 weighted	T2 weighted
Cervix (stroma)	Dark	Dark
Adrenal	Intermediate	Moderately bright
Brain		
CSF	Dark	Very bright
Grey matter	Intermediate to dark	Intermediate to bright
White matter	Bright	Intermediate to dark
Cortical bone	Very dark	Very dark
Liver	Intermediate	Intermediate to dark
Fat	Bright	Bright
Ovary		
Stroma	Dark	Intermediate
Follicles	Dark	Bright
Uterus		
Endometrium	Dark	Bright
Myometrium	Dark	Intermediate
Serous fluid	Dark	Bright
Pancreas	Intermediate to bright	Intermediate to dark

images from a three-dimensional distribution of concentrations of radioactivity in the body. These technologies are rarely used in pregnancy because of the risk of radiation injury to the fetus.

Clinical Applications of Diagnostic Imaging by Anatomic Site of Cancer in Pregnancy

Cervical Cancer

Invasive carcinoma of the cervix is the most common malignancy associated with pregnancy, occurring in approximately 1:2200 pregnancies.[12] The staging of cervical cancer is determined predominantly by clinical examination of the cervix and parametrium. During pregnancy, this examination may be difficult to perform accurately because of the presence of the fetus. Thus, non-imaging techniques that avoid ionizing radiation have a major role in the evaluation of such patients.

Ultrasonography can be used to evaluate the cervix. The normal cervix has a medium echogenicity and there are two recognizable layers. The endocervical canal is hypoechoic, while the cervical stroma gives a medium echo texture. Although cervical enlargement, irregular borders, and decreased echogenicity may represent signs of tumor, the limited field of cervical ultrasonography makes it unsuitable for full staging of tumor extent.

MRI allows a full view of the cervix and pelvic organs as well as supportive structures, and may clarify the extent of tumor in patients who are otherwise difficult to examine. At the Yale-New Haven Medical Center, MRI is the preferred technique for delineating the local and regional extent of cervical cancer in order to plan management strategies for treating pregnant patients. Normal cervical anatomy is best seen on T2-weighted imaging and consists of a normal hypointense zone composed of cervical stroma, which is continuous with the junctional zone of the uterus. The centrally hyperintense signal within the cervix represents the endocervical canal. The parametrial tissues are generally hyperintense on fast spin echo T2-weighted scans. Cervical cancer is usually hyperintense to stroma on T2-weighted images. Imaging of small cancers are best accomplished with surface coils (such as endorectal or phased array coil), to increase signal to noise ratio. Using these techniques, tumor size, depth and extension outside the cervix, and the presence of enlarged lymph nodes may be evaluated. Parametrial invasion may be reliably excluded when a dark rim of fibrous stroma is seen to surround the cervix. However, the absence of this rim is not entirely reliable for the presence of parametrial invasion. The presence of abnormal signal within the parametria itself is more predictive of parametrial extension.[13,14] Figs 9.1 and 9.2 are illustrative examples of MR images obtained from patients with cervical cancer in pregnancy.

The accuracy of CT and MRI for evaluating regional lymph nodes is compromised by their failure to detect small metastases and because patients with bulky necrotic tumors often have enlarged reactive lymph nodes. In a Gynecologic Oncology Group (GOG) study that compared the results of radiographic studies with subsequent histologic findings in non-pregnant patients, Heller et al[15] found that 79% of the cases with paraaortic lymph node involvement were detected with lymphangiography, whereas only 34% were detected by CT. As described above, MRI is able to provide

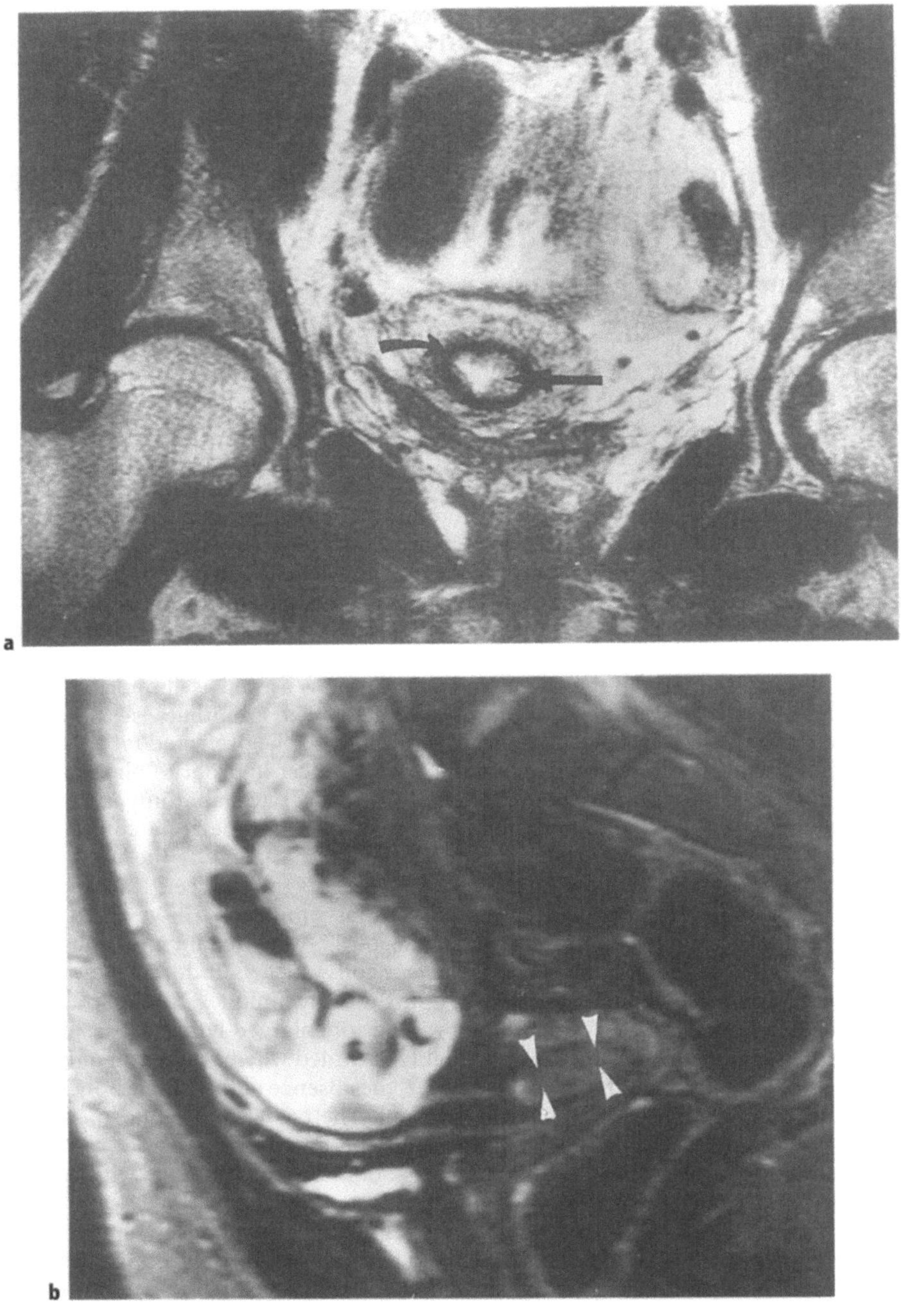

Fig. 9.1. **a** Sagittal T2 weighted MRI scan in a patient with squamous cell carcinoma in the second trimester of pregnancy. Arrow indicates tumor within the cervix. **b** Coronal T2 weighted MRI scan of the cervix in the same patient demonstrates cervical cancer (straight arrow), with an intact fibrous stroma (curved arrow), indicating no evidence of parametrial invasion.

useful information about the location and depth of invasion of tumors in the cervix,[16,17] but gives less accurate evaluation of parametrial involvement.[18]

Breast Cancer

Breast cancer is the leading cause of cancer deaths in the 15–44 year old age group.[19] Carcinoma of the breast is the second most common malignancy associated with pregnancy, complicating approximately 1 in 3,000 to 10,000 pregnancies.[20] Of patients with breast cancer 2–4% are pregnant at the time of diagnosis. Although the overall 5-year survival for breast cancer is 50%, this figure is halved in pregnancy mainly because the incidence of positive nodes is greater, and metastasis has usually occurred before therapy is begun.[21]

The pre-treatment evaluation of breast cancer in pregnancy should determine the clinical stage of disease and identify the best management strategy. A bilateral diagnostic mammogram should be obtained before surgical biopsy. The study can be performed with abdominal shielding. In general, mammography of the pregnant or postpartum patient demonstrates increased fibroglandular tissue consistent with preparation for the state of lactation. Breast ultrasonography can be performed alone or in conjunction with mammography, and it is especially useful in evaluating a cystic lesion. The use of MRI to identify the presence of mammographically occult multifocal carcinoma in non-pregnant patients is under evaluation. Some reports suggest that MRI might be able to identify additional foci of disease in 20–35% of patients, suggesting that this an attractive procedure in pregnant patients and in those desiring breast conserving therapy.[20-23]

The extent of further pre-operative work-up should be guided by the clinical stage of disease and the patient's symptoms. Bone scans are frequently used as pre-operative screening test for patients with invasive breast cancer, but the incidence of occult bony metastasis detected by scanning in patients with Stage I and II disease is less than 5%.[24] By contrast, bone metastasis are identified by scanning in 20–25% of asymptommatic women with Stage III disease, making this a worthwhile screening procedure in patients with locally advanced breast cancer.[24]

The yield of screening liver scans is even lower than that seen with bone scanning, and the test is of little benefit in the pre-operative evaluation of Stage I and II breast cancer.[25] Liver imaging should be reserved for patients with abnormal liver chemistries or signs or symptoms suggestive of hepatic metastasis. This evaluation is often performed using a CT scan in the non-pregnant patient. In pregnancy, the risk of ionizing radiation to the fetus needs to be considered in the overall management plan, and so MRI of the liver should be considered.

Lymphoma

Hodgkin's disease occurs at a frequency of 1 in 6,000 pregnant women.[26] Staging is determined by site of involvement as well as whether or not disease is present on both sides of the diaphragm. Anteroposterior and lateral chest radiographs should be ordered in all patients. Staging with thoracic CT can more precisely identify sites of initial involvement in the thorax than chest radiograph[27] and has considerable potential to alter clinical management.[28] Detection of pulmonary disease, pleural or pericardial involvement, apical cardiac nodal enlargement, and extension into the chest wall, as well as defining the extent of involved axillary lymph nodes, can be documented by thoracic CT. Although it appears that the ability of MRI to detect tumor in

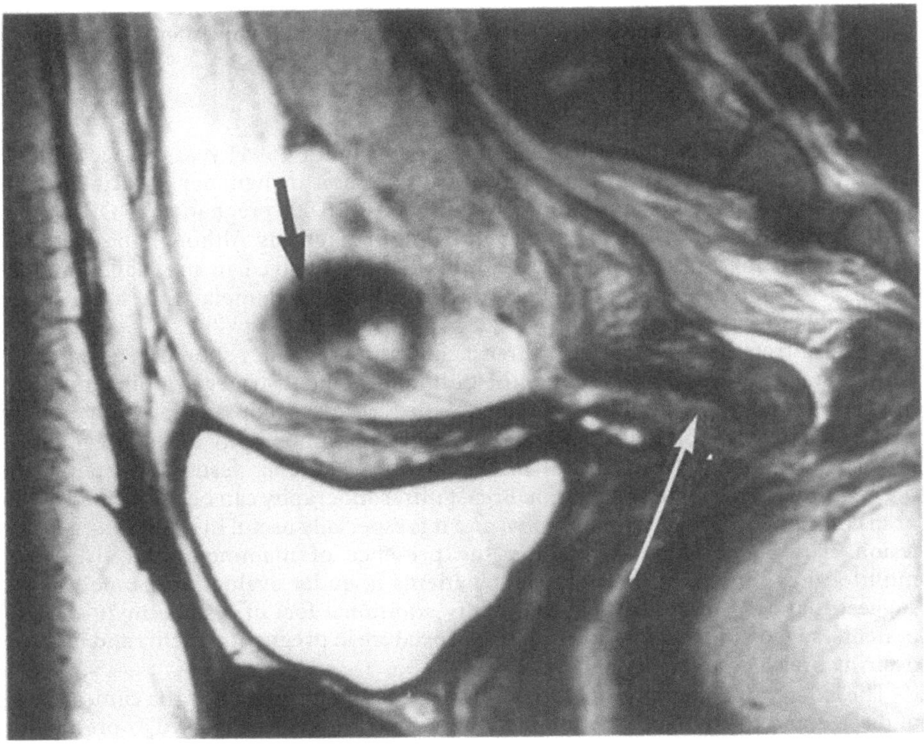

a

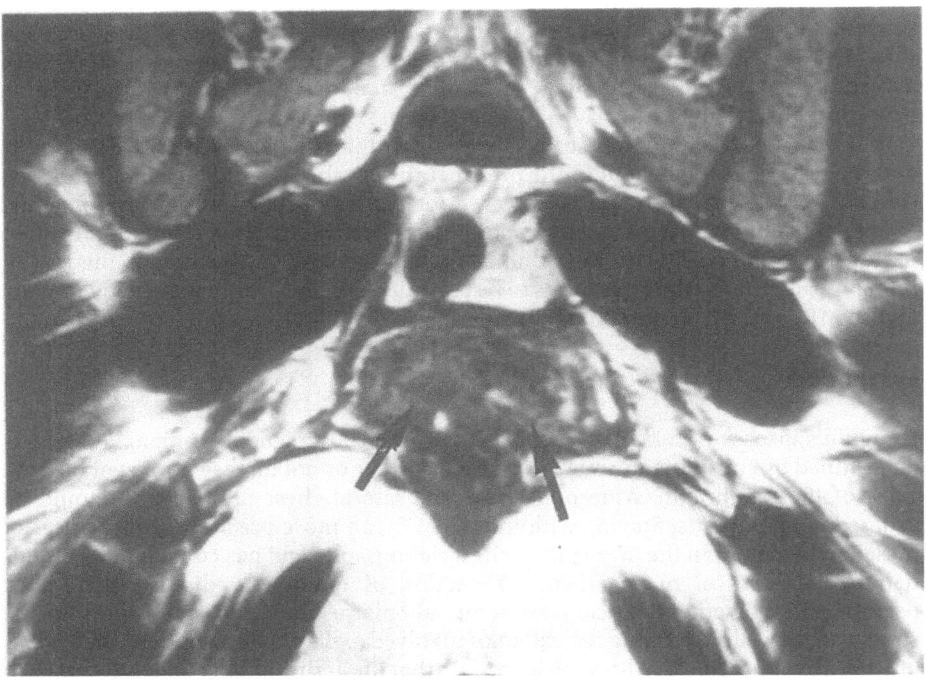

b

the mediastinum or hilar lymph nodes is not superior to that of CT scanning,[29] it is a reasonable substitute for thoracic CT in order to minimize the risk of radiation exposure to the pregnant patient. Ultrasonography may also be used to evaluate the presence of pericardial fluid, but under most circumstances its use is limited.

In the staging of Hodgkin's disease below the diaphragm, there is no single reliable study (CT, lymphography, MRI and gallium scanning) for detecting disease in normal-size nodes, and all studies have a 20–25% false negative rate in detecting occult disease in the spleen and upper abdominal nodes.[30] Head-to-head comparisons of bipedal lymphangiography (LAG) and CT suggest that LAG has an advantage over CT scanning in determining the presence of small lymphadenopathy because it provides useful information on lymph node architecture. CT scan, on the other hand, is better for the evaluation of adenopathy in the celiac axis, splenic hilus, porta hepatis, and mesentery, and relies almost exclusively on increases in the size of the nodes. CT may also demonstrate foci of Hodgkin's disease in the liver and spleen.

On balance, LAG and CT scanning should be used as complementary techniques in evaluating the extent of abdominal involvement of Hodgkin's disease. Gallium scanning may also complement LAG or CT, but its routine use in pregnancy is not recommended. Although information on the use of MRI for detecting abdominal Hodgkin's disease is limited, it should be considered in pregnancy. MRI is also potentially valuable in investigating bone marrow involvement and can help in directing imaging-guided biopsies.

Non-Hodgkin's lymphoma (NHL) occurring during pregnancy is rare.[31] As in Hodgkin's disease, radiographic staging should include chest radiographs, and CT or MR of the thorax, abdomen and pelvis. MRI is most valuable in evaluating the brain and spinal cord, as well as identifing focal areas of bone marrow involvement.[32]

Carcinoma of the Ovary

Ovarian cancer is associated with pregnancy in 1:12,000 to 1:25,000 births.[33] Although only 2–5% of all ovarian tumors in pregnancy are malignant, the identification of an adnexal mass in pregnancy should still prompt a diagnostic ultrasound evaluation. Although the morphologic indices that indicate the likelihood of malignancy have been defined in non-pregnant patients, they are usually applied for pregnant patients with adnexal mass.[34] Further, particular color Doppler flow patterns and resistive indices characteristic of malignant pelvic masses have been described.[35] However, resistive and pulsatility indices may not always be effective in distinguishing between benign and malignant ovarian masses, especially in the pregnant patient.[36]

CT scanning is useful in the pre-operative evaluation of the extent of disease in the non-pregnant patient. Since ovarian cancer is a surgically staged disease, the information obtained from clinical examination and ultrasound imaging of the pregnant patient should enable the physician to proceed with the next step of management without the need for CT scanning. Indeed, if sonography is equivocal, MRI can localize the mass to the ovary or uterus and provide a definitive diagnosis in approximately 50% of these cases and this strategy will minimize the risk of radiation exposure to the developing fetus.[37] Fig. 9.3 is an MRI in a patient at 21 weeks gestation with an ovarian mass.

Fig. 9.2. **a** Sagittal T2 weighted MRI scan in a 21 year old woman with poorly differentiated squamous cell carcinoma of the cervix at 16 weeks gestation. The white arrow shows tumor within the cervical canal. The black arrow indicates axial section through the fetal liver. **b** Coronal T2 weighted MRI in the same patient demonstrates no evidence of extension beyond the cervix.

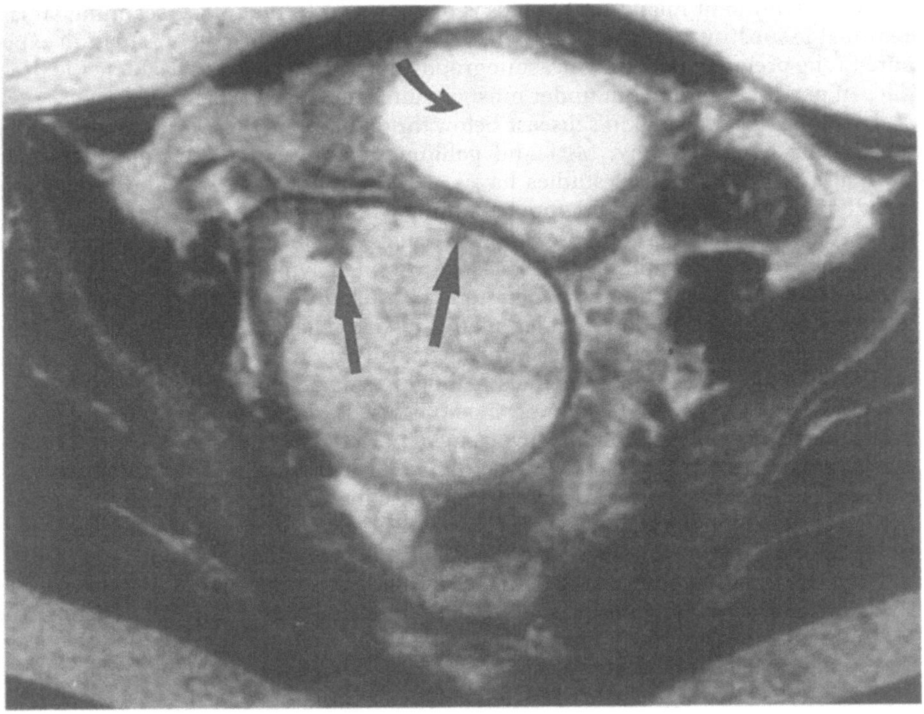

Fig. 9.3. Axial T2 weighted MRI in a patient at 21 weeks gestation demonstrates an ovarian mass with nodules and thickened septations (straight arrows). Curved arrow indicates amniotic fluid. At laparotomy, the patient had a papillary serous carcinoma of the ovary.

Conclusions

Clinical evaluation of the pregnant woman with cancer is difficult. Several diagnostic imaging modalities are now available to aid the clinician in determining the extent of disease so as to guide the choice of therapy. The choice of diagnostic imaging modality in pregnancy requires individualization with careful thought to the radiation hazards to the fetus, and overall effect of the disease on the course of pregnancy. Close interaction between the obstetrician, oncologist and diagnostic radiologist provides the optimal environment for the judicious use of diagnostic radiology. The specific question or questions to be addressed should be identified. The disease must be assessed and treated in the full light of its exact location and stage, with an understanding of the natural history within the context of pregnancy. The formation of the Radiology Diagnostic Oncology Group (RDOG) studies, by the National Institutes of Health and the National Cancer Institute, is an important step in the development of carefully designed, prospective, multi-institutional clinical research protocols for evaluating the accuracy of various imaging studies in oncology.[38] It is hoped that this group will provide research direction on the appropriate imaging modalities for the pregnant patient with cancer.

References

1. Donegan WL. Cancer and pregnancy. CA Cancer J Clin 1983; 33:194
2. Wingo PA, Tong T, Bolden S. Cancer statistics. CA Cancer J Clin 1995; 45:8–30
3. Michel C. Radiation embryology. Experientia 1989; 45:69
4. Mole RH. Irradiation of the embryo and fetus. Br J Radiol 1987; 60:17
5. Mole RH. The effect of prenatal radiation exposure on the developing human brain. Int J Rad Biol 1990; 57:647
6. Moore MM, Shearer DR. Fetal dose estimates for CT pelvimetry. Radiology 1989; 171:265
7. Bithel JF. Epidemiological studies of children radiated in-utero. In: Baverstock KF, Stather JW (eds) Low dose radiation: biological basis of risk assessment. London: Taylor & Francis, 1993.
8. Gilman EA, Stewart AM, Knox EG, Kneale GW. Trends in obstetric radiography, 1931–81. J Radiol Prot 1989; 9:93–101
9. Shu XO, Jin F, Linet MS, et al. Diagnostic X-ray and ultrasound exposure and risk of childhood cancer. Br J Cancer 1994; 70:531
10. Prasad N, Wright DA, Ford JJ, et al. Safety of 4T MR imaging: study of effects on developing frog embryos. Radiology 1990; 174:251
11. Rofsky NM, Pizzarello DJ, Weinreb JC, et al. Effect on fetal mouse development of exposures to MR imaging and gadopentetate dimeglumine. J Magn Reson Imaging 1994; 4:805
12. Hacker NF, Berek JS, Lagasse LD, et al. Carcinoma of the cervix associated with pregnancy. Obstet Gynecol 1982; 59:735–46
13. Kim SH, Choi BI, Lee HP, et al. Uterine cervical carcinoma: comparison of CT and MRI findings. Radiol 1990; 175:45
14. Kim SH, Choi BI, Han JR, et al. Pre-operative staging of uterine cervical cancer: comparison of CT and MRI in 99 patients. JCAT 1993; 17:633
15. Heller PB, Malfetano JH, Bundy BN, Barnhill DR, Okagaki T. Clinical-pathologic study of Stage IIB, III, and IVA carcinoma of the cervix: extended diagnostic evaluation for paraaortic node metastasis: a Gynecologic Oncology Group study. Gynecol Oncol 1990; 38:425
16. Hawnaur JM, Johnson RJ, Buckley CH, Tindall V, Isherwood I. Staging, volume estimation and assessment of nodal status in carcinoma of the cervix: comparison of magnetic resonance imaging with surgical findings. Clin Radiol 1994; 49:443
17. Martin AJ, Poon CS, Thomas GM, Kapusta LR, Shaw PA, Henkleman RM. MR evaluation of cervical cancer in hysterectomy specimens: correlation of quantitative T2 measurement and histology. J Magn Reson Imaging 1994; 4:779
18. Lien HH, Blomlie V, Iversen T, Trope C, Sundfor K, Abeler VM. Clinical Stage I carcinoma of the cervix: value of MR in determining invasion into the parametrium. Acta Radiol 1993; 34:130
19. Parker SP, Tong T, Bolden S, et al. Cancer statistics. CA Cancer J Clin. 1997; 47:5
20. Parente JT, Amsel M, et al. Breast cancer associated with pregnancy. Obstet Gynecol 1988; 71:861–4
21. Segreti EM. Management of the obstetric patient with malignancy. In: Sciarra JJ, (ed.) Obstetrics and Gynecology (vol 2). Philadelphia: Lippincott-Raven, 1997
22. Harms S, Flamig D, Hesley K, et al. MR imaging of the breast with rotating delivery of excitation of resonance: clinical experience with pathologic correlation. Radiology 1993; 187:493
23. Orel S, Schnall M, Powell C, et al. Staging of suspected breast cancer: effect of MR imaging and MR guided biopsy. Radiology 1995; 196:115
24. Khanusur T, Haick A, Patel B. Evaluation of bone scan as a screening work-up in primary and local-regional recurrence of breast cancer. Am J Clin Oncol 1987; 10:167
25. Namura Y, Kondo H, Yamagata J. Evaluation of liver and bone scanning in patients with early breast cancer, based on results obtained from more advanced cancer patients. Eur J Cancer 1978; 14:1129
26. Stewart HL, Monto RW. Hodgkin's disease and pregnancy. Am J Obstet Gynecol 1952; 63:570–8
27. Rostock R, Giangreco A, Wharam M, et al. CT scan modification in the treatment of mediastinal Hodgkin's disease. Cancer 1982; 49:2267
28. Hopper H, Diehl L, Lesar M, et al. Hodgkin's disease: clinical utility of CT in initial staging and treatment. Radiology 1988; 169:17
29. Tesoro-Tess J, Balzarini L, Ceglia E, et al. Magnetic resonance imaging in the initial staging of Hodgkin's disease and non-Hodgkin's lymphoma. Eur J Radiol 1991; 12:81
30. Mauch P, Larsen D, Osteen R, et al. Prognostic factors for positive surgical staging in patients with Hodgkin's disease. J Clin Oncol 1990; 8:257
31. Ward FT, Weiss RB. Lymphoma and pregnancy. Semin Oncol 1989; 16:397–409
32. Hoanne B, Shields A, Porter B, Shulman H. Detection of lymphomatous bone marrow involvement with magnetic resonance imaging. Blood 1991; 78:728

33. Chung A, Birnbaum SJ. Ovarian cancer associated with pregnancy. Obstet Gynecol 1973; 41:211
34. DePriest PD, Varner E, Powell J, et al. The efficacy of a sonographic morphology index in identifying ovarian cancer: a multi-institutional investigation. Gynecol Oncol 1994; 55:174
35. Kurjak A, Shalan H, Kupesic S, et al. An attempt to screen asymptomatic women for ovarian and endometrial cancer with transvaginal ultrasound and pulsed Doppler sonography. J Ultrasound Med 1994; 13:295
36. Taylor KJW, Schwartz PE. Screening for early ovarian cancer. Radiology 1994; 192:1
37. Kier, R, McCarthy SM, Scoutt LM, Viscarello RR, Schwartz PES. Pelvic masses in pregnancy. Radiology 1990; 176:709–13
38. Gastonis C, McNeil BJ. Collaborative evaluations of diagnostic tests: experience of the Radiology Diagnostic Oncology Group. Radiology 1990; 175:571–5

10. Pregnancy Derived Tumor Marker

Takeshi Maruo and Tetsuo Otani

Introduction

During pregnancy, a wide variety of proteins are produced by both the placenta and the fetus. While many of these proteins are identical to those produced by normal adult tissues, some are unique to either the placenta or the fetus. It is known that cancers produce placental or fetal proteins. Some of these proteins which can be detected in the serum or urine are used as tumor markers. The most well known tumor marker of placental origin is human chorionic gonadotropin (hCG). Fetus specific proteins that are used as tumor markers include alpha fetoprotein (AFP) and carcinoembryonic antigen (CEA). It should be noted, however, that these placental or fetal proteins are expressed in a small quantity by normal tissues. For instance, hCG is transcribed in the pituitary at a very low level, but still detectable by reverse-transcriptase polymerase chain reaction (RT-PCR) and other sensitive methods.[1] CEA is known to be expressed in normal colorectal membrane.[2] Therefore, caution must be exercised in interpreting the data when these proteins are used as tumor markers.

Ideal tumor markers should be organ specific, as such markers would be useful in identifying the origin of a metastatic tumor. It should also have quantitative relation with the magnitude of the tumor expansion, as it would help diagnosing the extent of the disease and monitoring the effectiveness of a therapy. hCG is one of the tumor makers which satisfies these requirements and is the main tool of the diagnosis and prognostic indicator of specific tumors, i.e. trophoblastic disease and gonadal germ cell tumors. On the other hand, placental alkaline phosphatase, which has poor disease specificity and sensitivity, is increased in sera in 40–100% of seminoma cases and still is useful in the management of some germ cell tumors.[3] Therefore, one should be aware of the usefulness and limitations of various tumor markers, use the most appropriate marker for the tumor, and interpret the data according to the characteristic of the marker.

Many other placental or fetal proteins such as pregnancy specific beta 1 glycoprotein (SP-1) have been identified and have been preliminarily investigated for their usefulness as tumor markers.[4] Nevertheless, in most cases, the information available is not sufficient to assess their specificity or sensitivity. Lately, pregnancy related tumor markers widely used in clinical practice are hCG, CEA and AFP.

Human Chorionic Gonadotropin (hCG)

Human chorionic gonadotropin is a glycoprotein hormone produced mainly by the trophoblast. It is composed of alpha and beta subunits that are linked non-covalently. There is only one hCG alpha gene in the entire human genome which is located on chromosome 6.[5] The alpha subunit is common among such glycoprotein hormones as hCG, TSH, FSH and LH. One alpha subunit gene is transcribed for the production of hCG, TSH, FSH and LH in the trophoblast and in the pituitary. It is the beta subunit that is unique to hCG and confers biological activity. The hCG beta gene is located on chromosome 1,[5] consists of 6 genes and is aligned in tandem with single LH beta gene.[6] It is believed that hCG beta gene family was derived by the mutation and multiplication of the LH beta gene. The biological activity of hCG and LH is quite similar and their amino acid sequences share more than 80% homology.

Human chorionic gonadotropin beta has carboxy terminal peptide which is absent in the LH beta. This carboxy terminal peptide is created because of the mutation in the termination codon which is present in the LH beta gene. Because of the absence of the termination codon, the gene is transcribed further downstream to the next termination codon, adding a 24 amino acid long carboxy terminal peptide sequence to the hCG beta mRNA. The carboxy terminal peptide of hCG beta makes the half-life of hCG longer than that of LH. Another difference between the LH beta and hCG beta gene is the CAP site where the transcription of the mRNA begins. LH beta utilizes CAP site with TATA and CAT box, but for unknown reason, the transcription of hCG beta gene starts 360–366 bases upstream. Since the nucleotide sequence between LH beta and hCG beta gene in this region is quite similar, the reason for the differential initiation of transcription is of significant interest.[7] There is a steroidogenic factor 1 (SF–1) responsive element just upstream of the LH beta CAP site which makes LH beta transcription responsive for SF–1.[8]. Since this region is transcribed into mRNA in hCG beta gene, hCG beta transcription does not respond to SF–1.

The biological function of hCG is to stimulate the luteal body to secret progesterone which in turn makes the endometrium thicker, optimizing for implantation and supporting the maintenance of pregnancy. In normal pregnancy, hCG can be detected at 6–9 days after conception and the serum level increases until about the 8–10th week of gestation when it reaches a peak and thereafter declines.[9] It is actually the beta subunit which peaks at 4–6th week of gestation. The production of the alpha subunit continues to increase until term.[9] Most hCG synthesis and secretion is by the cytotrophoblast in 4–5 week placenta, while in 6–12 week placenta, it is mostly produced by the syncytiotropoblast.[10]

It is reported that hCG cross-reacts with TSH receptor and stimulates thyroid function.[11] This function is supposed to be responsible for hyperthyroidism observed in patients with trophoblastic disease.

As noted above, small amount of hCG is transcribed in the pituitary. It had been reported by immunoassay that a hCG-like substance exists in the pituitary, but recent study by RT-PCR revealed that complete hCG mRNA is present in the pituitary.[12] This finding is of significant importance when using hCG as tumor marker especially in women over climacteric age. It is recommended to pre-treat those patients with estrogen before measuring the serum levels of hCG to suppress pituitary hCG.

Recent advances in monoclonal antibodies revealed that several forms of hCG are present in the human body. These include hCG dimer, free alpha subunit, free beta subunit and beta core fragment or urinary gonadotropin fragment (UGF). Among these various peptides, only hCG dimer has been proven to have biological activity.

However, there is a report that free alpha subunit of glycoprotein hormones stimulates prolactin production by endometrial cells and induces differentiation of endometrial stromal cells to decidualized cells.[13]

Recent reports suggests that a bacteria called *Xanthomonas maltophilia*[14] and a fungus called *Candida albicans*[15] also produce an hCG-like substance. It is reported that hCG in these species exert autocrine or paracrine activity.

Various methods were developed to measure the concentration of hCG. During the 1960s, radioimmunoassays for hCG were developed, but it had cross-reactivity with pituitary LH. In 1972, radioimmunoassay using specific antibody for hCG beta subunit was developed.[16] This assay lowered cross-reactivity with LH, but some cross-reaction still remained. Then enzyme immunoassay or radioimmunoassay was developed using specific antibodies raised against hCG beta carboxy terminal peptide which is unique to hCG.[17] The most recent assay is called sandwich assay and uses multiple monoclonal antibodies. These recent assays can measure hCG with the specificity of 0.2–0.5 mIU/ml without cross-reaction with pituitary LH.

Gestational trophoblastic disease includes hydatidiform mole, invasive mole, choriocarcinoma and placental site trophoblastic tumor. In the management of trophoblastic disease, with the possible exception of placental site trophoblastic tumor, hCG is an ideal tumor marker with high specificity and sensitivity. Serum level of hCG correlates with the expansion and mass of the tumor except for placental site trophoblast tumor, in which hCG may not be elevated. It is more accurate than any imaging or other clinical findings in the diagnosis of trophoblastic disease. As an index substance which is closely related to the growth of trophoblastic tumor, hCG is invaluable in the diagnosis and follow-up of trophoblastic disease.

Combination of hCG measurement and ultrasonography is powerful tool in the diagnosis of hydatidiform mole. After evacuation of hydatidiform mole, the serum concentrations of hCG declines rapidly. We prefer weekly assessment of hCG while some argue that assay of hCG at every 2 weeks is sufficient. It should fall in the normal range and become undetectable at 16 weeks following molar evacuation (Fig. 10.1). Once hCG levels become undetectable, the hCG measurement should be performed once a month for 6 months, and then every 2 months for a total of 1 year. If hCG remains undetectable after 1 year, the patient has less than 0.1% risk of recurrence of trophoblastic disease[18] and hence follow-up may be discontinued and pregnancy is allowed.

In about 20% of patients who underwent molar evacuation, further therapy becomes necessary for the suspect of persistent trophoblastic disease. Persistent trophoblastic diseases, which include invasive mole and choriocarcinoma, follow some kind of pregnancy, i.e. molar pregnancy, normal pregnancy or ectopic pregnancy. Although invasive mole usually occurs after a hydatidiform mole, it is evident that the percentage of choriocarcinoma proceeded by hydatidiform mole is approximately 50% and the half of cases of choriocarcinoma arise after a normal term delivery, a stillbirth, an abortion or an ectopic pregnancy. The presence of hCG in serum or urine reflects tumor burden and is a potential marker for assessing the efficacy of therapy in persistent trophoblastic disease.

Qualitative Aspect of hCG as Tumor Marker of Trophoblastic Disease

Fig. 10.2 shows hCG values in patients who were diagnosed as having invasive mole following evacuation of molar pregnancy. Following the evacuation of the original hydatidiform mole, the patient may remain symptom free for several weeks or even

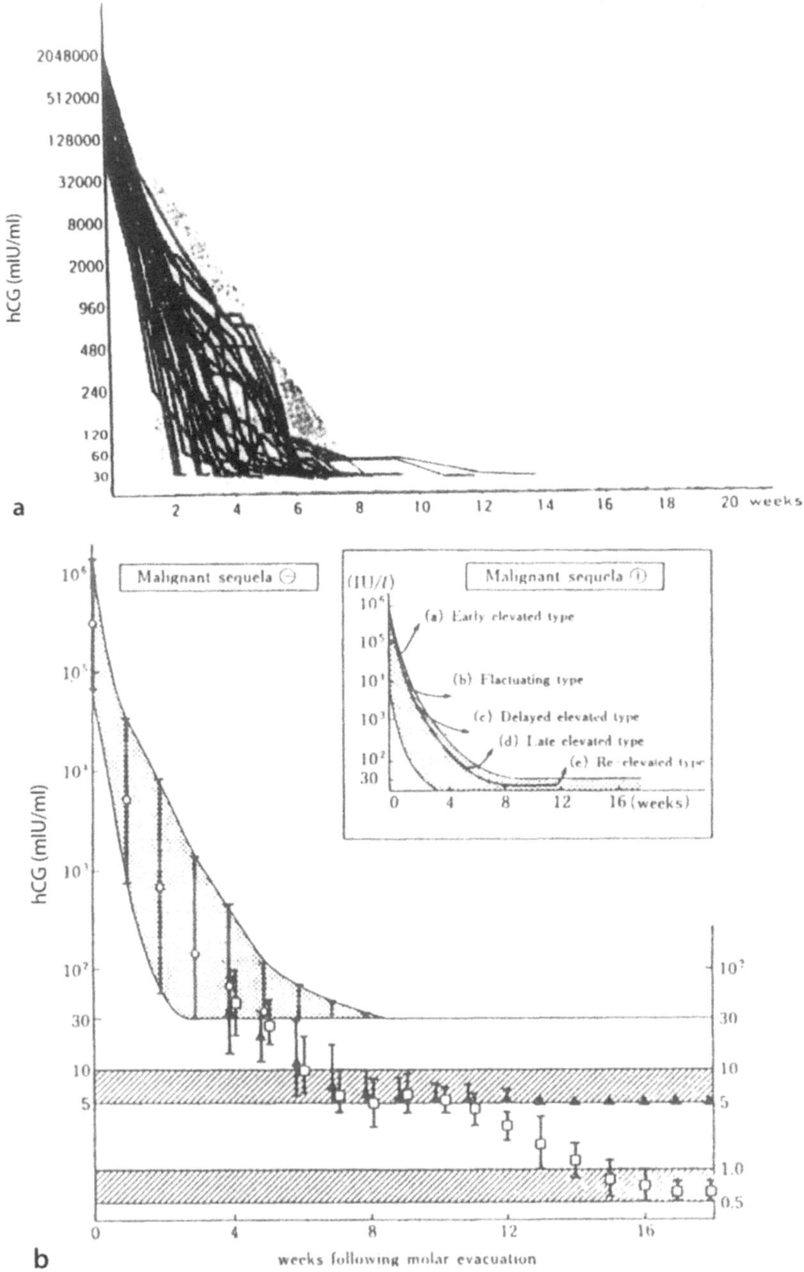

Fig.10.1 Normal regression curve of hCG following evacuation of molar pregnancy. Follow-up result (**a**) and the schematic illustration (**b**). Triangles, serum hCG by hCG beta RIA; squares, urinary hCG by hCG beta carboxy terminal peptide (hCG-beta-CTP) EIA.

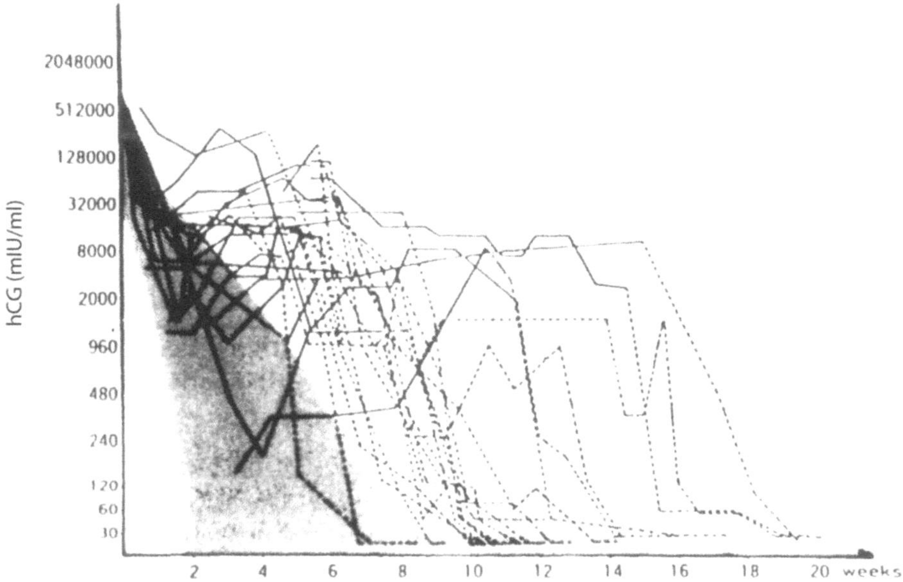

Figure 10.2. Follow-up of hCG levels in patients who were diagnosed as having invasive mole following evacuation of molar pregnancy. Solid lines, before hysterectomy; broken lines, after hysterectomy. In most patients with invasive mole, reincrease in hCG levels appeared during the initial three months following molar evacuation.

months before reelevation of hCG values. It should be noted that the reelevation of hCG values in patients with invasive mole usually occurs during the first 6 months following molar evacuation. Unlike invasive mole, reelevation of hCG values in patients with choriocarcinoma usually occurs after at least 6 months following the termination of the preceding pregnancy including hydatidiform mole. In those patients, hCG values usually reelevate after declining to undetectable levels for a certain period of time (Fig. 10.3).

In gestational trophoblastic diseases, the response to chemotherapy is quite good. In patients with no metastasis or with metastasis to lung only, the sustained remission rate is almost 100%. In those low risk women, single agent chemotherapy is effective. Methotrexate is the most commonly used agent. In high risk patients with metastasis to multiple distant organs, on the other hand, single agent chemotherapy achieves remission in only 20–40% of cases. However, combination chemotherapy, despite higher toxicity, yields a better outcome in these patients.[19] Fig.10.4 shows serum hCG pattern of a patient receiving several courses of combination chemotherapy because of recurrence of choriocaricinoma. Only the elevation of hCG values could detect the recurrence of choriocarcinoma.

It must be noted that a transient rise in the hCG value may be observed when chemotherapy is initiated. The exact cause for this phenomenon is not yet elucidated but several hypotheses exists. It may be because hCG already fabricated within the destroyed cells is released into circulation, or chemotherapy may induce differentiation of stem cells into more differentiated hCG producing cells.

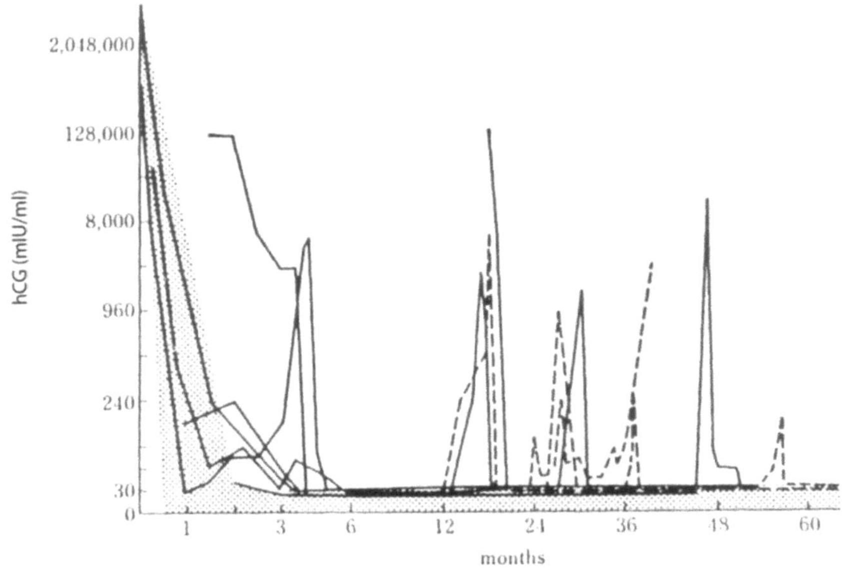

Figure 10.3. Follow-up of hCG levels in patients who were diagnosed as having choriocarcinoma following molar evacuation. In most patients with choriocarcinoma, reincrease in hCG levels appeared once after declining to the cut-off level for a certain period of time longer than three months after molar evacuation.

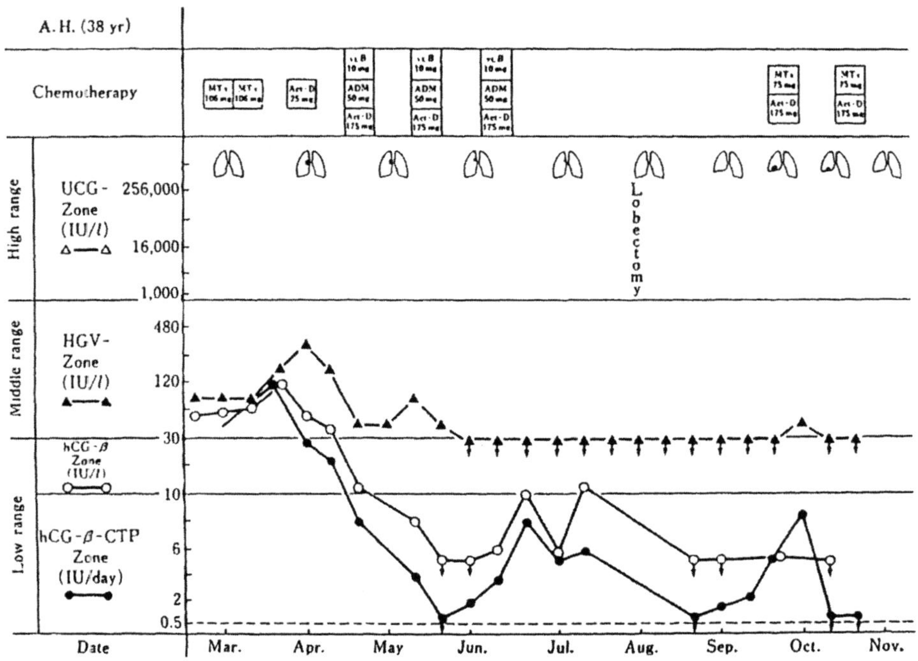

Figure 10.4. Follow-up of hCG levels in a patient with recurrent choriocaricinoma. Determination of hCG with hCG-beta-CTP-EIA was powerful for the early detection of the recurrence of the disease.

Qualitative Aspects of hCG as Tumor Marker of Trophoblastic Disease

There is a qualitative alteration in the biochemical structure of hCG during malignant transformation of the trophoblast. Amino acid analysis of urinary hCG preparations from normal gestation, hydatidiform mole, and choriocarcinoma has shown that there is no differences in amino acid composition of these three hCG preparations. However a great difference in carbohydrate composition among the hCG preparations from normal gestation, hydatidiform mole and choriocarcinoma has been demonstrated. Sialic acid content in choriocarcinoma hCG is extremely low or undetectable, whereas normal hCG and hydatidiform mole hCG contain approximately 8.5% sialic acid in the molecule. This suggests that the malignant transformation of the trophoblast may result in an alteration of the glycosylation process, especially in the sialylation of hCG (Table 10.1).

Both alpha and beta subunits contain two asparagine-linked sugar chains and, in addition, the beta subunit contains four serine-linked sugar chains. In the asparagine-linked sugar chains of normal hCG, all sialic acid residues occur exclusively as the NeuAc $\alpha 2 \rightarrow$ 3Gal grouping. Choriocarcinoma hCG possesses several prominent structural diffrences in the sugar chains as compared with normal hCG. More than 97% of the sugar chains of choriocarcinoma hCG are free from sialic acid, whereas the sugar chains of normal hCG are mostly sialyated. Choriocarcinoma hCG contains unusual biantennary complex type sugar chains. Furthermore, the occurrence of the Galß1–4G1cNAcß1 $\rightarrow$ 4man $\alpha 1 \rightarrow$ group is a characteristic feature of the sugar chains of choriocarcinoma hCG, as normal hCG does not contain any triantennary sugar chains. The total of fucosylated sugar chains of choriocarcinoma hCG is twice as much as normal hCG, indicating that fucosylation is also modified in choriocarcinoma (Table 10.2). In contrast, urinary hCG purified from patients with hydatidiform mole is found to have almost the same profile of sugar chains as that of normal pregnancy hCG.[20] It can therefore be concluded that the structural changes in the sugar chains of choriocarcinoma hCG observed are specific for malignant trophoblast.

Table 10.1 Carbohydrate composition of urinary hCG preparations from normal pregnancy

Carbohydrate	Normal pregnancy	Hydatidiform mole	Choriocarcinoma
Fucose	1.5	1.4	1.4
Galactose	5.3	9.0	7.6
Mannose	5.3	4.8	5.7
N-Acetyl galactosamine	3.6	3.6	3.9
N-Acetyl glucosamine	8.5	4.9	5.0
Sialic acid	8.6	8.5	Undetectable
Total carbohydrate	32.8	32.2	23.9

Table 10.2 Structural alterations in sugar chains of choriocarcinoma hCG.

1	Appearance of sugar chains free from sialic acid
2	Occurrence of triantennary sugar chains with Galβ1 $\rightarrow$ 4GlcNAcβ1 $\rightarrow$ 4man α1 $\rightarrow$ group
3	Increase in sum total of fucosylated sugar chains

Recently two methods have been developed to detect the structural change of sugar chains of choriocarcinoma hCG. One is based on the capability of the lectin from *Arachis hypogala* peanut (PNA) to bind to asialylated sugar chains and the other is an immunologic assay method using an antiserum (R141) generated against desialylated ßhCG-COOH-terminal peptide. In PNA-sepharose affinity chromatography, the entire portion of choriocarcinoma hCG containing no sialic acid is absorbed, whereas the major portion of urinary hCG from normal pregnant women and patients with hydatidiform mole is not absorbed on the column. When the PNA binding of urinary hCG from six patients with choriocarcinoma was studied, two of the six cases (33%) were highly bound to the PNA-sepharose column, suggesting that PNA-sepharose affinity chromatography is an effective means of detecting the incompletely sialylated hCG in patients with choriocarcinoma.

On the other hand, with the radioimmunoassay using the antiserum (R141) generated against desialylated ßhCG-COOH terminal peptide, no asialo-hCG immunoreactivity was found in patients with hydatidiform mole and invasive mole, whereas urinary hCG from one-third (33%) of patients with choriocarcinoma demonstrated asialo-hCG immunoreactivity (Table 10.3). Thus, this immunologic method to detect desialylated hCG also seems to be a useful means for the biochemial diagnosis of choriocarcinoma.[21] However, desialylation of sugar chains of hCG does not always appear in patients with choriocarcinoma. Development of a specific method to detect the prominent structure of sugar chains of Galβ1 $\rightarrow$ 4GlcNacβ1 $\rightarrow$ 4man α1 $\rightarrow$ group, characteristic of choriocarcinoma hCG, will be the next step in the biochemical diagnosis of choriocarcinoma.

Table 10.3. Detection of desialylated hCG in patients with hydatidiform mole, invasive mole, persistent trophoblastic disease, and choriocarcinoma using radioimmunoassay for deialylated β-hCG-COOH-terminal peptide

Diagnosis	Cases (n)	Asialo-hCG detected cases (n)
Hydatidiform mole	11	0
Invasive hydatidiform mole	5	0
Persistent trophoblastic disease	7	0
Choriocarcinoma	6	2
Totals	29	2

Human Chorionic Gonadotrophin as Tumor Marker of Germ Cell Tumor of the Testis

About 95% of testicular carcinoma are germ cell tumor of the testis. It can be classified into seminoma and non-seminomatous germ cell tumor. Seminoma accounts for about 35–50% of germ cell tumor of the testis. Non-seminomatous germ cell tumor can be further classified into embryonal carcinoma, teratocarcinoma, adult teratoma and choriocarcinoma.

About 11% of patients with seminoma are positive for hCG in serum. The source of hCG is trophoblastic giant cells found in seminoma tissues. About 45% of patients with non-seminomatous germ cell tumor of the testis are positive for hCG in serum. Trophoblastic giant cells and syncytiotrophoblasts produce hCG in these tumors.

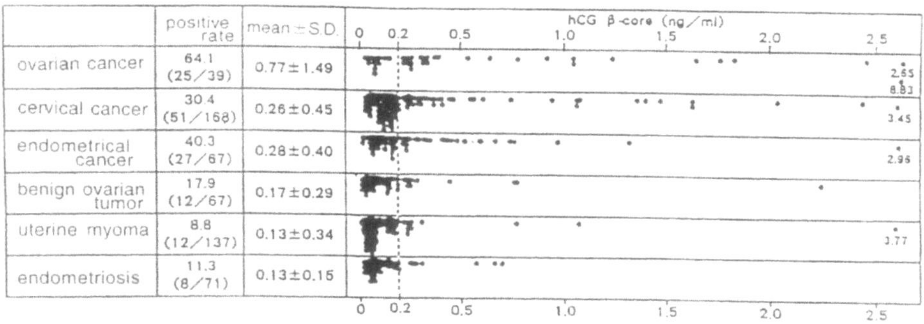

Figure 10.5 Distribution of urinary levels of hCG beta core fragment in patients with gynecologic tumors

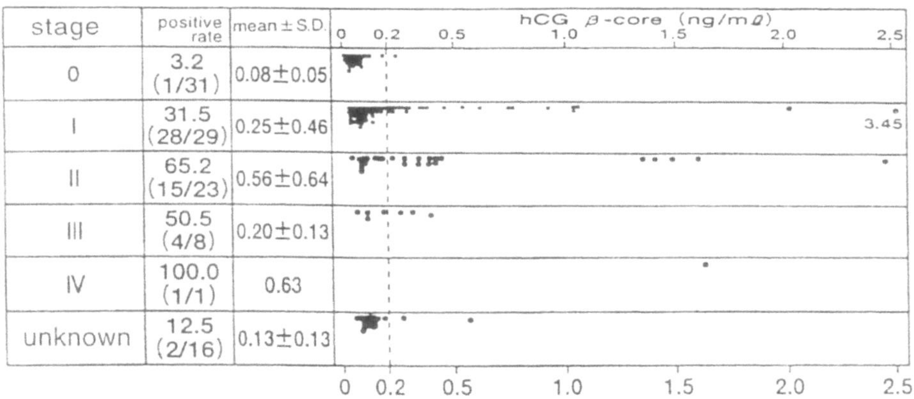

Figure 10.6. Urinary levels of hCG beta core fragment related to the stage of disease in patients with cervical cancer before treatment. There was no correlation between the urinary levels of hCG beta core fragment and the stage of the disease.

In patients with germ cell tumor of the testis, measurement of alpha fetoprotein (AFP) along with hCG provides a useful marker for monitoring the extent of tumor mass and metastasis.[22] After orchiectomy, serum levels of hCG and AFP reduce quickly if there is no residual tumor.[23] Care must be taken to use specific assay for hCG with antibody against hCG beta carboxyl terminal peptide since pituitary LH levels increase after orchiectomy which may cross-react with hCG assay with antibody against hCG beta. In monitoring the efficacy of chemotherapy or irradiation therapy, hCG is also useful. If the hCG concentrations increase in spite of therapy, the tumor is likely to be progressing. On the other hand, if the hCG concentrations decrease, the tumor is likely to be regressing. However, in 10% of cases, there is discordance between hCG level and tumor expansion.[24] It is supposed to occur when chemotherapy or irradiation therapy destroys hCG producing cells while other components of the tumor may continue to grow.

Human Chorionic Gonadotrophin Beta Core Fragment

While hCG can occasionally be found in the serum of patients with non-trophoblastic cancer, its clinical usefulness as a tumor marker is hampered by the existence of hCG-like substance in healthy subjects. Another problem with hCG as a tumor marker for non-trophoblastic cancer is that serum levels of hCG in those patients have no correlation with the stage of disease. Serial measurement of hCG in non-trophoblastic cancer has little prognostic value.

Recent evaluation of hCG beta core fragment or urinary gonadotropin fragment as tumor marker of non-trophoblastic cancer seems to be more promising. The beta core fragment of hCG is a substance composed of residues 6–40 and 55–92 of hCG beta subunit bound by disulfide bonds.[25] This beta core fragment is known to have a shorter half-life as compared with hCG and to be detected in urine. Although the origin of hCG beta core fragment is unknown, two different routes have been postulated. One possibility is that hCG beta core fragment is secreted directly by tumor tissues and the other is that it is a peripheral degradative product in the circulation or in the kidney.

In our study, 103 out of 274 patients (37.5%)with gynecologic cancer had urinary levels of hCG beta core fragment higher than 0.2 ng/ml, whereas among patients with benign gynecologic disease, urinary hCG beta core fragment level higher than 0.2 ng/ml were found in 32 out of 275 patients (11.2%) (Fig. 10.5). No correlation was noted between the urinary levels of hCG beta core fragment and the stages of the disease.[26] (Fig. 10.6).

In patients with ovarian cancer, beta core fragment in urine and CA125 in serum had similar positive rates of 61.1% and 66.7%, respectively. However, there was no correlation between urinary hCG beta core fragment values and serum CA125 values. When combination assay of hCG beta core fragment and CA125 were performed in patients with ovarian cancer, the positive rate increased to 83.3%. This suggests that the combination assay will be useful in screening patients with ovarian cancer which is a disease with no reliable means for the early diagnosis. Likewise, in patients with uterine cervical carcinoma, in which hCG beta core fragment in urine and SCC antigen in serum had the positive rate of 30.9% and 26.2%, respectively, combination assay of hCG beta core fragment and SCC antigen enhanced the positive rate to 43.6%. While with endometrial carcinoma, hCG beta core fragment showed the positive rate of 41.0% and CA19–9 had the positive rate of 42.6%, combined assay of these two markers increased the positive rate to 65.6%.[26]

Thus, combined assay of hCG beta core fragment in urine and other tumor-related marker in serum markedly increased the positive rate for predicting ovarian cancer, uterine cervical cancer, and endometrial cancer. This implies that hCG beta core fragment in urine becomes positive in patients with gynecological malignancies independently from such tumor-related markers in serum as CA125, CA19–9 and SCC. These data suggest that hCG beta core fragment deserves further consideration as a complementary marker to CA125, CA19–9 and SCC in the diagnosis of patients with gynecologic cancers. Since hCG beta core fragment values was not correlated with the clinical stage of the disease or tumor burden of malignancy, hCG beta core fragment seems unlikely to be adequate for monitoring the therapeutic effect of the treatment. Nevertheless, hCG beta core fragment may be a unique tumor marker which can be detected in urine in patients with a variety of malignancy.

Carcinoembryonic Antigen (CEA)

CEA is a glycoprotein of 180 KDa in size expressed in a variety of cancer tissues and the fetal intestine.[27] CEA is secreted into the mucous and acts as a cell adhesion molecule. Antibody to CEA has cross-reactivity with non-specific cross-reacting antigen (NCA) and normal fecal antigen (NFA). CEA has structural similarity with these molecules and is considered to be a member of the immunoglobulin superfamily.

Increased levels of CEA are often observed in the serum of patients with adenocarcinoma and squamous cell carcinoma, but the expression of CEA is not limited to malignant tissues. Normal colorectal membranes also express CEA. Conditions with increased serum CEA are summarized in Table 10.4.

Because of its increase in a wide range of conditions, CEA is hardly a specific tumor marker for the individual malignancy. Although elevation of CEA levels alone does not necessarily indicate the existence of malignant tumor, the presence of cancer should be suspected and suitable examination must be carried out if CEA levels in serum are abnormally high. Since CEA is a glycoprotein which is very rich in sugar chains and has a very long half-life, it may not be an ideal marker for the purpose of follow-up of the effect of therapy. Nevertheless, its elevation in a wide range of malignancies often makes it the only marker available. Indeed, it has been successfully used for follow-up of ovarian cancer and cervical cancer (Fig. 10.7). In ovarian epithelial cancer, CEA tends to be more prevalent in mucinous cystoadenocarcinoma than in serous cystoadenocarcinoma.

Table 10.4. Diseases and conditions associated with elevated serum CEA.

Malignant tumor
Cancers of gastrointestinal tract
Colorectal cancer, pancreatic cancer, gastric cancer, hepatoma, esophageal cancer
Cancers of gynecological region
Ovarian cancer, endometrial cancer, cervical cancer
Cancers of other regions
Lung cancer, breast cancer, thyroid cancer, renal cell cancer, testicular cancer
Benign disease
Hepatitis, liver cirrhosis, pancreatitis, gall bladder stone
Gastric ulcer, gastric polyp, inflammatory diseases of the gastrointestinal tract
Chronic respiratory disease, hypothyroidism, benign ovarian tumor, renal failure, diabetes mellitus, autoimmune disease
Others
Smoking, pregnancy

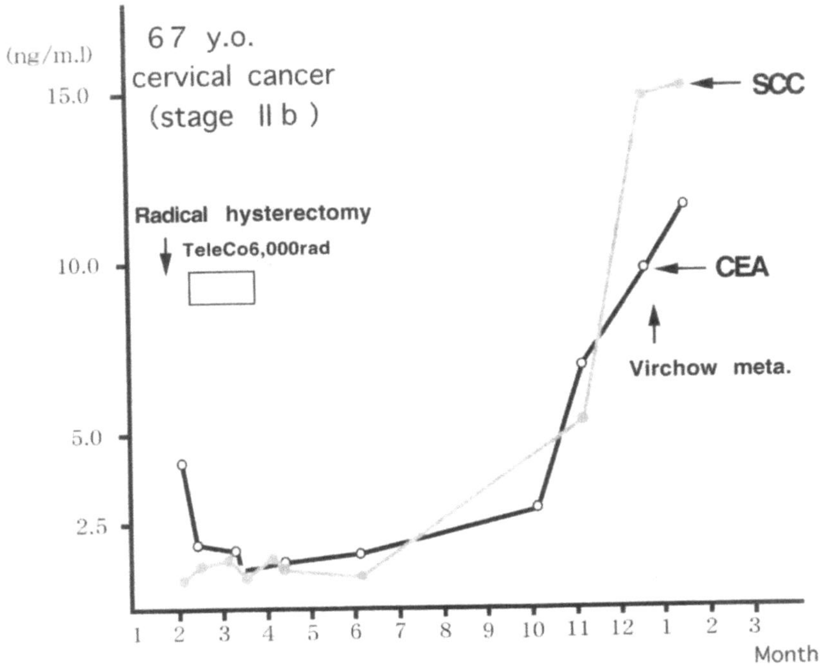

Figure 10.7. Follow-up of CEA and SCC levels in a patient with recurrent cervical cancer. Increase in CEA and SCC levels appeared prior to the clinical manifestation of recurrence of the disease.

Alpha Fetoprotein (AFP)

AFP is one of the oldest fetal proteins used as a tumor marker. It was first observed in the sera of mice bearing transplanted hepatocellular carcinoma.[28] Shortly afterwards, its presence in human patients with hepatocellular carcinoma was observed. Now, it is used clinically as a tumor marker of hepatocellular carcinoma and germ cell tumors of the gonads.

In the human embryo, AFP is first produced by the yolk sac and the liver and after the yolk sac disappears at the end of the first trimester, by the liver alone. It can be detected in the fetal serum at the 6th week of gestation, reaches a peak of 200–300 mg/dl at the 13th week and thereafter gradually declines. Serum levels of AFP decline to comparable levels to that of an adult at 250 to 300 days after birth.

AFP is a glycoprotein with a molecular weight of 70 Kda. Immunochemical data, amino acid sequence and gene analysis have shown that AFP is functionally and structurally related to albumin. AFP is produced not only in the fetal tissue but also in cancers, though only to a very limited extent in normal adult tissues. Thus, it reflects the re-expression of fetal genes in malignant cells, and serves as a tumor marker.[29]

In 20–70% of patients with germ cell tumor of the gonads, serum AFP levels are elevated.[30] Synthesis of AFP by germ cell tumors correlates with the existence of endometrial sinus elements analogous to the yolk sac. The serum AFP concentrations reflect the tumor burden of yolk sac tumor and thus its serial measurement is useful

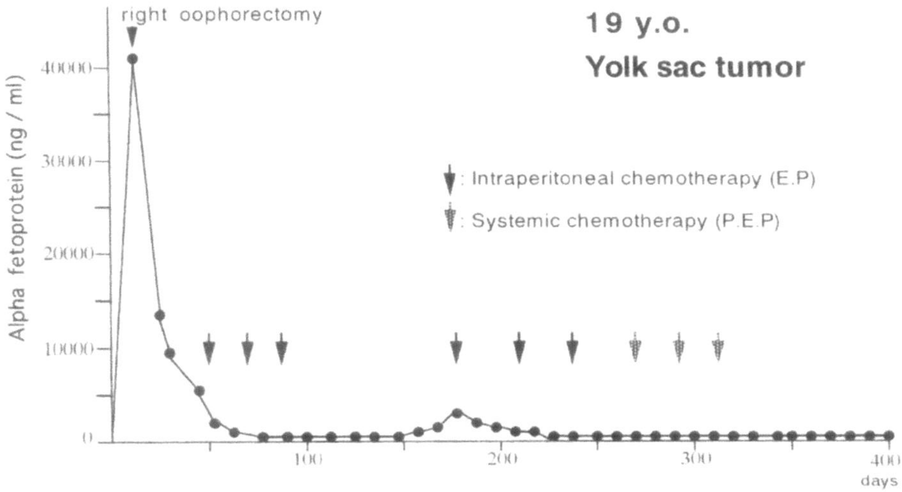

Figure 10.8. AFP levels in response to the treatment in a patient with yolk sac tumor. Serum AFP determination provides a potential means for monitoring the effects of individual therapy for yolk sac tumor and for early detection of the recurrence.

for monitoring the effect of therapy in those patients (Fig. 10.8). The half-life of AFP is about 5 days and deviation away from expected decline with treatment indicates resistance to the particular treatment. Like hCG, serum levels transiently increase after chemotherapy.

About 80–90% of patients with hepatocellular carcinoma have elevated serum AFP.[29] However, the levels of AFP do not correlate with the size of tumor. This is because AFP producing cells represent only a minor fraction of tumor cells. In spite of the fact that serum AFP is a sensitive marker for hepatocellular carcinoma, it cannot be solely relied upon. Both radiological examination and AFP measurement are needed to detect small liver cancers. AFP is elevated in 10–35% of patients with non-malignant liver diseases such as hepatitis, cirrhosis and tyrosenemia. In these benign patients, the elevation of AFP is usually slight.

Summary

The biological substances derived from pregnancy widely used as tumor markers are still limited to hCG, hCG beta core fragment, CEA and AFP. Other substances tested so far have failed to achieve clinical usefulness in screening malignancy and evaluating the effects of therapy in patients with malignant disease. However, the advent of new cytogenetic and molecular markers together with an improved evaluation of known substances may provide the basis for a more accurate assessment of tumor behavior, provide better diagnostic information and eventually allow better treatment to be discovered.

References

1. Birken S, Maydelman Y, Gawinowicz MA, Pound A, Liu Y, Hartree AS. Isolation and characterization of human pituitary chorionic gonadotropin. Endocrinology 1996;137: 1402–11.
2. Quentmeier A, Moller P, Schwarz V, Abel U, Schlag P. Carcinoembryonic antigen, CA 19-9, and CA 125 in normal and carcinomatous human colorectal tissue. Cancer 1987;60: 2261–6.
3. Horwich A, Tucker DF, Peckham MJ. Placental alkaline phosphatase as a tumour marker in seminoma using the H17 E2 monoclonal antibody assay. Br J Cancer 1985;51: 625–9.
4. Kuhajda FP, Bohn H, Mendelsohn G. Pregnancy-specific beta-1 glycoprotein (SP-1) in breast carcinoma. Pathologic and clinical considerations. Cancer 1984;54: 1392–6.
5. Naylor SL, Chin WW, Goodman HM, Lalley PA, Grzeschik KH, Sakaguchi AY. Chromosome assignment of genes encoding the alpha and beta subunits of glycoprotein hormones in man and mouse. Somatic Cell Genet 1983;9: 757–70.
6. Graham MY, Otani T, Boime I, Olson MV, Carle GF, Chaplin DD. Cosmid mapping of the human chorionic gonadotropin beta subunit genes by field-inversion gel electrophoresis. Nucleic Acids Res 1987;15: 4437–48.
7. Otani T, Otani F, Krych M, Chaplin DD, Boime I. Identification of a promoter region in the CG beta gene cluster. J Biol Chem 1988;263: 7322–9.
8. Keri RA, Nilson JH. A steroidogenic factor-1 binding site is required for activity of the luteinizing hormone beta subunit promoter in gonadotropes of transgenic mice. J Biol Chem 1996;271: 10782–5.
9. Braunstein GD, Rasor J, Adler D, Danzer H, Wade ME. Serum human chorionic gonadotropin levels throughout normal pregnancy. Ann J Obstet Gynecol 1976;126: 678–81.
10. Maruo T, Ladinel-Llave CA, Matsuo H, Manalo AS, Mochizuki M. A novel change in cytologic localization of human chorionic gonadotropin and human placental lactogen in first-trimester placenta in the course of gestation. Am J Obstet Gynecol 1992;167: 217–22.
11. Kraiem Z, Sadeh O, Blithe DL, Nisula BC. Human chorionic gonadotropin stimulates thyroid hormone secretion, iodide uptake, organification, and adenosine 3',5'-monophosphate formation in cultured human thyrocytes. J Clin Endocrinol Metab 1994; 9: 595–9.
12. Dirnhofer S, Hermann M, Hittmair A, Hoermann R, Kapelari K, Berger P. Expression of the human chorionic gonadotropin-beta gene cluster in human pituitaries and alternate use of exon 1. J Clin Endocrinol Metab 1996;81: 4212–7.
13. Moy E, Kimzey LM, Nelson LM, Blithe DL. Glycoprotein hormone alpha-subunit functions synergistically with progesterone to stimulate differentiation of cultured human endometrial stromal cells to decidualized cells: a novel role for free alpha-subunit in reproduction. Endocrinology 1996;137: 1332–9.
14. Carrell DT, Hammond ME, Odell WD. Evidence for an autocrine/paracrine function of chorionic gonadotropin in *Xanthomonas maltophilia*. Endocrinology 1993;132: 1085–9.
15. Caticha O, Li Y, Griffin J, Winge D, Odell WD. Characterization of a human chorionic gonadotropin-like protein from *Candida albicans*. Endocrinology 1993;132: 667–73.
16. Vaitukaitis JL, Braunstein GD, Ross GT. A radio-immunoassay which specifically measures human chorionic gonadotropin in the presence of human luteinizing hormone. Am J Obstet Gynecol 1972;113: 751–8.
17. Wehmann RE, Harman SM, Birken S, Canfield RE, Nisula BC. Convenient radioimmunoassay for urinary human choriogonadotropin without interference by urinary human lutropin. Clin Chem 1981;27: 1997–2001.
18. Bagshawe KD. Clinical application of hCG. Adv Exp Med Biol 1984;76: 313–24.
19. Ross GT, Goldstein DP, Hertz R, Lipsett MB, Odell WD. Sequential use of methotrexate and actinomycin D in the treatment of metastatic choriocarcinoma and related trophoblastic disease in women. Am J Obstet Gynecol 1965;93: 223–9.
20. Mizuochi T, Nishimura R, Derappe C, Taniguchi T, Hamamoto T, Mochizuki M, Kobata A. Structures of the asparagine-linked sugar chains of human chorionic gonadotropin produced in choriocarcinoma. Appearance of triantennary sugar chains and unique biantennary sugar chains. J Biol Chem 1983;258: 14126–9.
21. Takeuchi Y, Matsuura S, Nishimura R, Mochizuki M. The determination of the recognition site of an antiserum detecting desialylation on 0-glycosidic carbohydrates of hCG and its clinical applications. The relationship between the presence of asialo-hCG and malignant change in trophoblastic disease. Folia Endocrinol 1984;60: 1046–57.
22. Scardino PT, Cox HD, Waldmann TA, Mcintire KR, Mittemeyer B, Javadpour N. The value of serum tumor markers in the staging and prognosis of germ cell tumors of the testis. J Urol 1977;118: 994–9

23. Willemse PH, Sleijfer DT, Schraffordt Koops H, De Bruijn HW, Oosterhuis JW, Brouwers TM, Ockhuizen T, Marrink J. Tumor markers in patients with non-seminomatous germ cell tumors of the testis. Oncodev Biol Med 1981;2: 117–28.
24. Norgaard-Pedersen B, Schultz H, Arends J, Brincker H, Jacobsen GK, Lindelov B, Rorth M, Svennekjaer IL. Biochemical markers for testicular germ-cell tumors in relation to histology and stage: some experiences from the Danish testicular cancer (DATECA) Study from 1976 through 1981. Ann N Y Acad Sci 1983;417: 390–9.
25. Nam JH, Cole LA, Chambers JT, Schwartz PE. Urinary gonadotropin fragment, a new tumor marker. I. Assay development and cancer specificity. Gynecol Oncol 1990;36: 383–90.
26. Maruo T, Otani T, Mochizuki M, Nishimura R, Hasegawa K. Clinical significance of the measurement of urinary hCGß-core fragment in patients with gynecologic malignant tumors. Obstet Gynecol (Tokyo) 1991;117: 1197–208.
27. Golf P, Freedman SO. Specific carcinoembyonic antigens of the human digestive system. J Exp Med 1965;122: 467–81.
28. Abelev GI, Perova SD, Kharmkove NI, Postnikova ZA, Irlin IS. Production of embryonal alpha globulin by transplantable mouse hepatomas. Transplantation 1:174, 1963
29. Ruoslahti E. Alpha-Fetoprotein in cancer and fetal development. Adv Cancer Res 1979;29: 275–346.
30. Sell S. Cancer markers for the 1990s. Clin Lab Med 1990;10: 1–37.

11. Chemo and Radiation Therapy During Pregnancy

Muhammad Muslim, Jack Goldberg and Alexandre Hageboutros

General Principles

The simultaneous occurrence of pregnancy and cancer is fortunately rare, but presents a therapeutic challenge for the physicians. The immediate and delayed effects of diagnostic and therapeutic measures are potentially deleterious to the fetus. When termination of pregnancy is unacceptable, decisions regarding the use of chemotherapy and radiation therapy are complicated by high risk of abortion and fetal malformation. This risk is concentrated during the first trimester and varies with the type of treatment used. However, delay or modification of treatment could adversely affect maternal prognosis. Chemotherapy should not be delayed if cure or prolongation of the survival is a realistic goal such as in the treatment of lymphoma, leukemia, breast and ovarian cancer. If cure or significant palliation is not possible, the use of potentially teratogenic therapy should therefore be avoided during pregnancy.

In this chapter we will briefly review the data available for the use of chemotherapy and radiation therapy during pregnancy followed by recommendations for use of such treatment. The risks to the fetus considering gestational age versus benefits to the mother should be calculated. The risks to the fetus for various diagnostic radiology procedures are negligible if radiation doses do not exceed 0.1 GY (10 rads). See also Chapters 13, 14, 15.

Pharmacology

Adequate data on the pharmacokinetic studies of antineoplastic drugs during pregnancy will never be available. Pharmacokinetics can be altered by the physiological changes that occur during pregnancy. Absorption, distribution, metabolism and excretion of a drug are affected by this altered physiologic state. During pregnancy, the stomach empties more slowly with a decrease in gastrointestinal motility which could affect the rate and completeness of drug absorption. Total body water and plasma volume are increased in pregnancy which results in larger dilutional space for water soluble drugs. The albumin concentration decreases and plasma proteins are increased due, in part, to high estrogen levels. Thus drugs which are tightly bound to plasma protein and have low lipid solubility will be in higher concentration.[1]

The half-life of a drug depends upon its volume of distribution, metabolism and excretion.

An increased distribution volume will decrease the peak concentration of a drug following bolus administration and the half-life will be longer unless drug metabolism or excretion are also increased. The increase in renal blood flow, glomerular filtration rate and creatinine clearance may increase the clearance of the drugs excreted by the kidney. The concentration × time relationship (AUC which represent the total drug exposure over time), which determines therapeutic efficacy and toxicity of a drug, may thus be altered in pregnancy. Amniotic fluid may act as physiologic third space, potentially increasing the toxicity of particular agents (e.g. Methotrexate) by delaying drug elimination. In addition, hepatic oxidation by the oxidase system is more active during pregnancy.

Placental Transfer and Fetal Pharmacokinetics

Drugs that readily cross the placenta have a low molecular weight, high lipid solubility, are nonionized and loosely bound to plasma proteins. Most chemotherapeutic drugs possess these qualities and thus should easily cross the placenta. The immature fetal liver is capable of metabolizing a large number of substrates by oxidation, and the fetal kidney may be involved in the drug elimination. It should be noted that a drug excreted into the amniotic fluid may be ingested by the fetus and reabsorbed from the gastrointestinal tract, potentially increasing any adverse effect of the drug on the fetus, such as the antimetabolites which are excreted in the active form. The placenta is not only a route of drug elimination, but is also involved in excretion of waste products and toxins from the fetus.

At birth, the ability of the neonate to metabolize and excrete many drugs is underdeveloped. Therefore, chemotherapy administered shortly before birth may be particularly hazardous because of delayed metabolism and excretion of the newborn liver and kidney.[2]

Principles of Chemotherapy Administration During Pregnancy

All chemotherapeutic agents are theoretically teratogenic and mutagenic. Their use may result in spontaneous abortion, fetal death, fetal malformation or fetal growth restriction. It is difficult to differentiate teratogenic or mutagenic effects from those related to a suboptimum intrauterine environment or those resulting from a maternal toxicity such as neutropenia, infection, thrombocytopenia or organ toxicity.[3]

The effects of chemotherapy on the fetus are influenced by the particular drug and timing of exposure.[4]

Chemotherapy During First Trimester

The first trimester, especially the third to eighth week of development (5–10 weeks of gestational age), is the most critical with respect to exposure to chemotherapy. With the exception of brain and gonadal tissue, organogenesis is complete by 13 weeks of gestation.

If chemotherapy induces severe damage early in gestation, spontaneous abortion results. If, however, sublethal damage occurs between the second and tenth weeks of development, teratogenesis may occur. In one study fetal outcome after in utero exposure to chemotherapy were analyzed in 21 pregnant women. Of thirteen women who were exposed to chemotherapy during first trimester, four had spontaneous abortions and four had therapeutic abortions. Two of the five women whose pregnancies continued to term had major malformations in their infants.[5]

Approximately 10–20% of infants exposed to cytotoxic agents during the first trimester have major malformations as compared to a rate of 3% in general population. Generally, chemotherapy should be delayed until after the first trimester.[6]

Chemotherapy During Second and Third Trimester

After organogenesis is complete, the risk of developing birth defects induced by chemotherapy is decreased.[7] Central nervous system development is not complete and chemotherapy may continue to affect fetal growth and development.

From the data available, chemotherapy administered after organogenesis does not appear to result in significant teratogenic risk. Chemotherapy, however, may induce myelosuppression in the fetus and newborn infant. The Toronto Leukemia Study Group has reported that 33% of all infants exposed to chemotherapy in the last month of pregnancy had cytopenia at birth. Twenty-eight of the fifty-eight cases reviewed were born prematurely, and four had low birth weights for their gestational age. Only one child had obvious congenital malformations, and this child later developed a neuroblastoma. Long-term follow-up of seven cases showed normal growth and development and no increased malignancies.[8]

Premature birth and low birth weight for gestational age are probably the most common complications and are most likely underreported.

Chemotherapy Prior to Delivery

Chemotherapy administered shortly before delivery may not have been eliminated from the fetus by the time of delivery and prolonged drug levels may persist in the newborn who now lacks the placental route of excretion. Chemotherapeutics may not be excreted because the neonatal liver and kidneys have a limited ability to metabolize agents such as the vinca alkaloids or cyclophosphamide.[9]

Delayed Effects

The delayed effects of in utero exposure to chemotherapeutic agents are less well documented than the immediate birth defects. Clear cell vaginal carcinoma in daughters of women taking DES (diethylstilbestrol) serves as a reminder for the need for long term follow-up. In 1985 National Cancer Institute established a national registry for in utero exposure to chemotherapeutic agents. Of the first 210 cases studied, 29 were abnormal outcomes with a total of 52 birth defects. Although extensive generalization is not possible because of the small number of birth defects, the data are reassuring in that only two abnormal outcomes were associated with exposure after the first trimester. The data should be cautiously interpreted because of potential for bias.[10]

In one study, thirty-eight children who were exposed in utero to alkylating agents were followed for three to nineteen years. No child had any evidence of physical, intellectual or chromosomal abnormalities.[11]

Chemotherapy-induced second malignancies, impaired growth and development, intellectual impairment and infertility have been reported.[12] There have been no controlled studies demonstrating sustained ill effects on physical growth. There has been one reported case of mental retardation occurring in a child exposed in utero to cyclophosphamide and prednisone; 17 other cases of in utero exposure evaluated by neuropsychological testing showed normal development. The incidence of infertility after in utero exposure to chemotherapy is not known. It is well known that the age of exposure and the type of agent used are crucial determinants of later infertility.

Adjuvant chemotherapy for breast cancer has a significant effect on subsequent fertility. Approximately 50% of women less than 35 years of age resume menses after a full course of adjuvant chemotherapy. Cyclophosphamide is a major cause of ovarian failure.[13] Nitrogen mustard vincistine, prednisone, procarbazine (MOPP) chemotherapy regimens are associated with amenorrhea in more than one-third of patients. Adriamycin, Bleomycin, Vincristine, DTIC (ABVD) regimen seems to be less gonadotoxic with less than 5% of patients becoming amenorrheic.[14]

Incidence of second generation teratogenesis is an area that requires further longitudinal studies. From studies of children exposed to chemotherapeutics for childhood malignancies, no increased incidence of chromosomal aberrations or malformation in their progeny have been noted.

The issue of carcinogenesis is of great concern since it is well documented that alkylators are leukemogenic. There has been only one reported case of in utero exposure to chemotherapy associated with development of 2 cancers (neuroblastoma at age 14 and thyroid carcinoma at age 17). The twin sister of the patient with thyroid carcinomas had no evidence of malignancy.[15]

The use of common chemotherapeutic agents during pregnancy and their reported side effects on the fetus have been reported in various retrospective studies and are discussed below.

Alkylating Agents

Alkylating agents such as busulfan, chlorambucil, cyclophosphamide, and nitrogen mustard are associated with an increased incidence of congenital anomalies if administered during the first trimester. The rate of fetal malformation has recently been reported to be 14% when these drugs are used during the first trimester. When administered later in pregnancy, the incidence of fetal malformation decreased to 4%.[16]

Case reports describe cisplatin administration during the second and third trimester without adverse neonatal outcome.[17] A patient with endodermal sinus tumor of the ovary diagnosed in the 25th week of gestation received cisplatin, vinblastine, and bleomycin. She delivered a healthy infant by Caesarian section at 32 weeks gestation.

Antibiotic-like Agents

Turchi and Villasis reviewed 28 cases of anthracycline exposure in pregnancy. Twenty-three women were exposed to doxorubicin and five were exposed to daunorubicin. Four women received doxorubicin in addition to other agents during the first trimester without any malformation in the neonate. There were two maternal and two fetal deaths resulting from anthracycline chemotherapy. There were two spontaneous abortions, and one pregnancy terminated in patients receiving Anthracycline. Four of the five cases of infant mortality occurred in patients with hematological malignancies.[18]

There were no detectable effects of anthracycline exposure in utero on the newborns with follow-up to 54 months of age.

Bleomycin has been administered to mothers without any reported adverse effect.[19]

Actinomycin D has been administered during the second and third trimester also without reported congenital anomalies.[20]

Vinca Alkaloids

Although vincristine and vinblastine have caused malformation in animals, no reports have yet described fetal malformation in humans. Schapira reported no malformation in ten neonates with first trimester exposure to vinblastine.[21]

Antimetabolites

The folic acid antagonists are the agents most commonly associated with birth defects.[22]

Methotrexate is a known teratogen. Infants of women who received methotrexate for malignancies during the first trimester had multiple birth defects including cranial defects and malformed extremities.

Purine and Pyrimidine Analozes

Caligiuri reported six patients with first trimester exposure to Ara C (cytarabine) either alone or in combination with other agents. There were four normal infants and two with congenital malformation.[23]

Case reports exist of congenital anomalies in neonates exposed to 5-FU during the first trimester.[24]

Taxanes

To date there are no published reports of Paclitaxel administered during pregnancy. Paclitaxel is teratogenic in animals.

Table 11.1. Physiologic changes of pregnancy and their effects on drug pharmacokinetics.

Physiologic activity	Effect
Plasma volume	Peak plasma concentration
Gastric motility and emptying	Overall absorption of drug
Albumin	Protein free drug
Glomerular filtration rate	Elimination
Maternal hepatic Phase I enzyme activity	Drug activation

Table 11.2. Adverse effects of antineoplastic agents on the fetus and neonate.

Immediate	Delayed*
Spontaneous abortion	Carcinogenesis
Teratogenesis	Sterility
Organ toxicity	Retarded physical and/or mental growth and development
Premature birth	
Low birth weight	Teratogenic in second generations

*Potential long-term complications of in utero exposure to antineoplastic agents

Table 11.3. Chemotherapy during first trimester of pregnancy.

Class	No. of exposed patients	No. of fetal malformations
Alkylating agents		
Busulfan	22	2
Chlorambucil	5	1
Cyclophosphamide	7	3
Nitrogen mustard	6	0
Trimethylene melamine	4	0
	44	6 (14%)
Antimetabolites		
Aminopterin	52	10
Methotrexate	3	3
6-Mercaptopurine	20	0
Cytarabine	1	1
Fluorouracil	1	1
	77	15 (19%)
Plant alkaloids		
Vinblastine	14	1
Antibiotics		
Daunorubicin	1	0
Miscellaneous		
Procarbazine	1	1
Amsacrine	1	1
Cisplatin	1	0
	18	3 (17%)
Total	139	24 (17%)
Combinations	45	7 (16%)

Table 11.4. Chemotherapy during second and third trimester of pregnancy.

Class	No. of exposed patients	No. of fetal malformations
Alkylating agents	26	1
Antimetabolites	38	0
Antibiotics	1	0
Plant alkaloids	6	0
Combinations	79	1*
Total	150	2 (1.3%)

*One case of chromósomal gaps and rings in a phenotypic normal infant was noted following intensive antileukemic therapy.

Radiation Therapy During Pregnancy

Ionizing radiation can induce cell death or cytogenetic effects in mammalian cells through direct effects or indirectly through the production of free radicals damaging critical cellular structures, including the DNA.[25]

The major adverse effects of irradiation on the fetus may include premature cell death, mitotic delay, and disturbance of cell migration.[26]

The biologic effect of ionizing radiation on the fetal tissue depends primarily on:

1 The stage of gestation and

2 The radiation dose.[27]

Evidence of the effects of ionizing radiation on the fetus is derived from two sources:

1 experimental data in laboratory animals with short gestation periods (mouse or rat) and

2 observational data in humans inadvertently exposed to radiation and in the survivors of atomic bomb explosions.

There are limitations in interpretation of reported data with respect to the two main determinants of fetal radiation effect, namely dose and gestational age. Gestational stages of the animals and their specific organ sensitivities are often difficult to extrapolate to humans. It is difficult to reconstruct the precise dose of the radiation applicable to human exposure. Despite these limitations, the data available provide guidelines for the management of patients requiring radiation therapy during pregnancy.

The adverse effect of radiation to the fetus can be divided into four major categories:

1 lethal effects

2 teratogenic effects

3 growth retardation

4 structural, functional, and carcinogenic effects.

Radiation Effect and Gestational Stages

Preimplantation (Conception to Day 9–10)

In the preimplantation phase and immediate postimplantation phase, the incidence of lethal effects of radiation to the fetus is highest.[28] A dose-dependent all or nothing effect is observed in animal studies.[29] These experimental observations correlate well with the human experience of atomic bomb survivors in Hiroshima and Nagasaki.[30] There was a high incidence of both normal births and spontaneous abortions among humans exposed to in utero radiation within fifteen days of conception after atomic bomb exposure.

Organogenesis (Weeks 2–6) and Early Fetal Period (Weeks 12–16)

Radiation induced teratogenic effects (structural congenital malformations) and growth disturbances predominate in the period of organogenesis (weeks 2–6).[31] Experimental animal data reveal a wide variety of radiation-induced organ malformations during organogenesis.

In contrast to animal experience, data on human exposure show a striking predominance of central nervous system (CNS) abnormalities and growth effects. The induction of CNS changes is not limited to the organogenesis stage but can extend to later periods of gestation. In humans, CNS abnormalities and growth effects predominate over other organ malformation probably because development of CNS takes place throughout gestation. Other reported radiation induced abnormalities include ocular abnormalities (microphthalmus, pigmentary retinal degeneration, optic atrophy, cataracts, strabismus), genital, skeletal and rare visceral abnormalities.[32]

Microcephaly which may occur with and without mental retardation is thought to be caused by radiation effects on developing glial cells.[33]

Mental retardation is caused by the deleterious effect of radiation on the formation of brain cortex. It is frequently associated with microcephaly. The most sensitive period for radiation induced microcephaly is 8–15 weeks of gestation.[34]

Growth retardation has been documented in the human fetus following irradiation in early as well as late gestation.[35,36]

Late Fetal Stage (Weeks 20–25 to Birth)

The later fetal stage appears to be much more resistant to radiation, requiring higher doses to induce structural damage. However, more subtle mostly functional disorders, including bone marrow, liver and kidney abnormalities and sterility have been described. These functional abnormalities may not be obvious at birth and may not be manifested until late in life.[37]

There is also concern regarding malignancies and genetic abnormalities that may not become apparent for years, decades or generations. The long term sequelae throughout adult life and for future generations born to the fetus after in utero radiation exposure are largely a matter of uncertainty. Even the data accumulated in Japanese atomic bomb survivors are not sufficient to clarify the long term consequences.

Radiation Dose Guideline

Unfortunately the dose level at which radiation will produce no teratogenic effect in the embryo is difficult to determine. The available data suggest that acute or continuous exposure to the fetus of less than 0.1 GY (< 10 rad) does not result in gross malformation and growth retardation.[38]

A commonly employed guideline, therefore, recommends that the pregnant woman consider therapeutic abortion if a dose of 0.1 GY or greater has been received within the first trimester.[39]

Table 11.5. Diagnostic procedures and related maternal radiation exposure.

Procedure	Dose (m rads)
Chest X-ray	8
Pelvic X-ray	40
Bone scan	194
Mammogram	300
IVP	400
Upper GI series	560
Lymphangiogram	1100
CT scan	1000–5000

Diagnostic Procedures

Mammography should not be used as a screening test during pregnancy because increase in size, vascularity and glandular density of the breast may decrease the sensitivity of mammograms. However, mammography should not be avoided, if indicated, because with abdominal shielding, radiation exposure to the fetus is negligible. There are no reports of untoward effects of mammography on the mother or the fetus.[40]

In one study of 120 non-pregnant women under the age of 35 with a palpable malignant breast mass, 52% of the mammograms were negative and 11% were equivocal. In young women, palpable breast masses should be biopsied regardless of the result of mammogram.[41]

Ultrasound may be a useful diagnostic modality, and several series have shown increased accuracy in confirming the presence of breast mass. Ultrasound may be helpful in differentiating cystic versus solid masses and may confirm the presence of a mass when physical examination is equivocal and the woman complains of pain and tenderness.[42]

In a pregnant patient, the usual staging investigations of cancer have to be modified. A chest X-ray with abdominal shielding may still be performed. Ultrasound has no known adverse fetal effects and may be helpful for assessing fetal age and the presence of lymphadenopathy or other problems. Magnetic resonance imaging is preferred to computed tomography as it does not expose the fetus to ionizing radiation and, therefore, appears to be free from genetic hazard.

Radiography of the long bones can be performed in symptomatic women. Radionuclide bone scanning is relatively contraindicated in pregnancy because of the danger of fetal radiation exposure. However, it has been reported that bone scanning, if needed for documentation of osseous metastasis, can be performed safely with a decrease in radiation exposure to the fetus (below the maximum permissible fetal-gestational exposure) if adequate hydration is used to promote rapid washout of excreted Tc-99m, and if an indwelling urinary catheter is used for eight hours to prevent retention of radioactivity in the bladder.[43]

Summary

Treatment of cancer during pregnancy should be individualized for each patient. Chemotherapy should be avoided during the first trimester. If treatment must be given during the first trimester, folate antagonists (such as methotrexate) should be avoided at all costs. Chemotherapy can increase the cure rate or prolong survival for certain tumors seen during pregnancy such as lymphoma, leukemia, breast and ovarian cancer. Certain chemotherapeutic agents such as alkylating agents and vinblastine are less teratogenic even when used during first trimester. Pregnancy related physiological changes should be kept in mind when administering and dosing chemotherapy.

Chemotherapy is less teratogenic when administered during the second and third trimester. However, there may be greater risk of stillbirth, fetal growth restriction, premature birth and fetal myelosuppression. Parents should be informed of the possible early and delayed effects of treatment. The available data regarding use of chemotherapy during pregnancy is limited and consists of case reports and small series. It is difficult to provide reassurance to the parents of children exposed in utero to chemotherapy. Physicians who care for women receiving chemotherapy during pregnancy should ensure long term follow-up of the children born through those pregnancies.

A surveillance program similar to that recommended for survivors of childhood malignancies is needed. Special attention should be paid to physical and intellectual development and delayed malignancies. Physicians should take responsibility for reporting their findings to a central registry. An international registry maintaining the data may provide us with future guidelines for management of cancer during pregnancy.

Ionizing radiation should be avoided during pregnancy. Therapeutic abortion should be recommended if doses in excess of 0.1 GY (10 rads) is delivered during pregnancy. If radiation is unavoidable, such as in the treatment of lymphoma, special shielding techniques should be used to minimize the radiation exposure to the fetus. The decision regarding radiation therapy should consider the potential effects of radiotherapy on the fetus and neonate, and the stage and prognosis of the mother's disease, and risks and benefits to the mother.

References

1. Doll D. Antineoplastic agents and pregnancy. Sem Oncol 1989; 16;5:337–46
2. Powis G. Anticancer drug pharmacodynamics. Cancer Chemo Pharm 1985; 14:177–83
3. Mulvihill JJ. Pregnancy outcome in cancer patients. Cancer 1987; 60:1143
4. Petrek JA. Pregnancy associated breast cancer. Sem Surg Oncol 1991; 7:306
5. Zemlickis F. Fetal outcome after in utero exposure to cancer chemotherapy. Arch Intern Med 1992; 52
6. Gliland J. The effect of cancer chemotherapeutic agents on the developing fetus. Obstet Gynecol Surv 1983; 38:6
7. Nettleton J. Breast cancer during pregnancy: quantifying the risk of treatment delay. Obstet Gynecol 1996; 87:414

8. Reynoso EE. Acute leukemia during pregnancy. The Toronto Leukemia Study Group experience with long term follow-up of children exposed in utero to chemotherapeutic agents. JCO 1987; 5:1098
9. Sorosky JI, Soud AK, Buekers TE. The use of chemotherapeutic agents during pregnancy. Obstet Gynecol Clinics 1997; 24:3
10. Randall T. National registry seeks scarce data on pregnancy outcomes during chemotherapy. JAMA 1993; 269:323
11. Aviles A. Growth and development of children of mothers treated with chemotherapy during pregnancy. Amer J Hematol 1991; 36:243
12. Gradisher W. Ovarian function following radiation and chemotherapy for cancer. Sem Oncol 1989; 16;5:425–36
13. Sutton R. Pregnancy and offspring after adjuvant chemotherapy in breast cancer patients. Cancer 1990; 65:847–50
14. Bonadonna G. Modern treatment of malignant lymphomas. Amer Oncol 1994; 5 (Suppl. 2)
15. Garber J. Long term follow-up of children exposed in utero to antineoplastic agents. Sem Oncol 1989; 16;5:437–44
16. Glantz JC. Reproductive toxicity of alkylating agents. Obstet Gynecol Surv 1994; 49:709
17. Malone JM. Endodermal sinus tumor of the ovary associated with pregnancy. Obstet Gynecol1986; 68:865–95
18. Turchi JJ. Anthracyclines in the treatment of malignancy in pregnancy. Cancer 1988; 61:435.
19 Malone JM. Endodermal sinus tumor of the ovary associated with pregnancy. Obstet Gynecol 1986; 68:865
20. Glilland J. The effects of cancer chemotherapeutic agents on the developing fetus. Obstet Gynecol Surv 1983; 38:6
21. Schapira DV. Successful pregnancy following continuous treatment with combination chemotherapy before conception and throughout pregnancy. Cancer 1983; 54:800
22. Milunsky A. Methotrexate induced congenital malformations. J Pediat 1968; 72:790–5
23. Caligiuri MA. Pregnancy and leukemia. Sem Oncol 1989; 16:388
24. Stephens JD. Multiple congenital anomalies in a fetus exposed to 5-FU during the first trimester. Amer J Obstet Gynecol 1980; 137:746
25. Hall EJ. The physics and chemistry of radiation absorption: Radiobiology for the Radiologist, ed. 4. Philadelphia: Lippincott, JB. 1994
26. Brent RL. The effect of embryonic and fetal exposure to X-rays, microwaves, and ultrasound. Counseling the pregnant and non-pregnant patients about these risks. Sem Oncol 1989; 16:347–368
27. Doll DC. Management of cancer during pregnancy. Arch Inter Med 1988; 148:2058–64
28. Rugh R. The impact of ionizing radiation on the embryo and the fetus. Amer J Radiol 1963; 89:182–90
29. Dekaban AS. Abnormalities in children exposed to X-radiation during various stages of gestation. Tentative timetable of radiation injury to the human fetus, Part I. J Nucl Med 1968; 9:471–7
30. Plummer G. Anomalies occurring in children exposed in utero to the atomic bomb in Hiroshima. Pediatrics 1952; 10:687–92
31. Brent RL. Irradiation in pregnancy. Gynecology and Obstetrics, Vol. 2. New York: Harper and Row, 1981
32. Wood JW. In utero exposure to Hiroshima atomic bomb. An evaluation of head size and mental retardation 20 years later. Pediatrics 1967; 39:385–92
33. Miller RW. Small head size after atomic radiation: Teratogen update: Environmentally induced birth defect risk. New York: Alan R. Liss, 1986
34. Otake M. In utero exposure to A-bomb radiation and mental retardation: A reassessment. B J Rad 1984; 57:409–14
35. Committee on the biological effects of ionizing radiations BEIR III: The effect on population of exposure to low levels of ionizing radiation. Washington, DC National Academy of Sciences, 1980
36. Burrow G. Study of adolescents exposed in utero to the atomic bomb, Nagasaki, Japan. JAMA 1965; 192:357–364
37. Stewart A. Malignant disease in childhood and diagnostic irradiation in utero. Lancet 1956; 2:447
38. Kinlen LJ. Diagnostic irradiation, congenital malformations and spontaneous abortions. B J Rad 1968; 41:648–54
39. Becker MH. Management of Hodgkin's disease coexistent with pregnancy. Radiol 1965; 85:725–8
40. Mayr N. Radiation therapy during pregnancy. Obstet Gynecol Clinics 1998; 25:2
41. Max MH. Breast cancer in 120 women under 35 years old. Am Surg 1984; 50:23–5
42. Parente JT. Breast cancer associated with pregnancy. Obstet Gynecol 1988; 71:861–4
43. Baker J. Bone scanning in patients with breast carcinoma. Clin Nuc Med 1987; 12:519–24

12. Management of Cancer in Pregnancy (Case Reports)

Matthew L. Anderson, Giancarlo Mari and Peter E. Schwartz

This chapter will discuss malignancies diagnosed during pregnancy at the Yale-New Haven Medical Center. Examples of both gynecologic and non-gynecologic cancers will be reviewed, highlighting the relevant diagnostic and management aspects of each case.

Gynecologic Malignancies

Case 1: Mucinous Cystadenoma

A 35-year-old woman, $G_3P_1SAb_1$, with an unremarkable medical and obstetrical history, underwent routine screening for maternal serum alpha-fetoprotein (MS-AFP) at 15 weeks of gestation. At that time, her measured AFP was found to be 12 ng/ml, consistent with an elevated Down's Syndrome risk of 1 in 191. After counseling, an amniocentesis was performed to assess amniotic fluid levels of AFP and obtain cells for fetal karyotyping. Both of these tests were ultimately normal. However, a left-sided adnexal mass, 7.2 × 6.3 × 6.0 cm, was discovered incidentally during a targeted obstetrical ultrasound. A second ultrasound, performed two weeks later, demonstrated modest growth in the dimensions of this cyst, which was now 8.1 × 7.4 × 8.2 cm. The options of needle aspiration versus exploratory laparotomy were discussed with the patient. Instead, the patient sought a second opinion, where a third ultrasound was performed. This ultrasound confirmed the presence of a septated mass anterior to the bladder, measuring 6.2 × 8.2 × 8.0 cm. Pelvic MRI also identified a 10 × 7 × 8 cm septated, cystic lesion in the left ovary, displacing the cervix to the left. There was no evidence of hydronephrosis, lymphadenopathy or ascites. Tumor markers, including liver function tests and serum CA-125 were also normal.

At 19 weeks of gestation, the patient underwent exploratory laparotomy and left salpingo-oophorectomy (Fig. 12.1). Intraoperatively, no evidence of other pelvic or abdominal disease was observed. The patient recovered well, with no evidence of preterm labor or fetal compromise during the intraoperative or postoperative period. Pathologic examination of the mass revealed a benign, mucinous cystadenoma. She

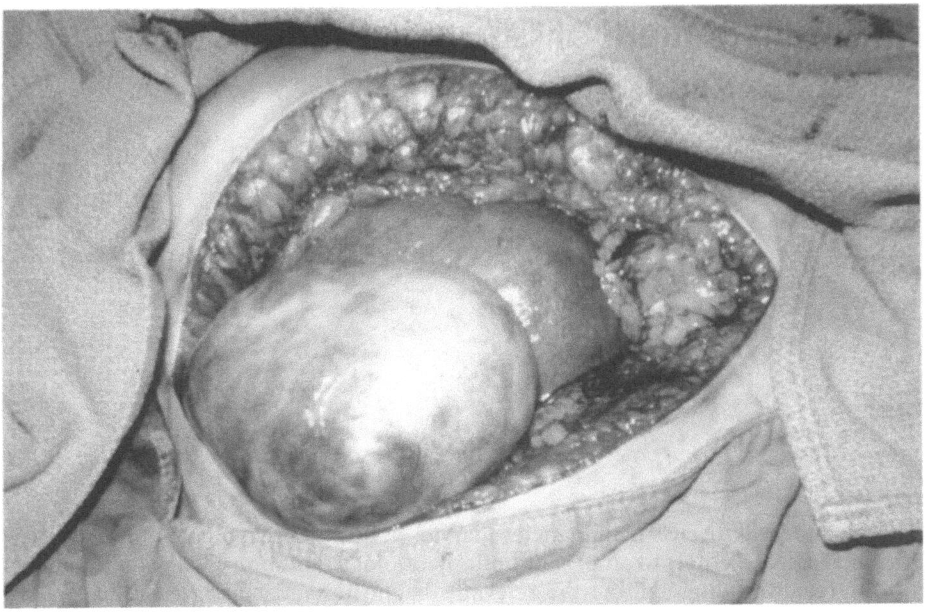

Figure 12.1. Laparotomy at 19 weeks of gestation revealed a large, multiloculated adnexal mass, ultimately identified as a benign mucinous cystadenoma

was discharged home on the fifth postoperative day and ultimately delivered a live infant at term without complications. Both mother and child remain well.

Discussion

Adnexal masses complicate as many as 1 in 190 pregnancies.[1] More than one-third of all adnexal masses are found in pregnant women.[2] As the resolution of obstetrical ultrasound continues to improve, adnexal masses will be detected during pregnancy with increasing frequency. Traditionally, a number of criteria have been used to decide whether surgical exploration is necessary. These criteria include a size greater than 6 cm, a solid or complex appearance, failure of the mass to resolve after with first trimester and the presence of bilateral abnormalities. After considering the size and complex nature of this patient's mass as well as its persistent nature, laparotomy was performed at 19 weeks of gestational age. Surgical exploration was well timed, as pregnant women tend to tolerate surgery best in the second trimester. During the second trimester, the risk of fetal loss associated with surgical procedures is reduced, when compared to the first trimester. Furthermore, the smaller size of the gravid uterus is less of an impediment to abdominal exploration, when compared to the third trimester.

Ultimately, this patient tolerated laparotomy well and delivered a healthy infant at term. Pathologic examination of the extirpated adnexae revealed a mucinous cystadenoma. In some respects, the benign nature of this patient's mass is not surprising. No more than 5% of adnexal masses detected in pregnant women ultimately prove to be malignant.[3] However, the use of traditional criteria for performing laparotomy often results in unnecessary surgery for patients with benign adnexal lesions. Recent evidence suggests that the characterization of adnexal blood flow by

Doppler ultrasound appears to be useful in distinguishing benign from malignant ovarian masses.[4] In particular, identification of high impedance Doppler flow is consistent with a benign etiology, while low impedance flow suggests a malignant lesion. If it had been available, Doppler ultrasound may have allowed for the conservative management of this patient until a healthy infant could be delivered at term.

Case 2: Serous Cystadenoma

A 25-year-old woman, G_2P_1, with an unremarkable medical and surgical history, presented at 34 weeks of gestational age with a two-day history of right upper quadrant abdominal pain. She denied significant gastrointestinal or genitourinary symptoms. However, physical examination revealed moderate to severe right upper quadrant abdominal pain without rebound, tenderness or guarding. The uterine fundus was found to deviate to the left. To further evaluate this finding, transabdominal ultrasound was performed. This revealed a 20 cm, septated adnexal mass adjacent to the uterus, distinct from the normal-appearing gallbladder and liver. An MRI was performed, which confirmed the presence of a unilateral adnexal cyst without septations (Fig. 12.2).

For the next several days, the patient was observed as an inpatient. Liver function tests and other tumor markers, including a serum CA-125 level were found to be normal. An amniocentesis was performed to assess fetal lung maturity. However, the

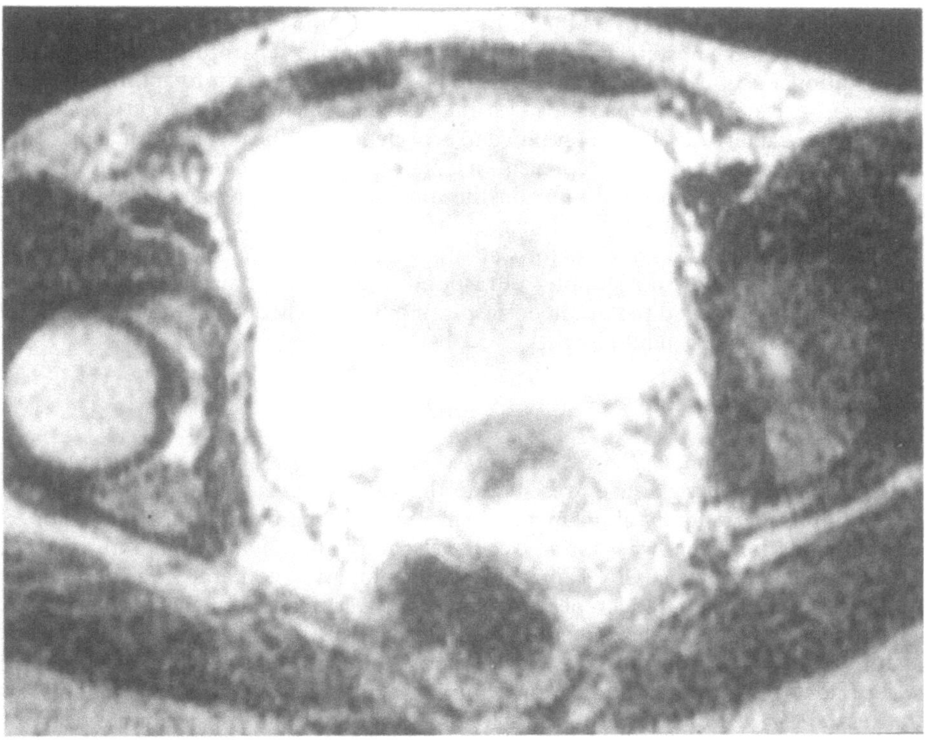

Figure 12.2. Pelvic MRI demonstrating a unilocular adnexal cyst. Surgical exploration later revealed a mucinous cystadenoma.

ratio of lecithin to sphingomyelin was unfavorable. The patient was started on a course intramuscular steroids. One week later, at 35 weeks of gestation, the L/S ratio in the amniotic fluid was 2.3. Exploratory laparotomy was subsequently performed. A large (20 cm) simple cyst was found in the right ovary and removed by a unilateral oophorectomy. Abdominal exploration revealed no other intraabdominal disease. A Cesarean section was performed during the laparotomy, resulting in the delivery of a male infant with Apgar scores of 7 and 8. The surgery otherwise proceeded in an uncomplicated fashion. She recovered without complications and was discharged home on postoperative day 5 in a stable condition. Following delivery, the infant required respiratory support with continuous positive airway pressure for several days, but otherwise did well and was discharged home in a healthy condition. The final pathology report revealed a serous cystadenoma.

Discussion

This patient presented with a large adnexal mass causing significant abdominal discomfort. Because surgery in the third trimester is often associated with premature labor and delivery, laparotomy was delayed until fetal lung maturity could be documented. In the interim, a course of intramuscular steroids was administered to further promote fetal lung maturity. Similar to the previous case, the benign nature of this patient's cyst suggests that size alone may be poorly predictive of the benign or malignant nature of an adnexal lesion. Use of Doppler ultrasound, if it had been available, may have prevented laparotomy or allowed the surgeons to comfortably delay laparotomy until term.[4] Given the difficulties the infant encountered immediately after delivery, some obstetricians would advocate delaying laparotomy until 39 weeks of gestational age, even with a mature ratio of amniotic lecithin to sphingomyelin. However, excision of this patient's cyst may have been necessary, regardless of its Doppler characteristics, if she continued to experience significant abdominal discomfort. Percutaneous aspiration represents a less invasive alternative to laparotomy and is likely to become more common in the management of pregnant patients with benign adnexal masses. Although there is currently no consensus regarding its use, aspiration could be considered for patients with a simple cystic mass with high impedance blood flow on Doppler ultrasound, regardless of size. The use of both Doppler ultrasound and percutaneous aspiration will likely decrease the future need for laparotomy in pregnant patients.

Case 3: Cervical Cancer

A 26-year-old woman, G_5P_1, with a history of mitral valve prolapse, tobacco use and prior intravenous drug abuse presented to the Yale-New Haven Medical Center for evaluation of persistently abnormal Pap smears. Approximately four years prior to her consultation, she was found to have condylomatous atypia and cervical intraepithelial neoplasia (CIN-I) on colposcopic biopsy. Cryotherapy was performed at that time. One year later, a repeat Pap smear was performed, which was interpreted as evidence of a high grade intraepithelial lesion (HGSIL). Colposcopic biopsies were again performed, the results of which were consistent with CIN-I. Repeat cryotherapy was performed without complications. Similar results were again noted on a follow-up PAP smear, at which time, a "condyloma" was noted on the posterior cervical lip. Cryotherapy was performed for a third time.

The patient again became pregnant and a Pap smear was performed at 8 weeks of gestation. Although squamous atypia was noted on this smear, no further evaluation was completed. The patient experienced an uneventful delivery at term. A Pap smear was not performed with her postpartum visit. One year later, the patient again became pregnant. At her initial prenatal visit, she reported intermittant post-coital bleeding. Physical examination revealed a large cervical lesion, which appeared most consistent with a condyloma. A Pap smear was performed and interpreted as squamous atypia. However, colposcopy revealed a large mass which involved the entire posterior cervix. Biopsies were consistent with small cell carcinoma of the cervix.

After counseling, the patient underwent a Type III radical hysterectomy with bilateral pelvic lymphadenectomies and periaortic lymph node sampling at 15 weeks of gestation. Her postoperative recovery was significant for a brief fever, which resolved on intravenous ampicillin and gentamicin. The final pathology revealed a well-differentiated squamous cell carcinoma of the cervix involving more than 70% of the cervical thickness. Pelvic and periaortic lymph nodes were negative for metastases, although lymph vascular space invasion was noted. For this reason, she underwent three cycles of chemotherapy with cisplatin, methotrexate and bleomycin. Subsequent follow-up with interval CT scans and pelvic examinations have been unremarkable. Recently, the patient was noted to have atypical squamous cells of undetermined significance (ASCUS) on vaginal smear. A colposcopic evaluation was negative for malignancy or dysplasia. She otherwise remains well.

Discussion

This case emphasizes the need for prompt and thorough evaluation of cervical dysplasia in both pregnant and non-pregnant women. Further evaluation of the patient's second Pap smear, reported as a high grade intraepithelial lesion (HGSIL), should have most likely been performed by cone biopsy. This procedure may have identified and treated an area of more severe dysplasia or even early invasive cancer likely missed on colposcopy. Subsequently, multiple opportunities were also missed for appropriate follow-up, despite contact with health care providers.

The asymptomatic nature of this patient's lesion as well as the delay in its initial diagnosis are also typical of many cases of cervical cancer diagnosed during pregnancy.[5] At the time of actual diagnosis, clinical findings were consistent with a Stage Ib cervical cancer. Cone biopsy was no longer appropriate for either diagnosis or treatment at that time. As a result, she was offered and underwent a radical hysterectomy with staging lymphadenectomies. A delay in therapy to achieve fetal viability was considered, but declined by the patient. Given our current understanding, combination chemoradiation could also be considered for this patient.[6,7] However, an evaluation of the efficacy of these regimens in pregnant women has not yet been performed. Regardless, the patient has since recovered well with an apparent cure of her disease.

Case 4: Borderline Ovarian Malignancy

A 28-year-old woman, G_1P_1, with a five year history of tobacco use, was found to have bilateral ovarian masses at her initial prenatal evaluation. A sonogram confirmed the presence of these masses, which appeared complex with multiple septations (Fig. 12.3). At 16 weeks of gestation, she underwent exploratory laparotomy with bilateral salpingo-oophorectomy and peritoneal biopsies. Pathologic examination of these surgical specimens revealed borderline papillary serous carcinoma in both ovaries.

Pelvic washings were also positive for malignant cells and the biopsy of the uterine serosa further indicated that this organ was involved by disease. For the remainder of her pregnancy, the patient was managed conservatively and ultimately delivered a live infant at term. Delivery necessitated Cesarean section for cephalopelvic disproportion, during which, pelvic washings and random peritoneal biopsies were again performed. Cells compatible with a borderline carcinoma of low malignant potential were found in the pelvic washings. Psammoma bodies consistent with borderline papillary serous carcinoma were also observed in excrescences from the serosa of the uterus, urinary bladder and right uterosacral ligaments. No evidence of malignancy was observed in biopsies taken from the diaphragm, pelvic side walls, anterior peritoneum and omentum.

Six weeks after her Cesarean section, the patient underwent a total abdominal hysterectomy with complete surgical staging. Evidence of microscopic residual disease was noted on the uterine serosa. Postoperatively, she was started on cyclic hormone replacement therapy with estradiol and medroxyprogesterone acetate for the relief of estrogen withdrawal symptoms. Since that time, the patient has continued on hormone replacement without recurrence of her symptoms. She remains clinically free of disease until the present time, thirteen years after her initial diagnosis.

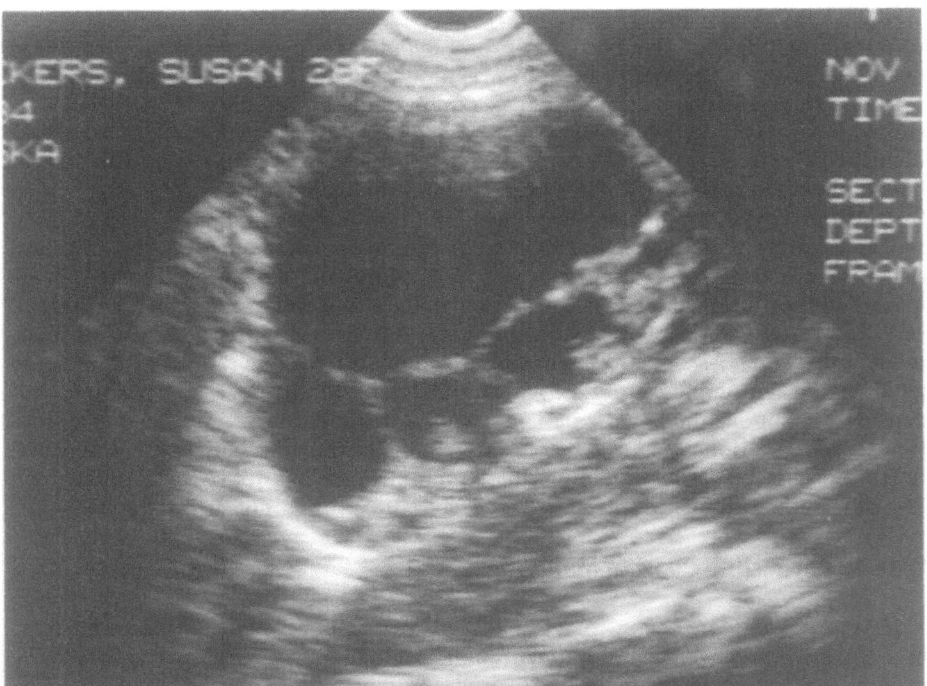

Figure 12.3. A complex adnexal mass detected by ultrasound. For this patient, laparotomy performed at 15 weeks of gestation revealed bilateral adnexal masses histologically consistent with epithelial ovarian carcinoma of borderline malignant potential.

Discussion

Epithelial ovarian carcinomas of borderline malignant potential are the most common ovarian malignancies diagnosed during pregnancy.[8] For this patient, surgical excision and staging of her carcinoma was performed stepwise, with an exploratory laparotomy and bilateral salpingo-oopherectomy completed soon after the identification of her adnexal mass. As mentioned earlier, the second trimester is optimal for surgical exploration of the gravid abdomen. A bilateral salpingo-oophorectomy was considered safe, because the placenta no longer requires ovarian gonadotropins for support of the pregnancy after the first trimester. Peritoneal biopsies were used to assess the extent of disease, both at the time of the patient's initial laparotomy and at the time of her Cesarean section. After the delivery of a live infant at term, the patient underwent a complete hysterectomy, bilateral lymphadenectomies and omentectomy. A delay in performing more definitive therapy for this patient was possible because of the borderline malignant potential of her carcinoma. However, if necessary, chemotherapy could have been initiated while the patient was still pregnant with minimal impact of the viability of the fetus.[9,10]

Lastly, the minimal tumor burden which characterized this patient has likely contributed to the patient's disease-free survival and permitted the use of hormone replacement therapy. Hormone replacement therapy is increasingly accepted for patients with borderline ovarian carcinoma with no evidence of focally invasive disease and minimal disease otherwise.[11] Use of hormone replacement in all likelihood improves quality of life with minimal impact on the patient's ultimate survival.

Non-Gynecologic Malignancies

Case 5: Non-Hodgkin's Lymphoma

A 27-year-old woman, G_2P_1, presented at 32 weeks of gestation with right upper quadrant abdominal pain and constipation. Despite conservative medical interventions, the patient's pain failed to resolve and she was referred to a gastroenterologist three days later. At that time, she also noted a lump in her right neck which, on examination, was suggestive of cervical lymphadenopathy. An abdominal ultrasound performed to evaluate her pain revealed a solid retroperitoneal mass 14 × 10 cm in dimensions. On CT scan, this mass displaced the right kidney and extended across the patient's midline (Fig. 12.4). A cervical lymph node biopsy was performed; microscopic examination of excised nodes revealed non-Hodgkin's lymphoma. Further evaluation, including a bone marrow biopsy, was unremarkable. Her serum lactate dehydrogenase was 411 mg/dl.

After discussing management options with the patient, a Cesarean section was planned for 34 weeks of gestational age followed by chemotherapy. In the interim, her abdominal pain continued to worsen. She also developed persistent nausea, vomiting and anorexia, resulting in a 4–5 lb weight loss. These symptoms necessitated several admissions for parenteral nutrition and pain relief. At 34 and 35 weeks of gestational age, she received intramuscular betamethasone to promote fetal lung maturity. Lung maturity could be documented by amniocentesis one week following the second adminstration of steroids. Cesarean delivery at that time resulted in the delivery of a live female infant with Apgars 7 and 9. Intraoperative inspection of the abdomen revealed a large, irregular retroperitoneal mass and mild splenomegaly, but normal

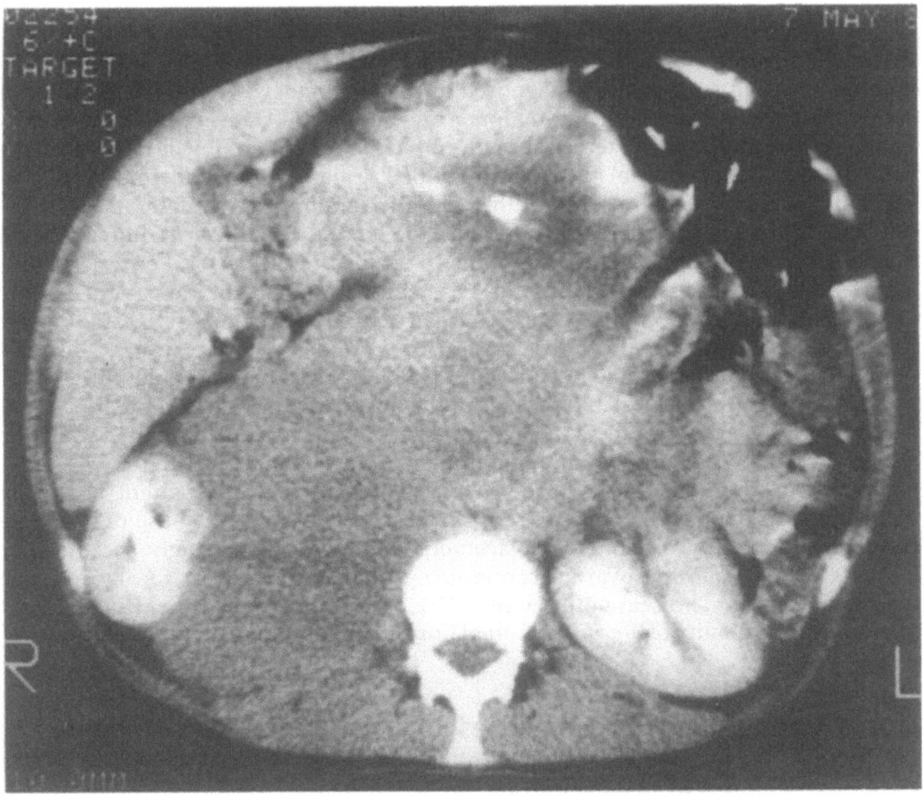

Figure 12.4. An abdominal CT scan demonstrating a large retroperitoneal mass, laterally displacing the patient's right kidney. The etiology of this mass was found to be non-Hodgkin's lymphoma.

liver and diaphragm. No lympadenopathy was palpable. The patient recovered rapidly from her Cesarean section and several weeks following her delivery, started on combination chemotherapy with methotrexate, bleomycin, adriamycin, prednisone and cyclophosphamide (MACOP-3). She has continued without recurrence for more than 12 months after her initial diagnosis and therapy.

Discussion

Only seventy-five cases of non-Hodgkin's lymphoma have been described in pregnancy.[12] As a result, limited data is available concerning the impact of pregnancy on the natural history of this disease or its prognosis in gravid women. Choice of treatment depends on both the grade and extent of disease. In general, diffuse intermediate- and high-grade non-Hodgkin's lymphomas are aggressive tumors and therapy should not be delayed.[13] Previously, therapeutic abortion followed by chemotherapy was routinely recommended for these patients. However, therapy for the patient described in this case was delayed several weeks to improve fetal viability with delivery, despite the intermediate grade of her tumor. The successful treatment of non-Hodgkin's lymphoma with combination chemotherapy has been described in women who subsequently gave birth to healthy infants.[12] The majority of these women were alive, without evidence of disease recurrence, four to nine years after delivery. Since chemotherapy appears to be a viable option for patients even close to term, the delay experienced by this patient may not have been necessary. There is no evidence that this delay, however, has had an adverse impact on this patient's outcome.

Case 6: Meningioma

A 30-year-old woman presented at 28 weeks of gestation with a 2 month history of left-sided frontal headache and diplopia. At the time of her initial evaluation, these symptoms had been occurring intermittently for more than two months and had particularly worsened during the two weeks prior to her referral. During this time, she also began to experience a left-sided decrease in visual acuity. On physical examination, significant left-sided cranial nerve findings, including a partial third nerve palsy, ocular proptosis, mydriasis and an inferior-outer quadrantanopsia were documented. Decreased sensation was also detectable across the first division of the left fifth cranial nerve.

To evaluate these findings, an MRI was performed, which revealed a large tumor at the left optic nerve at the cavernous sinus (Fig. 12.5). Angiogram confirmed the loca-

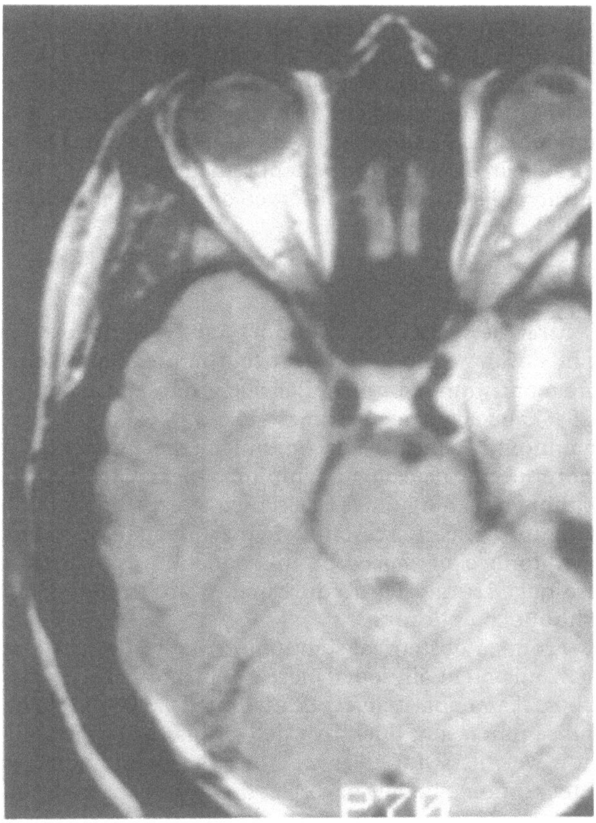

Figure 12.5. Head CT demonstrating a large intracranial mass compressing the left cavernous sinus. The patient subsequently underwent craniotomy with partial excision of an infiltrating meningioma.

tion of this tumor, which was partially thrombosed during angiography. Partial excision of this tumor was undertaken by craniotomy at the pterional skull base. Intraoperatively, however, tumor was found to be diffusely infiltrating the fifth and seventh nerve roots. A portion of the tumor remained in situ at the conclusion of the surgical procedure. Postoperatively, the patient's vision was unchanged. She experienced a grand mall seizure on postoperative day 3 and was placed on phenobarbital. A seventh nerve palsy became progressively appreciable. Although her gait and coordination were normal, she continued to experience recurrent grand mal seizures. For the remainder of her pregnancy, the patient's seventh nerve palsy slowly resolved. She vaginally delivered a live female infant at term without complications. However, her left visual acuity continued to worsen, eventually leaving the patient with left-sided blindness. Following delivery of the infant, radiation therapy was initiated, which resulted in left temporal and frontal encephalomalacia. Two months postpartum, the patient underwent hydroxyapatite cranioplasty and re-exploration at the site of her prior craniotomy. Intraoperatively, no evidence of recurrent tumor could be found. However, a fluid collection over a Marlex mesh placed with her prior craniotomies was identified and drained. Gram stain of this fluid showed gram negative rods, for which she received intravenous ceftazidime and vancomycin postoperatively. The patient recovered rapidly.

Unfortunately, initial control of the patient's seizures proved difficult, requiring multiple changes in her medication regimen. However, for the past five years, she has remained essentially free of seizures on felbamate and, more recently, topamax. She has tolerated these medications without evidence of hematologic or hepatic toxicity despite continued use. She has also undergone a left-sided orbital decompression, creation of a superior conjunctival flap and reconstruction of the left lateral canthus to treat an exposure keratopathy of her left cornea. For cosmetic purposes, dissection and advancement of her levator aponeurosis has also been performed. Despite this complicated course, the patient remains essentially healthy. No evidence of recurrent intracranial disease was observed on a follow-up MRI performed seven years after her initial craniotomy.

Discussion

Central nervous system tumors rarely complicate pregnancy. Histologically, the kinds of these tumors which occur in pregnant women are similar to those in non-pregnant women of a similar age group and include gliomas (32%), meningiomas (29%) and acoustic neuromas (15%).[14] Most individuals experience a combination of symptoms, such as headache, which reflect increased intracranial pressure as well as more specific neurologic symptoms specific to the intracranial location of the tumor. Although meningiomas are known to express functional estrogen and progesterone receptors, it is not certain whether pregnancy is causally related to the worsening symptoms experienced by this patient.[15] Nonetheless, she successfully tolerated a prolonged surgical procedure in the third trimester and delivered a live infant at term without complications.

From an obstetrical standpoint, many specialists recommend a Cesarean section to avoid potentially lethal increases in intracranial pressure during the second stage of labor. If a vaginal delivery is attempted, labor should be as pain-free as possible.[16] For the same reason, operative delivery is recommended to shorten the second stage. However, it is not clear whether anesthetic management or operative obstetrical interventions actually have a favorable impact on the outcome of labor and delivery in these patients.

Case 7: Colon Cancer

A 42-year-old woman, $G_5P_2Ab_2$, with a history of glaucoma and gestational diabetes, began to experience rectal bleeding during the second trimester of her pregnancy. After delivering a live infant in an uncomplicated fashion, these symptoms continued, despite conservative medical management. They were also increasingly accompanied by crampy abdominal pain and a visible narrowing of her stool. Colonoscopy was performed, which revealed carcinoma of the sigmoid colon, for which she underwent a partial colectomy. A preoperative CT scan indicated the presence of two liver lesions, which were also identified intraoperatively as metastatic carcinoma. Surgical staging was consistent with a modified Duke's C2 cancer. The patient received six cycles of chemotherapy with 5-fluorouracil (5-FU) and leucovorin.

Six months later, she again began to experience lower abdominal pain and cramping associated with nausea and vomiting. A CT scan was performed, which revealed an 18 × 12 cm heterogenous pelvic mass and ascites. The size of the hepatic lesions had also increased somewhat. An exploratory laparotomy was performed, which revealed a moderate amount of ascites and a smooth encapsulated tumor replacing the left ovary. This mass was both solid and cystic and was removed along with her left ovary without complications. At that time, there was no evidence of other intra-abdominal or pelvic disease. Pathologic examination of the surgical specimen was consistent with a metastatic adenocarcinoma. The patient was subsequently started on chemotherapy. Despite these efforts, her disease continued to progress and she eventually expired as a result of metastatic colon cancer less than two years after the initial diagnosis.

Discussion

Colon cancer occurs rarely in pregnant women, complicating only 1 out of every 13,000 live births.[17] Similar to many pregnant women diagnosed with colon cancer, this patient began to experience a number of symptoms, including abdominal pain and distension, rectal bleeding and a narrowing of stool caliber. However, the nonspecific nature of these symptoms can delay appropriate evaluation, as it most likely did for this patient. Her diagnosis was not clearly established until the postpartum period. Once identified, the appropriate surgery was performed. Unfortunately, liver metastases could be identified even at the time of her initial laparotomy.

In other respects, it is difficult to state that this patient's pregnancy contributed to her ultimate demise, as pregnancy does not appear to affect the natural history or survival of colorectal carcinomas.[18] For colon cancer diagnosed after 20 weeks of gestational age, definitive surgical therapy can be delayed until fetal maturity.[19] Patients willing to accept a therapeutic delay should understand, however, that an increase in tumor size and metastases may occur.

References

1. Hogston P, Lilford RJ. Ultrasound study of ovarian cysts in pregnancy: prevalence and significance. Br J Obstet Gynecol 1986;93: 625–8
2. Buttery BW, Beischer NA, Fortune DW, Macafee CA. Ovarian tumors in pregnancy. Med J Aust 1973; 1:345–9
3. Creasman WT, Rutledge F, Smith JP. Carcinoma of the ovary associated with pregnancy. Obstet Gynecol 1971; 38:111–6

4. Van Nagell JR, Ueland F. Ultrasound evaluation of pelvic masses: predictors of malignancy for the general gynecologist. Curr Opin Obstet Gynecol 1999; 11:45–9
5. Mikuta JJ. Invasive carcinoma of the cervix in pregnancy. South Med J 1967; 60:843–7
6. Morris M Eifel PJ, Lu J, Grigsby PW, Levenback C, Stevens RE, Rotman M, Gershenson DM, Mutch DG. Pelvic radiation with concurrent chemotherapy compared with pelvic and para-aortic radiation for high-risk cervical cancer. NEJM 1999; 340:1137–43
7. Rose PG, Bundy BN, Watkins EB, Thigpen JT, Deppe G, Maiman MA, Clarke-Pearson DL, Insalaco S. Concurrent cisplatin-based radiotherapy and chemotherapy for locally advanced cervical cancer. NEJM 1999; 340:1144–53
8. Degani R, Shohan Z, Atar E. Ovarian carcinoma during pregnancy: a study of 23 cases in Israel between the years of 1960 and 1984. Gynecol Oncol 1989; 33:326
9. Henderson CE, Elia G, Garfinkel D, Poirier MC, Shamkhani H, Runowicz CD. Platinum chemotherapy during pregnancy for serous cystadenocarcinoma of the ovary. Gynecol Oncol 1993; 49:92–4
10. Metz SA, Day TG, Pursell SH. Adjuvant chemotherapy in a pregnant patient with endodermal sinus tumor of the ovary. Gynecol Oncol 1989; 32:371–4
11. Ural W. Hormone replacement therapy in patients with cervical and ovarian cancers. Gynakol-Geburts Rundschau 1998; 38:89–92
12. Aviles A, Diaz-Maqueo JC, Garcia EL, Guzman R. Non-Hodgkin's lymphoma and pregnancy: presentation of 16 cases. Gynecol Oncol 1990; 37
13. Ward FT, Weiss RB. Lymphoma and pregnancy. Semin Oncol 1989; 16:397–409
14. Roelvink NCA, Kamphorst W, August H, van Alphen M, Rao BR. Pregnancy-related primary brain and spinal tumors. Arch Neurol 1987; 444:209–15
15. Speirs V, Walsh E, Fraser WD. Constitutive co-expression of estrogen and progesterone receptor mRNA in human meningiomas by RT-PCR and response of in vitro cell cultures to steroid hormones. Int J Cancer 1997; 72:714–9
16. DeAngelis LM. Central nervous system neoplasms in pregnancy. Adv Neurol 1994; 64:139–52
17. Woods JB, Martin JN, Ingram FH, Odorn CD, Scott-Conner CE, Rhodes RS. Pregnancy complicated by carcinoma of the colon above the rectum. Am J Perinatol 1992; 9:102–10
18. Bernstein MA, Madoff RD, Caushaj PF. Colon and rectal cancer in pregnancy. Dis Colon Rectum 1993; 36:172–8
19. Nesbitt JC, Moise KJ, Sawyers JL. Colorectal carcinoma in pregnancy. Arch Surg 1985; 120:636–9

13. Transplacental Carcinogenesis: Role of Chemicals, Radiation and Viruses

Orna Diav-Citrin, Asher Ornoy and Richard K. Miller

Introduction

During the early 1960s, experimentalists were becoming more concerned about the unique sensitivity of the conceptus to induction of cancer following in utero exposure.[1,2] Reports appeared that linked in utero exposure to ethylnitrosourea (ENU) and the induction of brain tumors, schwanoma and gliomas in adult rat offspring, lung tumors in mice and Wilms (renal) tumors in opossum pups.[3,4,5] Rice and associates[6] demonstrated that ENU given during pregnancy could result in the induction of choriocarcinoma in the mother *Patas* monkey. These were among the first reports of chemical induction of tumors in both offspring and mothers following in utero exposure. Of special note is that ENU has a biological half-life in the body of approximately 8–10 minutes. These examples of the unique sensitivity of the unborn to not only structural anomalies but also tumorigenesis has further raised interest in understanding the malleability of the developing organism in response to therapeutic, occupational and environmental exposures.

The age of the developing embryo and fetus of maximal susceptibility to the teratogenic or carcinogenic effects, or both, of an agent do not necessarily coincide, as noted for ENU,[3] when the maximum sensitivity for carcinogenicity appears to be during the fetal period. Another example is ionizing irradiation where the threshold for teratogenic versus carcinogenic effects do not coincide, but the age of the fetus for maximal susceptibility for carcinogenicity and teratogenicity appears similar.[7,8]

This review has selected known human transplacental carcinogens and also included information raising the question whether other exposures may also be associated with perinatal carcinogenesis. The authors hope this chapter will stimulate continuing discourse on this important subject. However, such discourse needs to be balanced with the accumulating evidence for and against a particular perinatal exposure producing tumorigenesis. The selected exposures to be discussed are for Diethylstilbestrol, Phenytoin, Zidovudine, radiation and viruses.

Diethylstilbestrol

Diethylstilbestrol (DES) has been widely used since its introduction in the 1940s. One of the first uses for this synthetic trans-stilbene estrogen was to prevent pregnancy loss.[9] Agricultural use was as a growth promoter in cattle production. DES was also used as an abortifacient. Today its use has been dramatically restricted. No longer is it used to prevent pregnancy loss because DES was found to be a transplacental carcinogen and teratogen in humans[10-13] approximately 25 years after its introduction into woman's health care. Even more time passed before it was demonstrated to be a transplacental carcinogen in animals species: mouse,[14-17] rat[18,19,20] and hamster.[21] It is noteworthy that across species the female reproductive tract tumors have been identified, especially vaginal clear cell adenocarcinoma in women exposed in utero to DES. As noted in Table 13.1, there are many similarities between the tumors and malformations noted in the female reproductive tract following DES exposure in utero. Avoiding the period of lower reproductive tract development for DES is consistent with reducing the risk for both vaginal tumors but also adenosis and reproductive tract malformations in rodents and in the human.[13,18]

DES has provided a rich field for investigating mechanisms of teratogenic and carcinogenic action (Table 13.1). Such animal and human observations place DES among the agents which through signal transduction mechanisms (hormones) can modify not only the receptor (estrogen) but also its expression, uterine lactoferrin .[22] More recent evidence has implicated chromosomes 3 and 6 as sites for gene control resulting in not only carcinogenesis but also teratogenesis.[23] It is especially noteworthy that investigative teams are identifying in animal models that exposure to DES in one generation can lead to clear cell vaginal adenocarcinoma in the next generation.[24,25,26]

Recent investigations have coupled the effects of diethylstilbestrol in the developing mouse female reproductive tract with down regulation of Wnt7a resulting in abnormal smooth muscle proliferation.[16] Wnt7a is normally expressed in the luminal epithelium of the uterus. Following DES exposure in utero, low levels of Wnt7a transcripts were detected at birth. Such alterations in the reproductive tract following DES exposure is consistent with knock out mice lacking Wnt7a having malformed female reproductive tracts.[15]

All of these investigations implicate the role of gene control and modification by estrogenic agents which may be more effective because of not only their estrogenic properties but their pharmacokinetics and metabolism.[19,20,28] Thus in the human, further questions are being raised about the gene–environmental interactions based upon the collective experience with diethylstilbestrol during pregnancy.[23]

Phenytoin

Phenytoin (hydantoin, diphenylhydantoin, Dilantin) is a known human teratogen.[29] An association between phenytoin therapy and malignant lymphoma had been reported in adults.[30,31] There is increasing evidence to incriminate phenytoin as a possible human transplacental carcinogen. Combined teratogenesis and oncogenesis can be viewed as a reaction to a special type of injury: teratogenesis being the more primitive reaction with a gradual shift to oncogenesis with time.

Table 13.1. Female abnormalities following prenatal exposure to diethylstilbestrol in man and in rat/mouse.

	Human	Rat/Mouse
Vagina		
	Adenosis	Adenosis
	Adenocarcinoma	
Adenocarcinoma		
	Squamous cell dysplasia	Squamous cell carcinoma
		Hyperkeratosis
		Hypospadias
		Calculi
		Vaginitis
Cervix		
	Hoods	
	Stenosis	
	Incompetence	
Uterus/ Fallopian tube		
	T-shaped uteri	Endometrial hyperplasia
	"Withered" fallopian tube	Uncoiled tubes
External genitalia		
		Patent vagina at birth
		Persistent cleft phallus
		Perineal excoriation
Functional abnormalities		
	Menstrual irregularities	Noncycling
	Spontaneous abortion	
	Ectopic pregnancy	
	Premature delivery	

A number of case reports suggest that prenatal phenytoin exposure is associated with an increased incidence of neuroblastoma and other neuroectodermal childhood neoplasms (Table 13.2). The association between neuroblastoma in infants and children following prenatal exposure to phenytoin was first raised in 1976.[32] The first cases were described in infants and children with fetal phenytoin syndrome but later publications reported neuroblastoma in children without dysmorphic features. Two of the described cases are in infants and children with features of both fetal phenytoin–alcohol syndromes. Later studies suggested an association with non-ectodermal tumors as well (Table 13.3). As shown in Tables 13.2 and 13.3, additional defects exist in many of the infants diagnosed with a malignancy after prenatal exposure to phenytoin. A causal relationship between prenatal phenytoin and tumors is supported by the oncogenic potential of phenytoin in adults. An association between phenytoin therapy and malignant lymphoma has been suggested in treated adults. Retrospective data to date, however, did not support this association. Koren and

Table 13.2. Neuroectodermal tumors associated with fetal exposure to phenytoin

Reference	Tumor	Site	Age at diagnosis	Gender	Drugs	Maternal age	Length of Maternal AET	Anomalies/Malformations
Pendergrass and Hanson[32]	Neuroblastoma	Abdomen	3 years	F	DPH and PHB	24 years	10 years	FHS
Sherman and Roizen[46]	Neuroblastoma	Adrenal	7 days	M	DPH and PHB	N/A	Since 8 years of age	FHS, hypospadias
Ramilo and Harris[47]	Neuroblastoma	Suprarenal	35 months	N/A	DPH and E-OH	N/A	N/A	FHS and FAS, VSD
Allen et al[99]	Neuroblastoma	Pelvis	1st day	M	DPH, PHB and primidone	30 years	25 years	FHS, VSD, EHDN
Ehrenbard and Chaganti[34]	Neuroblastoma	Metastatic (Stage IV)	31 months	M	DPH, primidone and diazepam	25 years	7 years	FHS
Koren et al[33]	Neuroblastoma	Abdomen	4 weeks		DPH and cigarettes	18 years	15 years	Proband's half brother with FHS
Al-Shammri et al[35]	Neuroblastoma	Metastatic (Stage IV)	30 months	M	DPH and CBZ	N/A	8 years	
Seeler et al[36]	Ganglioneuroblastoma	Adrenal	35 months	M	DPH and E-OH	27 years	1 year	FHS and FAS, VSD, eventration of the right hemidiaphragm
Jimenez et al[37]	Melanotic neuroectodermal tumor	Cheek	6 months	M	DPH and PHB	25 years	Throughout gestation and 5 years previously	FHS
Lipson and Bale[38]	Ependymoblastoma	Brain	28 months	F	DPH and methyl-PHB	N/A	'Many years'	Genetic carrier of OTC def.

AET, antiepileptic therapy; N/A not available; DPH, diphenylhydantoin or phenytoin; PHB, phenobarbital; E-OH, ethyl alcohol; CBZ, carbamazepine; FHS, fetal hydantoin syndrome; FAS, fetal alcohol syndrome; VSD, ventricular septal defect; EHDN, early hemorrhagic disease of the newborn; OTC def., ornithine transcarbamylase deficiency.

Table 13.3. Non-ectodermal tumors associated with fetal exposure to phenytoin.

Reference	Tumor	Site	Age at Diagnosis	Gender	Drugs	Maternal age	Length of Phenytoin Therapy	Anomalies/Malformations
Blattner et al[39]	Malignant mesenchymoma	Liver and retroperitoneum	18 years	M	DPH	N/A	Since 16 years of age	Left cleft lip and palate
Taylor et al[40]	Wilms' tumor	Extrarenal: scrotal	6 months	M	DPH, PHB and CBZ	23	Since 11 years of age	FHS, VSD
Cohen[41]	Wilms' tumor	Renal	N/A	N/A	DPH	N/A	N/A	FHS
Kousseff[42]	Soft tissue masses (cystic hygromas?)	Subcutaneous	Hardly noticeable at birth but gradually increased in size	M	DPH	N/A	N/A	FHS
Bostrom and Nesbit[43]	Hodgkin disease	Right cervical lymphadenopathy	31/2 years	F	DPH diazepam or lorazepam and E-OH	N/A	N/A	FHS and FAS
Sholler et al[44]	Rhabdomyosarcoma	Cardiac: left ventricular	5 years	F	DPH	N/A	N/A	
Murray et al[45]	T-lymphocyte Lymphoblastic lymphoma	Anterior mediastinum	21/2 years	M	DPH	33 years	Since 9 years of age	

N/A, not available; DPH, diphenylhydantoin or phenytoin; PHB, phenobarbital; CBZ, carbamazepine; E-OH, ethyl alcohol; FHS, fetal hydantoin syndrome; VSD, ventricular septal defect; FAS , fetal alcohol syndrome.

associates[33] reviewed medical records of 188 cases of childhood neuroblastoma. In none of the medical charts was the mother mentioned as having epilepsy or as being treated with phenytoin. The authors calculated that this would exclude an association between prenatal exposure to phenytoin in more than 1.5% of all cases of neuroblastoma.

Thus, a cluster of case reports suggest that phenytoin may be a human transplacental carcinogen. Ehrenbard and Chaganti[34] estimate the incidence of neuroblastomas to be 1 in 7,100 live births. A malignant tumor could be a rare but non-random event in infants and children prenatally exposed to phenytoin. The association between prenatal exposure to phenytoin with neural crest tumors and especially with neuroblastoma seems stronger than with other neoplasms.[35–40] Further studies are required firmly to establish a cause and effect relationship as well as to shed light on the mechanisms underlying this relationship. Since the potential transplacental oncogenic effect of phenytoin is based on a cluster of case reports with an unknown denominator (total number of exposed cases), it is impossible to derive a true risk rate. The anticipated absolute transplacental oncogenic risk of phenytoin is probably low.[41–47]

Zidovudine (AZT)

Anti-HIV therapies, especially AZT, have been a breakthrough for treatment and survival not only of adults but especially the offspring of mothers who have been infected. The most seriously and rapidly progressing subset of the HIV-1 infected population are children.[48,49] The numbers worldwide continue to indicate that both women and children are the most rapidly growing subsets of the population. For many in the United States and other developed countries, the vertical transmission of HIV has apparently been brought under control. In some clinical reports, the transmission rate from mother to baby has fallen from 25–40% in untreated pregnant women to as low as 1–4% in pregnant women treated with anti-HIV therapies. Such successes, due to these pharmacologic interventions containing this devastating disease, were first demonstrated in the Pediatric AIDS Clinical Trial Group (PACTG) 076 Study[49,50] using AZT and have been further refined and defined by the US Public Health Service. Based upon the original PACTG 076 findings, anti-HIV therapies have been remarkably successful in reducing the incidence of HIV-1 in babies born to mothers who are HIV-1 positive. One certainly finds it difficult, if not impossible, to withhold AZT from these pregnant women for the sake of their children. Yet what is the risk-to-benefit ratio we are determining for these therapeutic interventions?

For those who are infected (potentially 25–40% of babies from untreated mothers), the therapy is life saving. Approximately one-third of infected babies rapidly progress to CDC Clinical Category C or death between birth and 18 months.[49] In Africa, an entire generation is being decimated with 33% of the pregnant mothers being HIV positive and 33% of their children becoming infected. However, a significant number of babies of HIV-1 positive mothers will not be infected. One therefore continues to be anxious about any side effects and developmental toxicities associated AZT, which is why a number of these agents are listed as category C in the Physician's Desk Reference[50] because of animal studies reporting developmental toxicity at high doses of the agents. In many instances, the desire to prevent the vertical transmission of HIV-1 to the babies has expanded the therapeutic window to attempt success in HIV positive pregnant women with practically any combinations of anti HIV therapies

(RT inhibitors and protease inhibitors). Of particular concern is that many pregnant women are receiving their anti-HIV therapies throughout pregnancy. Thus, embryogenesis is now a major component of the treatment paradigm.

Clinically, growing experience with AZT during pregnancy from the PACTG 076 trials has demonstrated that this RT inhibitor may not be another thalidomide, at least through the first five years of life, for the children exposed in utero.[51,52] However, the original PACTG 076 trial did not initiate therapy until after 14 weeks of gestation. Today, many women are conceiving while on anti-HIV therapies and continue those therapies throughout their pregnancies. Controversy surrounds the use of antiretrovirals and the production of mitochondrial disease. Blanche and associates[53] reported on two neurologically related deaths due to mitochondrial dysfunction among uninfected infants born to mothers receiving combination AZT and lamivudine in an open label clinical trial, and an additional series of six living children exposed to AZT alone or to AZT/lamivudine, who had either clinical or laboratory findings suggestive of mitochondrial dysfunction. On the other hand, Fowler[48] reported an extensive review of all deaths among uninfected and indeterminate children from >20,000 perinatal HIV mother–infant pairs followed in NIH and CDC supported studies in the US and found no deaths among uninfected children that were similar to the two due to progressive neurologic disease and mitochondrial disease. Dialogue continues concerning the mechanistic possibilities for these anti-HIV actions.[54,55] Both human and animal studies must continue to examine possible risks not only to the conceptus but also the child.

Of particular interest have been reports in two different rodent species demonstrating tumors of the female reproductive tract following high dosages of AZT given prenatally to the mothers.[56,57] The direct application to human therapy especially during pregnancy has not been resolved. Obviously additional investigations must be undertaken. These current studies[56,57] emphasize the importance of acknowledging the potential risks to the unborn from these life-saving anti-HIV therapies. The risk-to-benefit ratio continues to be toward treatment with AZT since the risk of infection from HIV-1 is so high and HIV-1 is so deadly in those infected perinatally. Yet in this population of newborns, more than 60% of the newborns will not be infected but exposed to these anti-HIV therapies. Thus, these carcinogenesis studies sensitize all of us to the delicate balance that must be struck between benefit and possible risk to the unborn.

Ionizing Radiation

Human populations that have had high exposures to ionizing radiation have an increased incidence of cancer.[58] There is substantial evidence that exposure to high-dose ionizing radiation has the potential to induce leukemia and solid tumors in various adult populations (i.e., occupational exposure, radiation therapy patients, Japanese survivors of atomic bomb explosions). Miller[59] found a subsequent leukemia incidence of 1 in 1,000 in children who were under 10 years of age and were within 1500 meters of the epicenter of the atomic bomb explosion. Yoshimoto and associates[60] found that among 1,630 individuals exposed in utero to the atomic bombs, there were two cases of childhood cancer in the first year of follow-up. High-energy radiation during pregnancy may have various effects during different times of development (embryolethality, teratogenicity, growth-retardation, neurodevelopmental effect, and carcinogenicity). It is difficult to determine which mechanisms are most important for radiation induced embryopathologic disorders. Different pathogenic mechanisms may have an impact on the developing human at different stages of gestation.[58]

Evidence that diagnostic radiography (acute low dose radiation) might pose a carcinogenic risk to the human fetus was initially suggested by Stewart et al in 1956.[61] In this British case-control study, the mothers of children who had died of cancer remembered having an abdominal or pelvic X-ray during the related pregnancy with a higher frequency than did the mothers of matched control children who did not die of cancer. Abdominal radiographic examination during pregnancy was estimated to be double the risk for the child to develop cancer (both leukemia and other malignant disease). The study was criticized in that the reported difference could have been the result of recall bias. Similar results were reported in an extended series 2 years later.[62] MacMahon[63] supplied further evidence for the association reporting similar findings in the United States based on hospital records of exposure that were not susceptible to recall bias. Subsequently, Hewitt et al and Knox et al[64,65] showed that recall bias had relatively little impact on the results of the British study. The British study, now known as the Oxford Survey of Childhood Cancers (OSCC), was continued and expanded to include over 15,000 case-control pairs.[66] A recent comprehensive review summarized the available data.[67] The excess relative risk obtained from combining the results of various case-control studies has high statistical significance and suggests that, in the past, an abdominal X-ray of a pregnant woman produced a proportional increase in risk of about 40%. A causal relationship has been challenged on four grounds:

1. Children exposed in utero to radiation from the atomic bomb explosions in Hiroshima and Nagasaki have not experienced any corresponding increased risk of cancer.
2. The case-control studies of childhood cancer and intrauterine exposure to irradiation have an almost equal increase in relative risk of leukemia and for all solid tumors, while the increased risk of cancer in childhood among the Japanese irradiated by the atomic explosions when under 10 years of age has been limited to leukemia.
3. The excess risk estimated from the OSCC data, which mostly refer to exposure in the last month of pregnancy is substantially higher than that derived for childhood cancer following irradiation of young children.
4. Although twins were presumably more often exposed to irradiation in utero, they do not have a significantly increased risk of childhood cancer compared to singletons. A causal relationship is supported by evidence indicating an appropriate dose–response relationship and by animal experiments. An appropriate increase in relative risk is observed with the increase in the number of X-ray exposures and hence, presumably, the dose of radiation experienced by the fetus. A statistically significant decline in the relative risk was demonstrated within the OSCC for births between 1940 and 1965, that closely parallels the exponential decline in fetal dose that occurred during the same period. Animal studies in rats and beagle dogs found that in utero irradiation increases the lifetime risk of cancer. A causal relationship between diagnostic exposure of the fetus to ionizing radiation and risk of childhood cancer supports the hypothesis that there is no threshold dose below which no effect is produced. Doll and Wakeford[67] conclude that radiation doses of the order 10 mGy (1 rad) received by the fetus in utero produce a consequent increase in the risk of

childhood cancer. The excess absolute risk coefficient at this level of exposure is approximately 6% per gray (100 rad), although the exact value of this risk coefficient remains uncertain. In summary, there is concern about the carcinogenic effect of low-grade ionizing radiation. The natural level of occurrence of cancer in average pregnancies, however, is much higher than the one associated with in utero irradiation. It is estimated that the current practice of radiology in the United States increases the spontaneous frequency of cancer by less than 1%.[68]

Viruses

Several viruses are being linked with malignant disease. Among them are Epstein–Barr virus (Burkitt's lymphoma), hepatitis virus (hepatocellular carcinoma), cytomegalic virus (Kaposi's sarcoma), herpes simplex virus and genital papilloma virus.[69–71] The possible associations between maternal viral infections during pregnancy and malignant diseases during childhood remain open questions, and have been addressed in several studies.[71-73]

Possible transplacental viral carcinogenesis in man has been implicated but not necessarily proven for several viruses: Epstein–Barr virus (EBV), varicella zoster virus, hepatitis B virus, cytomegalic virus (CMV), mumps and influenza virus.[69-74] Most published studies are epidemiological in nature reporting an association of intrauterine infection mainly with acute lymphoblastic leukemia (ALL), the most common malignant disease in children, and with hepatocellular carcinoma.[72–74] We will examine the epidemiological evidence that exists for the possible association between specific prenatal viral infections and childhood tumors.

Epstein–Barr Virus (EBV)

There is an association between postnatal infection with Epstein–Barr virus, a herpes group virus, and Burkitt's childhood lymphoma. This virus was recovered in tumor cells[75,76] and has been described as a possible etiologic agent in several other malignancies, including Hodgkin's disease[77] and nasopharyngeal carcinoma.[78] EBV is known to persist in B lymphocytes and to cause "immortalization" of the infected cells, probably predisposing them to malignant transformation.[75,79] In a prospective seroepidemiological study performed on sera from 45,000 people in Uganda, the results indicated an association between Burkitt's lymphoma and both neonatal and perinatal EBV infection.[76] However, the results are considered by the authors to be only preliminary and more studies are obviously required for definitive conclusions.

In a recent study performed in Scotland in more than 400 children with various malignant tumors, an association was reported only between the occurrence of solid tumors with maternal EBV infection during pregnancy and the use of antibiotics.[77] No association was found with other risk factors such as eclampsia, excessive vomiting or the mode of delivery.[77] In this study, a negative association was observed between neonatal infections and childhood acute lymphoblastic leukemia (ALL). This is in contrast to other studies where a positive correlation between intrauterine infection and childhood ALL was observed.[69,70,74]

In another recent study performed in Germany, the rate of ALL increased with the decrease in maternal age (less than 20 years), increase in birth weight and with hormonal treatment for infertility.[78] However, the possible association of intrauterine infection and ALL was not reported.

In light of the above mentioned associations between postnatal EBV infection and malignancies, it is surprising that little evidence appears to exist in the literature regarding possible association between in utero infection with EBV and childhood malignancy. Even in general epidemiologic studies relating intrauterine infections with childhood malignancy, EBV was rarely observed.[72,73]

Varicella Zoster Virus

Stewart et al[61] were apparently the first to report that the mothers of 2 of 677 children with leukemia had herpes zoster during their pregnancy as opposed to one mother in the control group. Similar findings were reported later in other, relatively small, cohorts.[79–81] Adelstein and Donovan[81] found that 2 of the 270 children born to women who had varicella infection during weeks 23 and 25 of pregnancy developed leukemia as opposed to the expected rate of 1:3600 children to have leukemia. Similarly, Vianna and Polan[82] found 3 children with leukemia of 63 children born to mothers who had varicella during pregnancy. These mothers had varicella during the fourth to sixth month of gestation. Another description of a possible association was in the study by Till et al[33] who reported that in their series of children with malignancy, two children with ALL, the mothers had varicella zoster infection at 24 and 25 weeks of pregnancy. There were several other similar reports. The above described data provided limited statistical power to indicate that most varicella zoster infections related to childhood leukemia occurred after the 20th week of gestation, a period of pregnancy when the virus is not considered to be teratogenic.[84] It should be noted that the number of cases was small and that all of these studies were retrospective.

Cytomegalic Virus (CMV)

Little evidence exists to associate CMV with malignancy induction in general. However, the etiologic association of CMV with Kaposi's sarcoma, especially in patients with AIDS,[85] appears to be well-established. Also in AIDS patients with Kaposi's sarcoma, human herpes virus-8 was also recovered.[86]

In contrast to the possible etiology of CMV with human cancer, there appears to be little evidence that primary or recurrent CMV infection during pregnancy is associated with an increased rate of malignancy in the offspring. In one study, Fine et al[73] reported a preponderance of malignancy among children and adults who had a proven viral infection while in utero, but CMV was detected in few cases. In the study published by Roman et al,[87] a significant increase in documented viral infection during pregnancy was observed in mothers of children who developed leukemia and non-Hodgkin's lymphoma, but here again CMV was not the dominant virus.[87] In the large survey published by Stewart et al,[74] none of the 13 mothers who had viral infection during pregnancy and their children having died of childhood leukemia, had CMV.

We should remember, however, that most cases of primary or recurrent CMV infection in adults cause no significant clinical symptoms. In epidemiological studies like those performed by Roman et al,[87] and others,[73,74] there may still be many women who had CMV during pregnancy but appear in the non-infected group of mothers as they did not report CMV infection and were not screened.

Human Papillomavirus

This virus is known to cause genital warts, which in chronic untreated cases may undergo malignant transformation, causing squamous cell carcinoma of the skin and mucous membranes, including adenocarcinoma of the larynx.[88–92] The possibility of transmission of papilloma virus to the fetus in utero, or during birth, was studied in neonates and young children. Transmission of the virus to the newborn infant was described by many investigators,[86–88] but prenatal transmission seems to be rare. The rate of transplacental transmission varies from low[90] to relatively high[88,89] or very high.[78] To the best of our knowledge, there are no reports on the possible association between prenatally acquired papilloma virus and later development of cervical or laryngeal intraepithelial neoplasia. There were no reports found describing clinically evidenced intrauterine infection with papilloma virus.

Hepatitis B Virus

Hepatitis B virus may progress to active hepatitis and liver cirhosis. With more advanced disease stage, hepatocellular carcinoma of the liver may develop with increasing frequency.[92-94] Prevention of hepatitis B by active immunization interrupts persistent viral infection and thus decreases the danger of hepatocellular carcinoma.[92]

In a study of 51 children with hepatocellular carcinoma performed in Taiwan, hepatitis B transmission was suggested to have occurred in many of the children during the perinatal period or at early childhood.[93]

Hepatitis B virus is known to pass the placenta during pregnancy. No increase in the rate of congenital anomalies has been found. However, chronic active hepatitis has been described.[94-96] This may lead during childhood to hepatocellular carcinoma.

Hepatitis C virus can apparently be transmitted to the fetus only when the pregnant mother is also co-infected with HIV.[97] It is also yet unclear whether transplacental infection with hepatitis C virus may result in liver malignancy during childhood. Additional investigations are certainly required to establish a confirmed relationship to cancer (hepatocellular carcinoma and hepatitis B).

Summary

Many questions remain unresolved concerning the relationships between transplacental carcinogenicity in the human and exposure to a wide variety of chemicals, viruses and other agents.[98] However, based upon both animal and human investigations, it is absolutely clear that the conceptus can be sensitive to many agents (ENU, DES, X-radiation) resulting not only in an increased incidence of birth defects but also childhood and adult onset tumors. As with DES, the challenge to the medical community is to discover these associations, which may be at low incidence, and then to interpret the risk-to-benefit ratio for both mother and baby. The field of perinatal virology and cancer risk provides another complicated problem. It is hoped that with enhanced attention to these problems of perinatal carcinogenesis, confirmed associations will be established or the hypotheses disproven. Currently, with the exception of DES, it is difficult to provide patients with definitive counseling concerning risks and interventions.

References

1. Tomatis L, Mohr U. (eds) Transplacental Carcinogenesis. IARC Publications, Lyon, 1973.
2. Rice JM, (ed.) Perinatal Carcinogenesis. National Cancer Institute Monograph 51, DHEW Publication, Bethesda, MD 1979.
3. Druckrey H. Chemical structure and action in transplacental carcinogenesis and teratogenesis. In Tomatis L, and Mohr U. (eds) Transplacental Carcinogenesis, IARC Publications, Lyon, 1973.
4. Rice JM. The biological behaviour of transplacentally induced tumours in mice. In Tomatis L, and Mohr U. (eds) Transplacental Carcinogenesis, IARC Publications, Lyon, 1973.
5. Jurgelski W Jr, Hudson PM, Falk HL, Kotin P. Embryonal neoplasms in the opossum: a new model for solid tumors of infancy and childhood. Science 1976; 193:328–32.
6. Rice JM, Williams GM, Palmer AE, London WT, Sly DL. Pathology of gestation choriocarcinoma induced in Patas monkeys by ethylnitrososurea given during pregnancy. Placenta 1981; (Suppl 3) 223–30.
7. MacMahon B. Prenatal X-ray exposure and childhood cancer. J Natl Cancer Inst 1962; 28:1173–91.
8. Hewitt D, Sanders B, Stewart A. Reliability of data reported by case and control mothers. Monthly Bull Ministry of Health and Public Health Laboratory Service 1966; 25:80–5.
9. Smith OW, Smith G, Hurwitz S. Increased excretion of pregnandediol in pregnancy from DES with special reference to the prevention of late pregnancy accidents. Am J Obstet Gynecol 1946; 51:411–21.
10. Herbst AL, Ulfelder H, Poskanzer DC. (1971) Adenocarcinoma of the vagina: association of maternal stilbestrol therapy with tumor appearing in young women. N Engl J Med 1971; 284:878–81.
11. Herbst AL (1981) Clear cell adenocarcinoma and the current status of DES-exposed females. Cancer 1981; 48:484–8.
12. Kaufmann RH, Adam E, Binder GL, Gerthoffer E. Upper genital tract changes and pregnancy outcome in offspring exposed in utero to diethylstilbestrol. Am J Obstet Gynecol 1980; 137:299–308.
13. Goldberg J, Falcone T. Effect of diethylstilbestrol on reproductive function. Fertil Steril 1999; 72:1–7.
14. McLachlan J, Newbold R, Bullock B. Long term effects on the female mouse genital tract associated with prenatal exposure to diethylstilbestrol. Canc Res 1980; 40:3988–99.
15. Miller C, Sassoon D. Wnt 7a maintains appropriate uterine patterning during the development of the mouse female reproductive tract. Development 1998; 125:3201–11.
16. Miller C, Degenhardt K, Sassoon D. Fetal exposure to DES results in deregulation of Wnt7a during uterine morphogenesis. Nature Genetics 1998; 20:228–30.
17. Walker B, Haven MI. Intensity of multigenerational carcinogenesis from diethylstilbestrol in mice. Carcinogenesis 1997; 18:791–3.
18. Baggs RB, Miller RK, Odoroff C. Carcinogenicity of diethylstilbestrol in the Wistar rat: Effect of postnatal oral contraceptive steroids. Canc Res 1991; 51:3311–5.
19. Henry EC, Miller RK. Disposition of Diethylstilbestrol and Estradiol in the fetal rat: correlation with teratogenic potency. Biochem Pharm 1986; 35:1993–2001.
20. Henry EC, Miller RK, Baggs RB. Direct fetal injections of Diethylstilbestrol and 17β-estradiol: a method for investigating their teratogenicity. Teratology 1984; 29:297–304.
21. Marselos M, Tomatis L. Diethylstilboestrol: II, Pharmacology, toxicology and carcinogenicity in experimental animals. Eur J Cancer 1993; 29A:149–55.
22. Newbold R, Hanson R, Jefferson W. Ontogeny of lactoferin in the developing mouse uterus: a marker of early hormone response. Biol Reprod 1997; 56:1147–57.
23. Hanselaar A, van Loosbroek M, Schuurbiers O, Helmerhorst T, Bulten J, Bernheim J. Clear cell adenocarcinoma of the vagina and cervix: an update of the central Netherlands registry showing twin age incidence peaks. Cancer 1997; 79:2229–36.
24. Walker B. Animal models of prenatal exposure to diethylstilbestrol. In Napalkov NP, Rice JM, Tomatis L, Yamaski H. (eds) Perinatal and multigeneration carcinogenesis. IARC Scientific Publications, Lyon, No. 96, 1989.
25. Walker B, Kurth L. Multigenerational carcinogenesis from diethylstilbestrol investigated by blastocyst transfers in mice. Int J Canc 1995; 61:249–52.
26. Walker B, Haven M. Cancer risk assessment, J Natl Med Assoc 1997; 89:21–6.
27. Newbold R, Hanson R, Jefferson W, Bullock B, Haseman J, McLachlan J. Increased tumors but uncompromised fertility in the female descendants of mice exposed developmentally to diethylstilbesterol. Carcinogenesis 1998; 19:1655–63.
28. Miller RK, Heckmann ME, McKenzie RC. (1982) Diethylstilbestrol: placental transfer, metabolism, covalent binding and fetal distribution in the Wistar rat. J Pharmacol Expt Therap 1982; 220:358–65.
29. Hanson JW. Fetal hydantoin effects. Teratology 1986; 33:349–53.
30. Anthony JJ. Malignant lymphoma associated with hydantoin drugs. Arch Neurol 1970; 22:450–4.

31. Hoover R, Fraumeni JF Jr. 1975. Drugs. In: Persons at high risk of cancer: an approach to cancer etiology and control. Fraumeni JF Jr (ed.) New York: Academic Press, 1975.
32. Pendergrass TW, Hanson JW. Fetal hydantoin syndrome and neuroblastoma. Lancet 1976; 2:150.
33. Koren G, Demitrakoudis D, Weksberg R, Rieder M, Shear NH, Sonely M, Shandling B, Spielberg S. Neuroblastoma after prenatal exposure to phenytoin: cause and effect? Teratology 1989; 40:157–62.
34. Ehrenbard LT, Chaganti RSK. Cancer in the fetal hydantoin syndrome. Lancet 1981; 2:97.
35. Al-Shammri S, Guberman A, Hsu E. Neuroblastoma and fetal exposure to phenytoin in a child without dysmorphic features. Can J Neurol Sci 1992; 19:243–5.
36. Seeler RA, Israel JN, Royal JE, Kaye CI, Rao S, Abulaben M. Ganglioneuroblastoma and fetal hydantoin-alcohol syndromes. Pediatrics 1979; 63:524–7.
37. Jiminez JF, Seibert RW, Char F, Brown RE, Seibert JJ. Melanocytic neuroectodermal tumor of infancy and fetal hydantoin syndrome. Am J Pediatr Hematol Oncol 1981; 3: 9–15.
38. Lipson A, Bale P. Ependymoblastoma associated with prenatal exposure to diphenylhydantoin and methylphenobarbitone. Cancer 1985; 55:1859–62.
39. Blattner WA, Henson DE, Young RC, Fraumeni JF Jr. Malignant mesenchymoma and birth defects. Prenatal exposure to phenytoin. JAMA 1977; 238:334–5.
40. Taylor WF, Myers M, Taylor WR. Extrarenal Wilms' tumour in an infant exposed to intrauterine phenytoin. Lancet 1980; 2:481–2.
41. Cohen MM Jr. Neoplasia and the fetal alcohol and hydantoin syndromes. Neurobehav Toxicol Teratol 1981, 3:161–2.
42. Koussef BG. Subcutaneous vascular abnormalities in fetal hydantoin syndrome. Birth Defects 1982; 18:51–4.
43. Bostrom B, Nesbit ME Jr. Hodgkin disease in a child with fetal alcohol-hydantoin syndrome. J Pediatr 1983; 103:760–2.
44. Sholler GF, Hawker RE, Nunn GR, Bale P, Bergin M. Primary left ventricular rhabdomyosarcoma in a child: noninvasive assessment and successful resection of a rare tumor. J Thorac Cardiovasc Surg 1987; 93:465–8.
45. Murray JC, Hill RM, Hegemier S, Hurwitz RL. Lymphoblastic lymphoma following prenatal exposure to phenytoin. J Pediatr Hematol Oncol 1996; 18:241–3.
46. Sherman S, Roizen N. Fetal hydantoin syndrome and neuroblastoma. Lancet 1976; 2:517.
47. Ramilo J, Harris VJ. Neuroblastoma in a child with the hydantoin and fetal alcohol sydrome. The radiographic features. Br J Radiol 1979; 52:993–5.
48. Fowler MG. Follow-up of children exposed to perinatal antiretrovirals. Teratology 2000; 61:395–6.
49. Rich KC, Fowler MG, Mofenson LM, Abboud R, Pitt J, Diaz C, Hanson IC, Cooper E, Mendez H, and the Women and Infants Transmission Study Group. Maternal and infant factors predicting disease progression in human immunodeficiency virus type 1-infected infants. Pediatrics 2000; 105:E8–18.
50. Physicians Desk Reference 2000.
51. Culnane M, Fowler MG, Lee S, et al. Lack of long-term effects of in utero exposure to zidovudine among uninfected children born to HIV-infected women. JAMA 1999; 354:1084–9.
52. Hanson IC, Antonelli TR, Sperling RS, et al. Lack of tumors in infants with perinatal HIV type 1 exposure and fetal/neonatal exposure to zidovudine. J AIDS 1999; 20:463–7.
53. Blanche S, Tardieu M, Rustin P et al. Persistent mitochondrial dysfunction and perinatal exposure to antiretroviral nucleoside analogues. Lancet 1999; 354:1084–9
54. Brinkman K, Smetink JA, Romjin J, Reiss P. Mitochondrial toxicity induced by nucleoside-analogue reverse transcriptase inhibitors is a key in the pathogenesis of antiretroviral-related lipodystrophy. Lancet 1999; 354:1112–5.
55. Walker UA, Setzer B, Volksbeck SI. Toxicity of nucleoside-analogue reverse-transcriptase inhibitors. Lancet 2000; 355:1096.
56. Ayers KM, Torrey CE, Reynolds DJ. A transplacental carcinogenicity bioassay in CD-1 mice with zidovudine. Fund Appl Tox 1997; 38:195–8.
57. Olivero OA, Anderson LM, Diwan BA, et al. Transplacental effects of 3'-azido-2', 3'dideoxythymidine (AZT): tumorigenicity in mice and genotoxicity in mice and monkeys. J Natl Cancer Inst 1997; 89:1602–8.
58. Brent RL. The effect of embryonic and fetal exposure to X-ray, microwave and ultrasound: counseling the pregnant and non-pregnant patient about these risks. Sem Oncol 1989; 16:347–68.
59. Miller RW. Delayed effects occurring within the first decade after exposure of young individuals to the Hiroshima atomic bomb. Pediatrics 1956; 18:1–18.
60. Yoshimoto Y, Kato H, Schull WJ. Risk of cancer among children exposed in utero to A-bomb radiations 1950–84. Lancet 1988; 2:665–9.
61. Stewart A, Webb J, Giles D, Hewitt D. Malignant disease in childhood and diagnostic irradiation in utero. Lancet 1956; 2:447.

62. Stewart A, Webb J, Hewitt D. A survey of childhood malignancies. Br Med J 1958; 1:1495–1508.
63. MacMahon B. Prenatal X-ray exposure and childhood cancer. J Natl Cancer Inst 1962; 28:1173–91.
64. Hewitt D, Sanders B, Stewart A. Reliability of data reported by case and control mothers. Monthly Bull Ministry of Health and Public Health Laboratory Service 1966; 25:80–5.
65. Knox EG, Stewart AM, Kneale GW, Gilman EA. Prenatal irradiation and childhood cancer. J Soc Radiol Prot 1987; 7:177–89.
66. Gilman EA, Stewart AM, Knox EG, Kneale GW. Trends in obstetric radiology, 1939–81. J Radiol Prot 1989; 9:93–101.
67. Doll R, Wakeford R. Risk of childhood cancer from fetal irradiation. Br J Radiol 1997; 70:130–7.
68. Hall EJ. Scientific view of low-level radiation risks. Radiographics 1991; 11:509–18.
69. Hoppe-Seyler F, Butz K. Molecular mechanisms of virus-induced carcinogenesis: the interaction of viral factors with cellular tumor suppressor proteins. J Mol Med 1995; 73:529–38.
70. Greaves M.F. Aetiology of acute leukaemia. Lancet 1997; 349:344–9.
71. Wiemels JL, Cazzaniga G, Daniotti M, Eden OB, Addison GM, Masera G, Saha V, Biondi A, Greaves MF. Prenatal origin of acute lymphoblastic leukaemia in children. Lancet 1999; 356:1499–1503.
72. Bithell JF, Draper GJ, Gorbach PD. Association between malignant disease in children and maternal virus infection. Brit Med J 1973; 24:706–8.
73. Fine PEM, Adelstein AM, Snowman J, Clarkson JA, Evans SM. Long term effects of exposure to viral infections in utero. Brit Med J 1985; 290:509–51.
74. Stewart A, Webb J, Hewitt D. A survey of childhood malignancies. Brit Med J 1958; 4:1495–1508.
75. Zerbini M, Ernberg I. Can Epstein–Barr virus infect and transform all the b-lymphocytes of human cord blood? J Genet Virol 1983; 64:539–47.
76. de-The, G. Is Burkitt's lymphoma related to perinatal infection by Epstein–Barr virus? Lancet 1977; Feb. 12:335–8.
77. Jarrett RF, MacKenzie J. Epstein–Barr virus and other candidate viruses in the pathogenesis of Hodgkin's disease. Sem Hematol 1999; 36:260–9.
78. Jordan MC, Jordan GW, Stevens JG, Miller G. Latent herpesviruses of humans. Ann Int Med 1984; 100:866–80.
79. McKinney PA, Juszczak E, Findlay E, Smith K, Thomson CS. Pre- and perinatal risk factors for childhood leukaemia and other malignancies: a Scottish case control study. Brit J Canc 1999; 80:1844–51.
80. Schüz J, Kaatsch P, Kaletsch U, Meinert R, Michaelis J. Association of childhood cancer with factors related to pregnancy and birth. Intl J Epidemiol 1999; 28:6312–639.
81. Adelstein AM, Donovan JW. Malignant disease in children whose mothers had chickenpox, mumps, or rubella in pregnancy. Brit Med J 1972; iv:629.
82. Vianna NJ, Polan AK. Childhood lymphatic leukemia: prenatal seasonality and possible association with congenital varicella. Am J Epidemiol 1976; 103:321–32.
83. Till M, Rapson N, Smith PG. Family studies in acute leukaemia in childhood: a possible association with autoimmune disease. Brit J Canc 1979; 40:62–71.
84. Enders G, Miller E, Cradock-Watson J et al Consequences of varicella and herpes zoster in pregnancy. Prospective study of 1739 cases. Lancet 1994; 343:1548–51.
85. Grody WW, Lewin KJ, Naeim F. Detection of cytomegalovirus DNA in classic and epidemic Kaposi's sarcoma by in situ hybridization. Hum Pathol 1988; 19:524–8.
86. Rezza G, Andreoni M, Dorrucci M, Pezzotti P, Monini P, Zerboni R, Salassa B, Congangeli V, Sarmati L, Nicastri E, Barbanera M, Pristera R, Aiuti F, Ortona L, Ensoli B. Human herpesvirus 8 seropositivity and risk of Kaposi's sarcoma and other acquired immunodeficiency syndrome-related diseases. J Natl Canc Inst 1999; 91:1468–74.
87. Roman E, Ansell P, Bull D. Leukaemia and non-Hodgkin's lymphoma in children and young adults: are prenatal and neonatal factors important determinants of disease? Brit J Canc 1997; 76:406–15.
88. Selacek TV, Lindheim S, Eder C, Hasty L, Woodland M, Ludomirsky A, Rando RF Mechanism for human papillomavirus transmission at birth. Am J Obstet Gynecol 1989; 161:55–9.
89. Puranen M, Yliskoski M, Saarikoski S, Syrjanen K, Syrjanen S. Vertical transmission of human papillomavirus from infected mothers to their newborn babies and persistence of the virus in childhood. Am J Obstet Gynecol 1996; 174:694–9.
90. Watts DH, Koutsky LA, Holmes KK, Goldman D, Kuypers J, Kiviat NB, Galloway DA. Low risk of perinatal transmission of human papillomavirus: results from a prospective cohort study. Am J Obstet Gynecol 1998; 178:365–73.
91. Pakarian F, Kaye J, Cason J, Kell B, Jewers R, Derias DW, Raju KS, Best JM. Cancer associated human papillomaviruses: perinatal transmission and persistence. Brit J Obstet Gynaecol 1994; 101:514–7.
92. Chen PJ, Chen DS. Hepatitis B virus infection and hepatocellular carcinoma: molecular genetics and clinical perspectives. Sem Liver Diseases 1999; 19:253–62.

93. Chang MH, Chen DS, Hsu HC, Hsu HY, Lee CY. Maternal transmission of hepatitis B virus in childhood hepatocellular carcinoma. Cancer 1989; 64:2377–80.
94. Tong MJ, Govindarajan S. Primary hepatocellular carcinoma following perinatal transmission of hepatitis B. Western J Med 1988; 148:205–8.
95. Inaba N et al. Placental transmission of hepatitis B e antigen and clinical significance of hepatitis B e antigen titers in children born to hepatitis B e antigen-positive carrier women. Am J Obstet Gynecol 1984; 149:580–1.
96. Li L et al. Transplacental transmission of hepatitis B virus. Lancet 1988; 2:833–4.
97. Wejstal R, Widell A, Mansson, AS, Hermodsson S, Norkrans G. Mother-to-infant transmission of hepatitis C virus. Lancet 1995; 345:289–91.
98. Miller, RK. Perinatal toxicology: its recognition and fundamentals, Am J Indust Med 1983; 4:205–44.
99. Allen RW, Ogden B, Bentley FL, Jung AL. Fetal hydantoin syndrome, neuroblastoma, and hemorrhagic disease in a neonate. JAMA 1980; 244:1464–5.

Part II

Comparative Aspects of Pregnancy Development and Tumor Biology

14 Metabolism of Chemotherapeutic Drugs by Maternal and Conceptus Tissues

Mrinal K. Sanyal

Introduction

Tumor cells are genetically transformed clones of cells.[1-3] They divide vigorously under favorable conditions with doubling times ranging from several hours to years, invade host organs, attract blood vessels, secrete lysis materials and derive nutrients from the host. Tumors can be located in any body location, or metastasize by dispersal of cells to different areas, or may exist in the systemic blood circulation. The neoplastic tissue differentiation is pathological, capable of averting immune surveillance and acquiring mechanisms to destroy host tissues. Uncontrolled growth of cancer during pregnancy diverts resources from the mother and from the developing conceptus.

Pregnancy is a dynamic process associated with the development of the conceptus into placenta, fetal membranes and embryo-fetus. It is regulated by numerous metabolic processes.[4] Influences of various immunologic, endocrine and paracrine factors generated by these three interrelated components of the conceptus are central to the maintenance of normal pregnancy and fetal development. The cellular processes of receptor expression for potent biological products and drugs, changes in the membrane transport properties, and up or down regulation of numerous transcription and signal transduction factors also characterize differentiating tissues of the conceptus during pregnancy. The cellular differentiation of the conceptus is associated with the normal structural organization of tissues into organs for specialized functions, in contrast to disorganized growth in cancer.

Most cancer chemotherapeutic treatment procedures employ cytotoxic, hormonal and immunological agents or a combination of these agents.[5-7] At present, treatment is usually given at a highest tolerated dose, and the dose often is increased by using bone marrow transplantation to improve dose toleration and to overcome toxic effects. With the progress of cancer, the neoplastic cells become genetically heterogenous, and transform into a mixture of cells with different properties. Therefore, combination chemotherapy is often more effective compared to treatment with a single agent, as each drug has a different mechanism of action or attack upon a specific cell type of the neoplastic growth. An effective chemotherapy regimen is based on destruction of different neoplastic cell populations at the tolerated dose for the drug used. Adjuvant chemotherapy is application of drugs to eradicate a small population of neoplastic cells with a reduced probability of resistance early in the cancer development process or after an effective local treatment by surgical removal of the tumor, radiation or systemic chemotherapy. Neoadjuvant therapy uses drugs to reduce the tumor size prior to local treatment.

Thus, current cancer therapeutic procedures have a significant impact on the conceptus development and future wellbeing of the progeny produced. In this chapter, the interactions of the maternal system and the conceptus tissues with the chemotherapeutic drugs utilized will be discussed in relation to the growth and development of embryo-fetus. The focus of this chapter will be to describe some of the physiological and biochemical characteristics related to the metabolism of chemotherapeutic drugs since they affect both cancerous growth and the differentiating embryo-fetal tissues.

Cancer Chemotherapeutic Drugs and Mechanism of Action

The chemotherapeutic drugs are now classified on the basis of their mechanism of action and chemical derivations.[7,8] These are:

1. Antimetabolites (e. g., methotrexate, 5-fluorouracil, cytosine arabinoside) which inhibit biosynthesis or molecular polymerization of DNA by influencing both pyrimidine and purine bases
2. Alkylating agents (e. g., cyclophosphamide, ifosfamide, cisplatin and carboplatin) which produce cross-linking of macromolecules of DNA and DNA or DNA and protein, and adducts of reactive products of the drug with such macromolecules
3. Antibiotics (e. g., mitomycin C, bleomycin, doxorubicin and epirubicin, actinomycin D) which induce DNA strand breaks or intercalate to prevent unwinding of DNA helix for basic cellular activities
4. Mitotic inhibitors (e. g., vincristine, vinblastine, etoposide, teniposide, paclitaxel and docetaxel) which bind to microtubule preventing cell division
5. Natural and synthetic hormones or their inhibitors (e. g., tamoxifen, progestational agents, glucocorticoids, antiandrogens, and GnRH agonists) which bind with receptors or influence hormone responsive processes.

The antimetabolite drugs' affect on rapidly dividing cells is by abnormal substitution of nucleic acid bases into DNA rendering them incapable of replication. Methotrexate is a folic acid analog that competes with the naturally occurring dihydrofolate, thereby producing reduced folate levels in cancer cells. Since folates play an important role in purine biosynthesis, reduced folate causes cessation of DNA synthesis and death of the cancer cell. This drug can cross membranes and accumulate in body cavities and spaces, such as the pleural cavity, the "third space", from which it may be released slowly, thereby becoming a source of toxicity. Leucovorin (folinic acid), an end product of metabolism of methotrexate, is an antidote for such toxicity and also for rescuing normal cells affected by treatment with the drug. Similarly, 5-fluorouracil is a pyrimidine derivative suppressing thymidylate synthesis. Cytosine arabinoside is an analog of deoxycytidine, an inhibitor of DNA polymerase, arresting DNA synthesis and replication.

The alkylating drugs have to be activated in the maternal system. The reactive toxic metabolites are carbonium ions which cross-link macromolecules. Cyclophosphamide is activated by the mixed function oxidase enzyme system of the liver or other tissues into nitrogen mustard. Systemic toxicity for this drug can be regulated and reduced by using mesna (sodium 2-mercaptoethane sulfonate) which conjugates with the toxic metabolites to allow excretion in urine. Ifosfamide is a related alkylating compound with a side effect profile different from cyclophosphamide, and in general, it is less toxic. Cisplatin is a chlorinated platinum compound that may also cross-link with macromolecules for destruction of cancer cells. A major side effect of this drug is renal toxicity. A less reactive analog is carboplatinum which has similar cytotoxic effects, but with a reduced renal toxicity potential. The other cytotoxic compounds, melphalen, nitrogen mustard, and nitrosurea are used infrequently for specific cancers.

The antibiotics, actinomycin D and doxorubicin, are derived from the fungus *Streptomyces*, and they act by intercalation between DNA base pairs inhibiting RNA synthesis, and by interaction with DNA topoisomerase II to produce DNA strand breaks. Mitomycin C and derivatives of this class are promising bioreductive drugs. Bleomycin is a mixture of cytotoxic antibiotic peptides which produce similar DNA strand breaks by forming ferrous iron complexes with DNA. The derivatives of vinca plant alkaloids, vincristine and vinblastine, bind with tubulin subunits inhibiting spindle formation for cell division resulting in metaphase arrest. Etoposide and teniposide are semisynthetic glycoside derivatives of mandrake plant products. They bind to tubulin and DNA topoisomerase II inducing DNA breaks. Paclitaxel (Taxol) is an alkaloid of the yew tree, composed of complex of taxane ring structure. It also binds to microtubules preventing depolymerization, the opposite action of the vinca alkaloids.

Tamoxifen is a nonsteroidal antiestrogenic agent, which can bind competitively with estrogen receptors. The translocated receptor complex in the cell's nucleus inhibits both DNA and RNA synthesis. Tamoxifen inhibits estrogen-receptor-positive breast cancer and thereby benefits only one-third of patients with breast cancer. Recently, the possible prophylactic use of this drug has shown some success. Similar nonsteroidal antiandrogen derivatives are also used for prostate cancer treatment. Glucocorticoids have antitumor effects and are also useful in treatments of complications induced by cancer therapies.

Pregnancy Factors that Influence Cancer Chemotherapy

Physiology of Pregnancy

Human pregnancy is a specialized condition with innumerable maternal physiological adaptations for growth and development of the embryo-fetus.[9,10] There are three basic interacting compartments during pregnancy: maternal, placental and fetal. These collectively contribute to the progressive development and, finally, birth of the neonate. The changes in maternal body weight, plasma proteins and body fats are highly significant during pregnancy. In addition, adaptations in maternal physiology should be a consideration for cancer drug treatment during pregnancy. These adaptations include:

1 altered water and electrolyte balance which promote a rapid increase in the plasma volume to 40% above non-pregnant values at term

2 hemodynamic changes influenced by increased cardiac output altering the blood flow of the uteroplacental unit and other maternal organs

3 an increase of the renal glomerular filtration rate of the mother by more than 50% by the twelfth week of gestation.

Numerous hormones, growth factors, specific proteins and immunity products are expressed during pregnancy.[11-13] Some of them are mitogenic and may promote growth of the tumor during pregnancy. In addition, the conceptus is an allograft, and the invading trophoblast cells suppress the immune suppressive system. This process along with numerous cytokines may also influence the cancer process during pregnancy. At present, effects of such factors on the development, progress and suppression of cancer during pregnancy are of research interest, as they may arrest cancer progression.[14,15] It is known that some of the properties and products generated by cancer tissues are common to conceptus tissues (e.g. invasion into host tissues and expression of embryonic antigens). The strategies for treatment of pregnant patients based on such knowledge have remained to a great extent unexplored.[16,17]

Placental-Fetal Anatomy and Transport

Soon after nidation of the embryo on the maternal uterine epithelium, the embryonic trophoblast invades and establishes a chorioallantoic placentation with protruding and branching chorionic villi within the intervillus space that contains maternal blood. The fetal capillary system, trophoblast and mesenchymal cells of the villi participate in the gaseous exchange and transfer of the nutritional and hormonal materials from the maternal blood into the fetus (Fig. 14.1).[18,19] The vasculature for exchanges is not fully established until the twelfth week of gestation and exchanges prior to this period are by direct contact with decidual cells. The interface between the maternal compartment and the fetus is the trophoblast cell layer of the villi which is the critical anatomical structure that to a great extent is responsible for regulation of the transport of nutrients and entry of drugs into the fetal compartment. During the early stages of placental development, blood in the fetal capillaries is separated from that in the maternal intervillus space by endothelial cells of fetal blood vessels, subepithelial basement membrane (basal lamina), and coverings of the trophoblastic cell layer (Fig. 14.1).

Initially, the external villus layer is made of mononucleated cytotrophoblast cells which progressively differentiate into an outer layer of multinuclated syncytiotrophoblast cells. The core of the villus is a matrix of trophoblast cells (Langerhans cells), fibroblast cells, phagocytic Hofbauer cells and fetal capillaries.[20] In later stages of pregnancy, cytotrophoblast cells are sparse and form an inner layer along with fetal mesenchymal tissues. Exchanges between maternal and fetal systems occur mostly in areas where there is a thin syncytiotrophoblast layer and a basement membrane separating them. The exchange areas are located toward the surface of the villi. The areas of biosynthesis are in the body of syncitiotrophoblast and cytotrophoblast cells. The peripheral trophoblast surface area of the human placenta is approximately 1.2 m^2 at 14 weeks and increases to 13.4 m^2 at term.[21,22] The total trophoblast cell surface area available for exchanges and maternal interactions, estimated by electron microscopic morphometric analysis of the microvilli of the syncytiotrophoblast cell surface, increases by a factor of 9.47 during mid-gestation, from less than 20 m^2 at 22 weeks to 94 m^2 at 36 weeks of gestation, and then decreases slightly by the fortieth week. Anatomical features of the basement membrane have

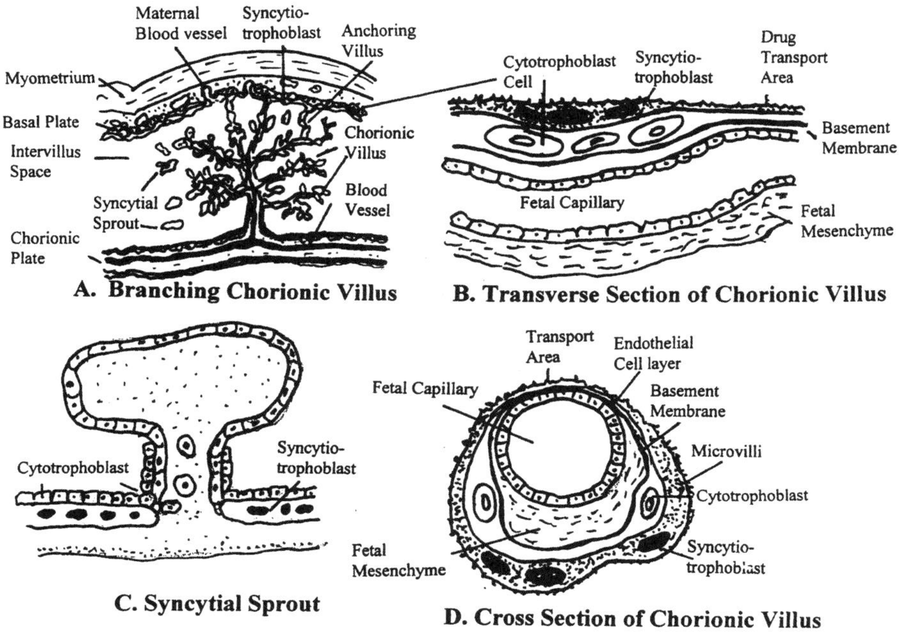

Fig. 14.1. **a** Branching chorionic villus. A diagrammatic representation of different structures associated with placental chorionic villus. The outer muscular layer is myometrium. The inner basal plate is highly vascularized and maternal blood vessels open into the intravillus space. The basal plate is also lined with layers of cytotrophoblast and syncytiotrophoblast cells facing the intravillus space. Within the intervillus space are the branching chorionic villi, some of which extend into the basal plate as anchoring villi. The branching villi are bathed within the intravillus space containing maternal blood pool. **b** Transverse section of the chorionic villus. A villus contains a capillary system surrounded by mesenchymal tissues. A basement membrane separates the inner cytotrophoblast cells and syncytiotrophoblast layer from the endothelial cells of the capillary. The cytotrophoblast cells are nucleated and secretory. The syncytiotrophoblast cells are multinucleated external to cytotrophoblasts with projected micropapillae which increase the surface for transfer of material from the maternal blood. In certain areas, the capillary system is opposed to the basement membrane and form thin areas which presumably are most effective in transport processes. **c** Syncytial Sprout. These structures are detached from the growing villus. They have a matrix surrounded by syncytial cells. The detached sprouts are released into the intervillus space and travel through maternal vessels. **d** Cross section of chorionic villus. The same structures of the transverse section are represented: the outer syncytiotrophoblast, inner cytotropblast, mesenchyme and fetal capillary with endothelium. (Adapted from Chard[12]; Williams[18])

been linked to smoking and to diseases such as pre-eclampsia and diabetes, and it may provide a barrier to drug transfer.[23]

Recent studies on the anatomy of the human placenta with the aid of scanning electron microscope have revealed the features of the syncytial sprouts (Fig. 14.1). They are mushroom-like outgrowths of the villus surface which provide the foundation for new villus formation during the first trimester of pregnancy.[24,25] These sprouts are proliferation areas connected by slender stalks. They may also fuse with the neighboring villi to form band shaped bridges. The syncytial sprouts of the mature placenta undergo degenerative changes. These sprouts often are detached and released into the maternal blood circulation. It is estimated that nearly 100,000 sprouts are shed daily in the maternal circulation. These sprouts often migrate from the placenta and settle in the maternal lung and disappear by lysis. Occasionally, they are neoplastic and a source of neoplastic disease.[18]

A number of factors may influence transplacental transfer of drugs.[26,27] The physiological factors of maternal hemodynamic changes of greater blood flow and volume, increased kidney filtration rates, and augmented metabolism and concentrations of nutritional substrates are important. Additionally, dissociation, receptor binding and metabolic characteristics of the drug in the maternal organs and placental tissues define the nature of placental transport, active or passive. In general, lipid soluble drugs and agents readily transfer across the placental barrier.[28] The placental transfer of cancer drugs is broadly regulated by dissociation potentials of the drug into ions, water and lipid solubilization properties, and cell surface receptor systems for its internalization. Metabolite production and binding of metabolite with carrier proteins or ligands for removal are also central to their transport into the fetal compartment. For example, antibiotics are poorly lipid soluble drugs and do not enter cells readily, whereas metabolized cytotoxic drugs with teratogenic potential bind to macromolecules and readily diffuse into the fetal compartment. The water soluble molecules up to 100 Da molecular weight, and lipid soluble drug molecules of 1000 Da may readily cross the placental barrier. A most important consideration in assessing the potential for birth defects of chemotherapeutic drugs is the possibility of their transfer into the fetus. At present, the placental transfer properties for a vast majority of cancer drugs are unknown. This gap in our knowledge is a major limitation for rational cancer treatment during pregnancy.

In addition to the placenta, the human fetal tissue is a major site for drug metabolism. Fig. 14.2 shows the early development of fetal organs.[29] Liver buds appear by the fourth week of development (Streeter Stage XII) and differentiate into two distinct lobes by the eighth week (Stage XX). A most noteworthy feature at this period is the loss of the right umbilical vein and the formation of the ductus venosus. The umbilical vein is the direct link for the incoming placental effluent into the heart. In addition, the portal sinus and blood vessels arising from it supply the right and left lobes of the liver. The hepatic veins carry blood from the liver into the inferior vena cava, and finally into the heart. The fetal circulation is regulated by umbilical blood flow and hypoxic conditions.[30] It is estimated that approximately 40% of fetal cardiac output is distributed to the placental circulation, and the same amount is returned to the heart via the umbilical vein. A portion of the return supplies the liver and the remainder passes through the ductus venosus into the inferior vena cava. The fetal liver also receives blood from the portal vein and hepatic artery. The hepatic arterial blood is equally distributed between the right and left lobes, whereas, the left lobe is exclusively supplied by the umbilical venous blood.

Pharmacokinetics of Cancer Drugs

Handling of drugs during gestation is markedly different from that of the non-pregnant state because of the progressive physiological changes that characterize the human pregnancy.[31-34] The developing conceptus is in close contact with the maternal tissues. The trophoblast villi are bathed within the maternal blood, and pharmacokinetic information about the drugs being used would be useful for optimal adjustment of the doses. Cancer treatment during pregnancy is highly complex as these drugs have a low therapeutic index and they affect both cancer cells and normal maternal and placental-fetal cells. The level of exposure of the cancer drugs toxic to trophoblast cells, and the mechanisms of toxic action on such cells, are unknown. It is

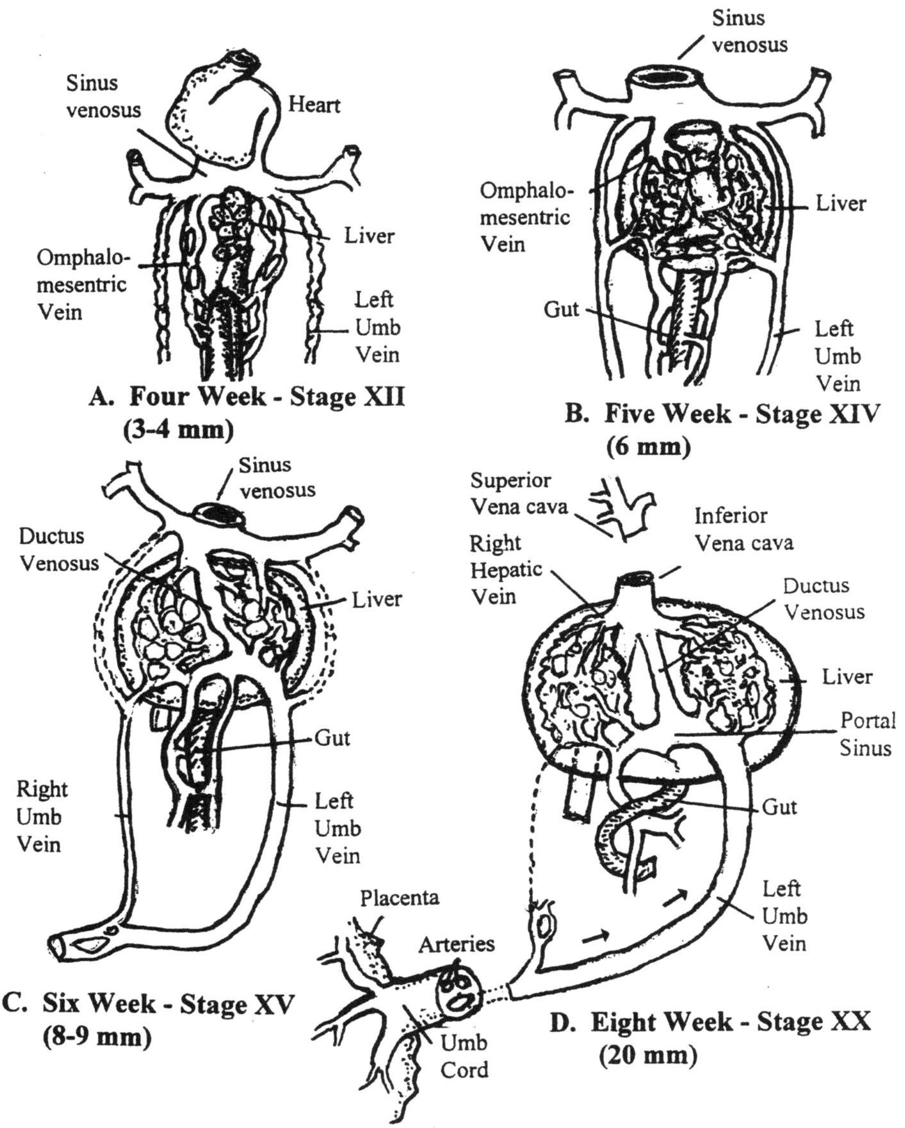

Fig.14.2. Diagrammatic representations of development of fetal vascular system during the organogenesis stage. Most notable feature in this process is the initial loss of both right and left anterior umbilical (Umb) veins, and later in development the right posterior umblical vein atrophies. The placental effluents are carried by the left umbilical vein primarily into the right liver lobe. The portal sinus develops the ductus venosus for direct drainage of oxygenated placental blood into the heart at the time of fetal distress. The umbilical cord from the second trimester onward has two arterial vessels and one venous vessel. (Redrawn from Patten[29])

likely that proliferating cells of the chorionic villi are destroyed at high doses, and thereby the transport mechanisms of nutrients and toxins into the fetal compartment are altered. Entry of toxic agents into fetal compartment leads to anomalous development.

Phamacokinetic values include the rate of absorption of the drugs, their distribution to various organs including the conceptus, and finally biotransformation and excretion potentials in the patient. Doses and routes of administration are chosen based on tumor burden, level of cell heterogeniety, drug resistance, and patient specific factors of drug metabolism. Concentration of the drug in the maternal system is the most critical factor during therapy. Therefore, the efficacy of the drug is regulated by bioavailability, detoxification, and clearance potentials by kidney and biliary routes. Standardized protocols considering the drug toxicity potential to the conceptus during cancer therapy at present are not available.

Metabolism of Cancer Chemotherapeutic Drugs

Cytochrome P450 (CYP-gene family)

Expression of Cytochrome P450 enzymes, which are phase-1 enzymes, is the principal enzyme system involved in biotransformation of cancer chemotherapeutic agents into activation- and detoxification-products.[35] In phase-1 reactions, functional hydroxyl and amine groups are introduced into the drug molecule by oxidation, reduction and hydrolysis to make it polar and more potent for killing of cancer cells. In addition, availability of such chemical groups allows conjugation with various ligands (e.g. glutathione) by the phase-2 enzymes for detoxification and systemic elimination.[36,37] The phase-1 reactions are catalyzed primarily by cytochrome P450 oxidases, which are iron containing hemoproteins, and by NADPH conjugated cytochrome P450 reductases. The oxidation reaction involves the utilization of molecular oxygen for the formation of hydroxylated drug derivatives, and the reductive processes leading to generation of reactive free radicals. These enzymes are widely distributed in mammalian organ tissues, but the liver is the most active site for metabolism of various drugs and xenobiotic agents. These enzymes are also present in conceptus tissues (placenta and fetus), and presumably participate in the metabolic processing of chemotherapeutic cancer drugs.

The cytochrome P450 enzymes are highly versatile and catalyze thousands of different chemical substrates. They exist in multiple forms or isoenzymes, identified with the root symbol CYP.[38-41] At present, nearly 500 genes for these enzymes, classified into 74 gene families, have been recognized. These enzymes participate actively in the metabolism of anticancer drugs and in drug interactions.[42,43] Among these, more than 90% of drug metabolism in humans is performed by the following enzymes: CYPs 1A2; 2C9, 10, 19; 2D6; 2E1; and 3A4. The CYPs, 2C, 2D and 3A are the most prevalent cytochrome P450 isoenzymes in human tissues involved in biotransformation of various drugs. It is now established that these enzymes show variable expression based on the genetic constitution of the patient. Differences in metabolism by these enzymes can be related to the effectiveness of the drug. The interindividual variation of metabolic activity due to genetic polymorphisms, and identification of specific metabolism phenotypes, will be important in designing the most effective cancer therapies with specific drugs.

A number of isoenzymes of CYP 2- A6, B1, B6, C8, C11 and C19 are known to be associated with toxic activation product formation from cyclophosphamide, and CYP3 A1 and A4 are the primary enzymes for activation of the analog ifosfamide.[44–51] The reactive alkylating products may cross-link with DNA strands and induce genotoxic effects. Isoforms of CYP associated with metabolism of other primary chemotherapeutic drugs: paclitaxel (CYP 2C8 and 3A4); vinca alkaloids (CYP 3A4); thio-TEPA (CYP 2B,C6 and C11) and tamoxifen (CYP 1A, 2C9, 2D6, 3A1 and 3A4); they are outlined in Table 14.1.[52–75]

Cancer chemotherapy employs multiple drugs simultaneously, and often additional drugs are used as adjuncts for controlling symptoms of side effects of the drugs used or other diseases simultaneously. Therefore, prevention of drug–drug interactions is an important aspect of clinical management of the cancer patient.[43] Use of different drugs in combination may contribute to the absence or excessive toxicity of the chemotherapeutic drugs. A primary mechanism of drug interaction involves the expression of specific CYPs for metabolism of the drug. Inhibition or amplification of CYP enzyme activities induced by these drugs leads to such undesired effects. Specific artificial metabolic substrates can be used to identify phenotypes (subjects) who show a reduced or extensive metabolism potential. The choice of appropriate drugs based on the CYP enzyme expression potential is an expanding area of investigation for the better treatment of cancer patients (Table 14.1).

Table 14.1. A partial list of cytochrome P450 isoenzymes associated with the metabolism of cancer chemotherapeutic drugs

Antineoplastic drugs	Cytochrome P450 isoenzyme	Absence of isoenzyme acitivty	Specific function of isoenzyme
Cyclophosphamide/isofosfamide	2A6	Reduced effect*	Activation
	2B1, 6	Reduced effect	Activation
	2C8,9,19	Reduced effect	Activation
	3A4	Reduced effect	Activation
	3A4,5	Increased toxicity**	Elimination
Tamoxifen	1A	Increased toxicity	Elimination
	2C9	Increased toxicity	Elimination
	2D6	Increased toxicity	Elimination
	3A1	Increased toxicity	Elimination
	3A4	Increased toxicity	Elimination
Taxol	2C8	Increased toxicity	Elimination
	3A4	Increased toxicity	Elimination
Vinca alkaloid	3A	Increased toxicity	Elimination
Thio-TEPA	2B1	Reduced effect	Activation
	2C11	Reduced effect	Activation

* Reduced therapeutic effect due to absence of activation of the drug for destruction of cancer cells.
** Increased toxicity due to absence of metabolism of the drug and absence of elimination by detoxification processes.

Bioactivation and Adduct Formation

The chemotherapeutic drugs, cyclophosphamide and its isomer, ifosfamide, that has less myelosuppression, are alkylating agents which require metabolic bioactivation by microsomal cytochrome P450s into toxic reactive agents.[44–48] The bioactivation process involves formation of a 4-hydroxy metabolite and open ringed aldophosphoramide, which then decomposes into phosphoramide mustard and acrolein.[49-51] They cross-link macromolecules and produce lesions in DNA strands. Genotoxicity includes increase in sister chromatid exchanges and break of meiotic synaptonemal complexes. Genetic damage induced by reactive metabolites are the primary mechanisms of cytotoxicity in cancer cells.

Doxorubicin (Adriamycin) and other antineoplastic anthracyclin drugs containing a quinone moiety are metabolized by NDPH-cytochrome P450 reductase to form semiquinone, a reactive free radical.[52–53] The free radicals intercalate with cellular DNA and also interact with the enzyme topoisomerase II causing breaks in double strands of DNA and subsequent cell death. Doxorubicin crosslinks with 5′-GC sequences which are abundantly present in the transcription factor binding sites, promoter and enhancer regions of genes. Mitomycins also undergo a similar bioreduction to be reactive cytotoxic agents. A new analog of mitomycin, KW2149, is activated in the human serum, in contrast to cellular activation, and appears to be a promising drug for cancer treatment.[54–56] Cisplatin is a chlorinated platinum compound, and in an aqueous environment, chloride ions are displaced from the electrophilic species.[57-59] These react with various cellular elements, including DNA, the primary target of cell toxicity. A number of DNA adducts of cisplatin have been identified. These adducts are in the major groove of DNA. The primary molecular mechanism of the genotoxic effect of the drug is the formation of adducts of cisplatin to DNA which prevents DNA replication.

Detoxification of Drugs

Detoxification of drugs is an important metabolic step that regulates bioavailability and drug actions in the patient. A widely used breast cancer drug, tamoxifen, is detoxified by several CYPs, and an absence of metabolism leads to increased toxicity (Table 14.1).[60-62] Similarly, the effect of paclitaxel (taxol), a plant derived product that inhibits cancer growth by promoting and stabilizing microtubule assembly, depends on metabolism by CYPs. This drug interacts with tubulin and inhibits cell replication in the late G_2 stage of the cell cycle. In vitro studies with human liver slices and microsomes revealed that it is metabolized into several products.[63-68] Hydroxylation of the C-6 alpha position of the taxol ring produces the primary detoxification product that is detected in bile. In addition, C-3 and C-13 hydroxylated metabolites of taxol are generated as minor metabolites. Similar metabolic detoxification processes have been described for the microtubule inhibitors, vinca alkaloid,[69-72] and thio-TEPA.[73-75]

Detoxification of chemotherapeutic drugs by an initial metabolism by CYPs and subsequent conjugation with ligands is a major pathway for elimination. Enzymes associated with conjugation are: glutathione S-transferase (GST), UDP glucuronidase, carboxyesterase and a number of transferases (sulfo-, methyl- and acetyl). Epoxide hydrolase is often considered a detoxifying enzyme, especially for a wide variety of xenobiotic agents. GST is expressed in four isoforms, α, μ, π and θ in humans, and their expression is important in detoxification of the electrophilic metabolites produced by the chemotherapeutic cancer drugs.[76-79] In addition, expression of P-glycoprotien (encoded by multidrug resistance gene, MDR1) reduces the efficacy of cytototoxic drugs, and the excision repair enzymes also detoxify the adduct producing cancer drugs.[80-83] Therefore, a combination of functions of both activation and detoxification enzymes regulate the effectiveness of chemotherapeutic drugs.

Metabolism of Drugs and Xenobiotics by the Conceptus

Early Development and Organogenesis

As the conceptus grows during pregnancy, it progressively develops the capability for metabolizing different types of xenobiotics and drugs. It is known that mixed function oxidase activity may be expressed during the preimplantation stages of development.[84-86] Such enzyme expression during the prenatal period has been shown using different models.[87-89] Since organogenesis is the most critical stage for birth defects, numerous studies have been performed using the rat whole embryo culture system exploring the metabolic potential of the conceptus at this period.[90-97] In these experimental studies using the whole embryo culture system, it has been established that cancer chemotherapeutic drugs, such as cyclophophamide, may induce dysmorphogenesis, and bioactivation of the cyclophosphamide into an active metabolite by microsomes is essential for production of embryotoxicity. Human embryonic tissues are also responsive to metabolic conversion of such teratogens.[98-99]

The causes of birth defects and intrauterine toxicity is a multifactorial process and generation of toxic metabolites is a major factor in this process.[100-104] At present, the overall metabolic capability of the human conceptus at different stages of gestation for numerous chemotherapeutic drugs remains unknown. Cytochrome P450s (CYP gene family) are important enzymes in this regard, and their relative expression is important in cancer therapy. A differential expression potential of these genes in the fetal and placental compartments and comparison with adult expressions have been outlined in Table 14.2.

Metabolism by Fetal Tissues

As early as 1970, Yaffe et al described the presence of monooxygenase enzyme system in the human fetal tissues.[105] Numerous subsequent studies have shown that these enzymes are expressed and play a critical role in the bioactivation of drugs, procarcinogens and xenobiotics.[106-110] The human fetal liver expresses: CYPs 1A1, B1; 2C8, D6, E1; 3A4, A5, and A7 during the organogenesis phase of development.[104] Specific CYP isoforms are expressed differentially in adult and fetal tissues, and fetal stage specificities are also wide.[111-115]

CYP1A1 expression begins before 20 weeks of gestation, while CYP1A2 and CYP1B1 expression remains highly reduced in human fetal hepatic tissues.[104,116] CYP2C and CYP2C8 expression products are detectable at low levels in the fetal liver before 20 weeks of gestation. CYP2D6 gene is expressed as mRNA as early as 11 weeks of pregnancy; however, the functional protein is detectable only after 20 weeks' gestation.[104,117,118] A most interesting situation is observed with regard to the expression of CYP2E1, which is inducible by alcohol exposure.[119-121] Studies of Vieira et al showed that this cytochome isoenzyme is low during early prenatal development, and that expression begins by 16 weeks of gestation and dramatically increases after birth.[122]

Table 14.2. Differential distribution of human CYP-gene family in different compartments during pregnancy *

CYP-gene	Adult	Embryo/Fetus	Placenta
CYP1A1	Hepatic (low); extrahepatic tissues	Hepatic (> 20 week)Lung	Induced by smoke exposure (first trimester and term)
CYP1A2	Hepatic (high);	Hepatic (low) extrahepatic (umbilical vein endothelium)	Low; not induced by exposure
CYP1B1	Number of organs; hydroxylation of 17β–estradiol	Hepatic (low, first trimester); Extrahepatic tissues – brain, adrenal, kidney, lungs, heart	Low; not induced by exposure
CYP2A5	—	Adrenal	—
CYP2A6	Hepatic (individual variation)	—	—
CYP2A7	Hepatic (individual variation)	—	—
CYP2B6	Hepatic (low) hydroxylation at 16α and β	—	—
CYP2B7	Hepatic (low); *O*-deethylation	—	—
CYP2C8	Hepatic (high); drug metabolism	Hepatic (< 20 weeks)	—
CYP2C9	Hepatic (high) inducible with drugs; non-steroidal	—	—
CYP2C18	Hepatic	—	—
CYP2C19	Hepatic (variable expression)	—	—
CYP2D6	Hepatic (high); drug metabolizing (variable expression)	Hepatic (first trimester); Neurons (brain)	—
CYP2E1	Hepatic (high) and extrahepatic tissues; drug and environmental agent metabolism	Hepatic (after16 weeks) low before birth, high after birth; Brain (7–17 weeks)	Expressed in first trimester and term placenta; alcohol metabolism
CYP2F1	Lung	—	—
CYP2J2	Heart (high) and other organs; Arachidonic acid metabolism	—	—

CYP-gene	Adult	Embryo/Fetus	Placenta
CYP3A4	Hepatic (high) and many extrahepatic tissues (gut); exogenous and endogenous substrate metabolism; drug interaction potential; major form of CYP for drugs	Hepatic (first trimester)	Expressed in term, not in first trimester
CYP3A5	Hepatic and extrahepatic tissues; highly variable; 6β–hydroxylation; 2–hydroxylation of estradiol–17β	Hepatic (first trimester)	Expressed in term, not in first trimester
CYP3A7	Hepatic (absent or low)	Hepatic (high) embryonic stage to birth; shifts to CYPA4 after birth; steroid 6β– and 16α–hydroxylation; major form of CYP.Adrenal (high)	Expressed in first trimester, not in term (<17 weeks)
CYP4A9	Various organs; metabolize fatty acids and leukotrienes	—	—
CYP4 B1	Lung (not in liver)	—	First trimester and term
CYP5	Thromboxane synthesis	—	—
CYP7	Cholesterol-7α hydroxylation	—	—
CYP8	Prostacyclin synthesis	—	—
CYP11	Cholesterol side-chain cleavage, 11β-hydroxylation aldosterone synthesis	—	—
CYP17	Steroid 17α-hydroxylation	Adrenal	—
CYP19	Aromatization of androgens	—	Expressed in first trimester and term – enzymes for estrogen biosynthesis; xenobiotic metabolism
CYP21	Steroid 21-hydroxylation	—	—
CYP24	Steroid 24-hydroxylation	—	—
CYP27	Steroid 27-hydroxylation	—	—
CYP51	Synthesis of sterols	—	—

* Data from Hakkola et al.104 and others.

Both CYP3A4 and CYP3A5 are expressed at a reduced level in the fetal liver. CYP3A4 is a major form of cytochrome P450 in the adult human liver. In contrast, CYP3A7 is the most important form of CYP expressed in the fetal liver.[123-126] Its nucleotide sequence is 90% identical to the adult form CYP3A4. It represents nearly one-third of total CYP in the fetal liver, and shift of expression potential to CYP3A4 occurs immediately after birth.[127] Participation of the CYP3A7 isoenzyme in 6β- position hydroxylation of testosterone is a major function of this cytochome P450 isoenzyme. In addition, CYP3A7 catalyzes the formation of 16β-hydroxy-dehydroepiandrosterone-3-sulfate (DHEAS) from DHEAS. This is the precursor for estrogen biosynthesis in the human placenta.[104] Potential for such metabolism in various extrahepatic tissues and in the adrenal of the fetus is as yet unknown.

Metabolism by Placental Tissue

Human placental tissue is a major metabolic site.[128-130] However, the metabolic capability for drugs and xenobiotics is relatively lower compared to that in the liver. In many metabolic processes placenta and fetus complement each other, and the placental metabolic potential is influenced by maternal endocrine and paracrine systems.

Numerous studies of the human placenta have shown that human placenta expresses a cigarette smoke inducible cytochrome P 450 localized in the microsomal fraction.[131-138] Recent studies in this area extended these findings showing that CYP1A1 (aryl hydrocarbon hydroxylase) is an inducible CYP, and expressed abundantly in both first trimester and term placentas.[139-144] The expression of this enzyme system occurs in the trophoblast cell layer of the human chorionic villi at the interface between the mother and the fetus (Fig. 14.3).[142,144] The CYP is involved in both activation and detoxification of drugs and xenobiotics.

A most intriguing discovery is that the human placental villi also express detoxification enzyme glutathione S-transferase in trophoblast cells as shown for CYP1A1 and the epoxide hydrolase in stromal cells. The observation of expression of these enzymes in the placental tissues of the first trimester, the most sensitive period for birth defects, is highly significant (see Fig. 14.3).[142] Thus, it is likely that chemical agents and drugs entering into villi cells from the maternal blood are subjected to metabolism and detoxification by both phase-1 cytochrome P 450 (CYP1A1) and phase-2 enzymes present in chorionic villi tissues.[145-150] Whether such metabolic activities in the human placenta are correlated with the abnormal development of the embryo-fetus is at present unknown.[134]

The expression potential of CYP1A1 depends on a number of factors, in particular, the receptor system at the cell membrane and a cascade of cellular processes and genetic factors associated with such augmentation.[151,152] A study from our laboratory on benzo[a]pyrene metabolism potential of human placental microsomes from both smoker and non-smoker donors showed that in vitro benzo[a]pyrene metabolism is significantly augmented by maternal cigarette smoke exposure, but only in a subset of placental samples assessed by the cluster analysis of the data (5/32; 15%; procedures outlined in ref. 143). The reactive benzo[a] pyrene metabolite production in the same assay mixture (analyzed by their binding with exogenous DNA) was not correlated to the overall metabolic capability. A scatter plot depicting these results shows that samples with greater metabolic potential are readily identifiable on the right side of the scatter plot (Fig. 14.4). Induction of placental metabolic potential for this xenobiotic was not related to DNA binding reactive product formation. Therefore, it is possible that detoxified product generation from such agents in the human placenta

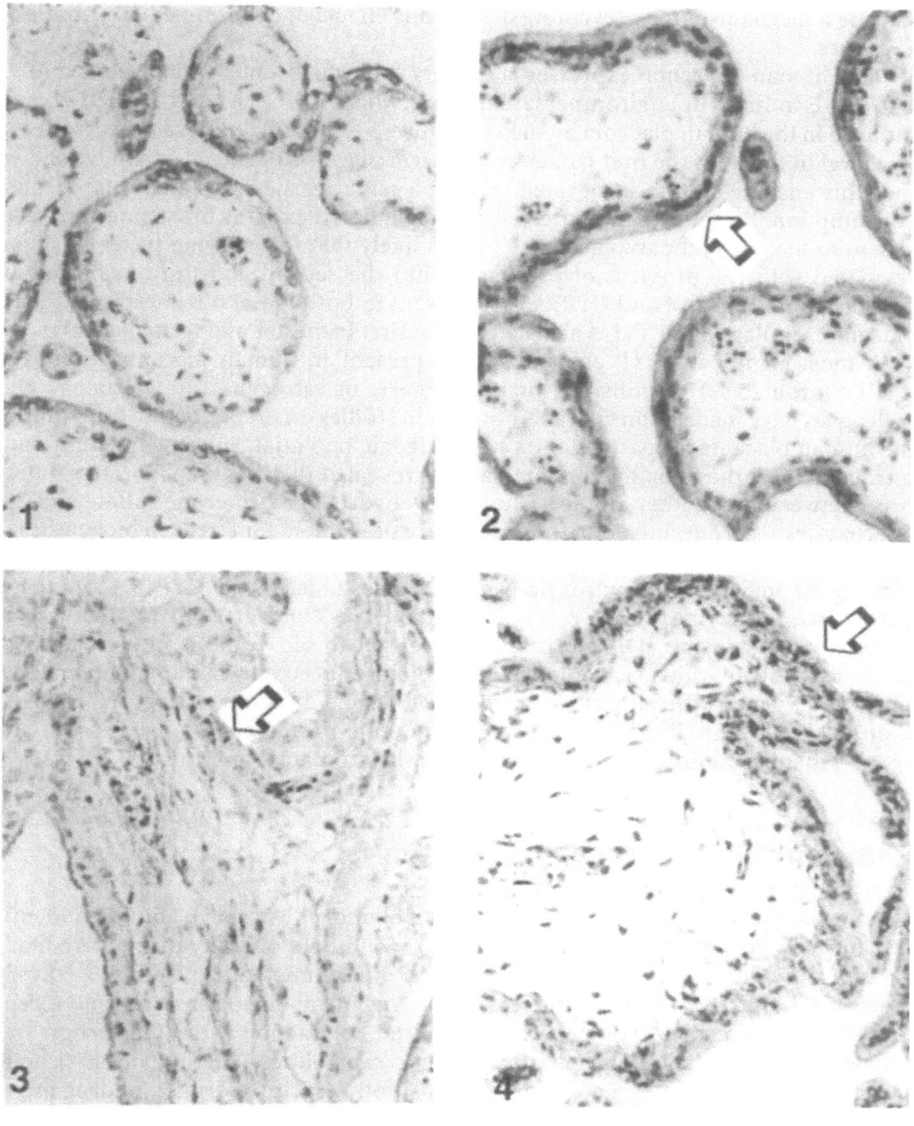

Figure 14.3. Immunocytochemical localization of the xenobiotic metabolizing enzymes in the trophoblastic cells of human chorionic villi at 10 weeks of pregnancy. **1** Control preparation of villi sample from a mother who smoked 30 cigarettes/day without antibody treatment. **2** Cytochrome P450 (CYP1A1) is localized in trophoblast cell layer of villi from a mother who also smoked 30 cigaretted/day. The trophoblast cell layer stained intensely with the antibody preparation MAb 1-7-1, indicating expression of this cytochrome isoenzyme (arrow). **3** The mesenchymal cells of the chorionic villi from a nonsmoker mother stained with an antibody preparation for epoxide hydrolase. The enzyme is differentially expressed in the mesenchymal cells (arrow). **4** Positive yellowish stain over the trophoblast cell layer of chorionic villi of a smoker mother (30 cigarettes/day) by an antibody prepared from glutathione S-transferase (arrow). This comparative study showed that the human first trimester placenta expresses these enzymes responsible for xenobiotic metabolism. It is likely that these enzymes participate in the metabolism of agents present in the maternal blood of placental intervillus space and provide a detoxification defense for the fetus toward xenobiotic exposure. Such metabolic potential in placenta may prevent transfer of toxic agents and drugs into the fetal compartment. Adapted from ref. 142.

may be a mechanism for preventing deleterious effects of environmental xenobiotic exposure.

The human placenta expresses a variety of cytochrome P450 isoenzymes.[104] CYP1A1 is induced by environmental exposure, whereas CYP1A2 and CYP1B1 are not induced in the human placenta by such exposure.[140] CYP2E1 is expressed (mRNA) at a low level in the both the first trimester and term placenta. Rasheed et al have shown that this enzyme system is elevated in the placental tissues after maternal alcohol consumption.[153,154] CYP3A7 is expressed in placental tissues of the first trimester, but is absent in the term human placenta .[104, 155] It is likely that this enzyme system is down regulated with the progress of pregnancy into the second and third semester. In contrast, both CYP3A4 and CYP3A5 are present in both the first trimester and term placenta. Similarly, CYP4B1 is also detected in first trimester and term placentas.

A most significant CYP enzyme system present in human placental tissues is CYP19 (aromatase) responsible for biosynthesis of estrogens.[156,157] Diczfalusy and colleagues have made a considerable advance in studies on the endocrine functions of the human placenta, in particular its steroidogenic potential. Subsequent studies on estrogen biosynthesis by the human placenta revealed that it is a cooperative enterprise between the mother and the fetus.[158-162] Dehydroepiandroterone sulfate and 16-hydroxy-testosterone and androstenedione are precursors for estrogen biosynthesis. These are largely provided by the fetus. The functions of both placental CYP17 (coding for enzymes 17α hydroxylase and 17,20 desmolase) and CYP19 (coding for aromatization enzymes of ring A of the steroid nucleus), and fetal CYP3A7 (coding for hydroxylation enzyme at 16 position), are central to biosynthesis of estrogens, in particular, estriol which is an important steroid produced during human pregnancy. The CYP19 gene is the largest cytochrome P450 gene. It is interesting that the first exon of CYP19 remains untranslated and alternate promoters are used in a tissue specific manner for initiating transcription of the aromatase enzyme.[163-165]

Pharmacogentics of Cancer Therapy

A large number of mutations and an array of polymorphisms have now been identified for CYP genes. Pharmacogenetics is a growing field of study of the hereditary basis of differences in responses to drugs and environmental exposures.[166-170] Every individual has a set of unique alleles encoding drug metabolizing enzymes and receptors that regulate efficacy of a specific drug used, interaction with other drugs, and activation, detoxification and pharmacokinetic capabilities. The individual genetic variability produces differences in drug disposition, toxicity to drugs and drug interactions. Monitoring of this variability to identify the appropriate drugs and drug doses may improve therapy for the patient. Numerous studies described the differences in various drug metabolism capability in human populations.[171,172] Based on these studies three categories of metabolizers have been identified: slow, rapid and ultrarapid.[173]

Among these enzymes, phase-1 monooxygenase cytochrome P450s (CYPs) which promote activation into reactive metabolites or hydroxylation for detoxification of drugs or xenobiotics have been center stage. Wide variations of CYP genes due to mutations or polymorphisms have been recognized. Identification of cancer susceptibility due to such hereditary changes in CYP genes has remained elusive.[174-179] However, individualization of drug therapy is beginning to take shape.[180-183] Required drug doses for an effective therapy can vary between individuals significantly, as

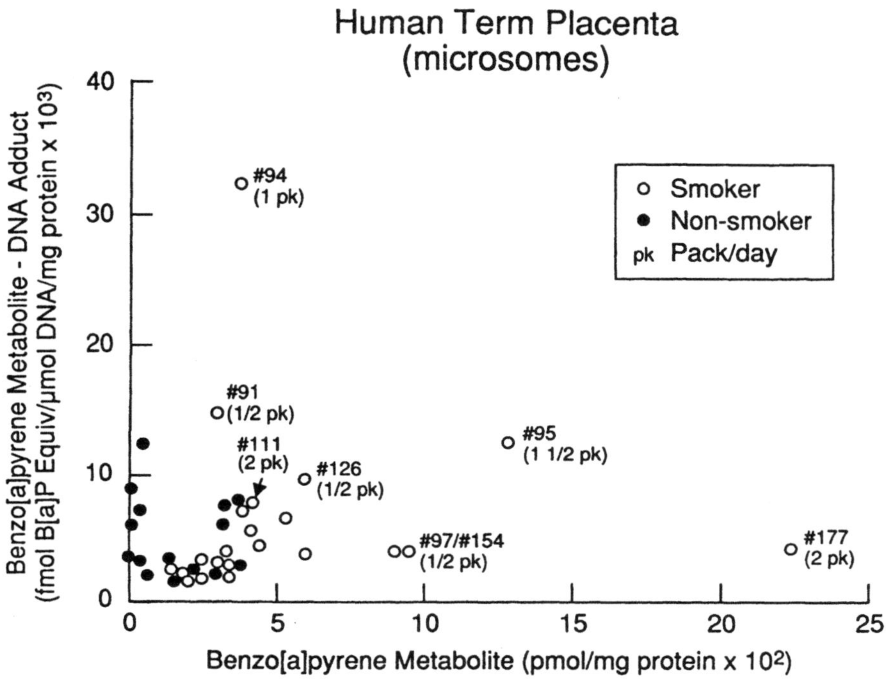

Figure 14.4. The relationship of overall benzo[a]pyrene (B[a]P) hydroxylase activity (B[a]P metabolism) and B[a]P-metabolite-DNA adduct production by the same term placental microsomal preparation under identical in vitro conditions. The estimates in placental samples of smoker donors could be classified into two groups: (i) nonresponsive phenotype which produced highly reduced quantities of metabolites with values similar to nonsmoker samples (left) and (ii) responsive phenotype with increased metabolic activity. In 4 responsive samples, metabolite values extend into far right-end of the plot (# 95, 97, 154 and 177) with reduced DNA-B[a]P-metabolite-adduct formation. Whereas, in 2 samples, relatively greater DNA-B[a]P-metabolite adducts were produced with reduced overall metabolite values at the left side of the plot. The material and method (incubation conditions) have been outlined before.[143] These data show that increased xenobiotic metabolism does not correlate with reactive product formation.

much as 200-fold. The metabolic characteristics of an individual with respect to chemotherapeutic drugs can be approximated by measurement of rate of metabolism relative to a well known drug's metabolic ratio.[184] This process is called phenotyping. Thus, by the use of both genotype and phenotype information, cancer therapy can be tailored to a specific individual for optimal efficacy.

These procedures can also be extended to the phase-2 enzymes, such as glutathione S-transferase, epoxide hydrolase and others.[185-187] At present, there is a need for development of such methods for fetal, amniotic and placental tissues which would be particularly useful in cancer therapy of pregnant women. Since the genetic profiles of the mother and fetus are different, cancer drug metabolism potential of both mother and fetus may determine the choice of therapy. Fetal derived tissues are readily available as amniotic cells and chorionic villi. They are potential source for such metabolic analysis.

Summary

Cancer chemotherapy is highly complex during pregnancy, as the physiology of the mother and the embryo-fetus progressively changes with the advancement of pregnancy. Since embryonic tissues resemble cancer tissues, the embryonic tissues are also the targets of current chemotherapeutic drugs. The embryo-fetus of the first trimester pregnancy is highly susceptible to anomalous development by such drugs. It is beginning to emerge that expression of drug metabolizing phase-1 enzymes, cytochrome P450 (CYP gene family), and several phase-2 enzymes in maternal and embryo-fetal systems may regulate the efficacy of the chemotherapeutic drugs and their potential for deleterious effects on embryo-fetal developments. The placental trophoblast layer, the interface between the maternal and fetal compartments, expresses these enzymes and participates in the activation and detoxification of drugs and their transfer into the fetus. The fetal tissues are also endowed with various CYP genes and their expression potential. The expression of these genes in the fetus may be different from that in the adult liver. In addition, these genes exhibit a wide range of polymorphisms which in the future will allow individualization of cancer therapy. A more effective therapy with reduced teratologic risks will be possible by in-depth characterization of drug-metabolism potential with genetic (genotypic/phenotypic) features in both maternal and fetal tissues.

Acknowledgments

My grateful thanks to Dr. Maurice J. Mahoney, Departments of Genetics, Obstetrics and Gynecology, and Pediatrics, Yale Medical School, for editing the manuscript, in-depth discussion and his thoughtful interpretation of the literature. I also thank Dr. F. Naftolin, Chairman, Department of Obstetrics and Gynecology, Yale Medical School for his support of the original studies described performed for over a period of more than ten years from my laboratory. My studies described in the article were performed with funding from the NIH (Es 05337), March of Dimes, State of Connecticut, Rockefeller Foundation and the Swebelius award.

References

1. Ruddon, R. Cancer Biology, 3rd edn, Oxford University Press, Oxford, 1995
2. Franks, L. M. and Teich, N. M. Introduction to Cellular and Molecular Biology of Cancer. 3rd edn, Oxford University Press, Oxford, 1997
3. Verschraegen, C. F., Dhingra, K. and Jones, L. A. Biology of Gynecologic Cancer. In: Kavanaugh, J. J., Singletary, S. E., Eoinhorn, N. and DePetriello, A. D. (eds), Cancer in Women Blackwell Science, Oxford, 1998: 3–29
4. Chamberlain, G. and Pipkin, F. B. (eds) Clinical Physiology in Obstetrics, 3rd edn, Blackwell Science, Oxford, 1998
5. Bertino, J. R. Antineoplastic Drugs. In: Smith C. M. and Raynard, A. M. (eds), Text Book of Pharmacology, W. B. Saunders, Philadelphia, 1992: 941–63
6. Devita, V. T. Principles in Cancer Management. In: DeVita, V. T. Jr., Hellman, S. and Rosenberg, S. A. (eds), Cancer Principles and Practice of Oncology, 5th edn, Volume 1, Lippincott-Raven, Philadelphia, 1997: 333–47
7. Moore, M. J. and Goldenberg, G. J. Antineoplastic Drugs. In: Kalant, H. and Roschlau, W. H. E. (eds), Principles of Medical Pharmacology, 6th edn, Oxford University Press, New York, 1998: 759–74

8. Valley, A. W. and Balmer, C. M. Cancer Treatment and Chemotherapy. In: DiPiro, J. T., Talbert, R. L., Yee, G. C. et al. (eds), Pharmcotherapy - Pathological Approach, Appleton & Lang, Stamford, CT, 1999: 1957–2012
9. Stock, M. K. and Metcalf, J. Maternal Physiology during Gestation. In: Knobil, E. and Neill, J.D. (eds), The Physiology of Reproduction, 2nd edn, Volume 2, Raven Press, New York, 1994: 947–83
10. Duvekot, J. J. and Peeters, L. L. H. Very Early Changes in Cardiovascular Physiology. In: Chamberlain, G. and Pipkin, F. B. (eds), Clinical Physiology in Obstetrics, 3rd edn, Blackwell Science, Oxford, 1998: 3–32
11. Ogren, L. and Talamantes, F., Placenta as an Endocrine Organ: Polypeptides. In: Knobil, E. and Neill, J.D. (eds), The Physiology of Reproduction, 2nd edn, Volume 2, Raven Press, New York, 1994: 875–945
12. Chard, T. Placental Metabolism. In: Chamberlain, G. and Pipkin, F. B. (eds), Clinical Physiology in Obstetrics, 3rd edn, Blackwell Science, Oxford, 1998: 419–35
13. Manyonda, I. T. The Immune System. In: Chamberlain, G. and Pipkin, F. B. (eds), Clinical Physiology in Obstetrics, 3rd edn, Blackwell Science, Oxford, 1998: 129–162
14. Sanyal, M. K., Brami, C. J., Bischof, P. et al. Immunoregulatory activity in supernatant from cultures of normal trophoblast cells of the first trimester. Am. J. Obstet. Gynecol. 1989; 161:446–453
15. Freedman, R. S., Kudelka, A. P., Verschraegan, C. F. and Platsoucas, C. D. Progress toward Tumor Specific Immunity in Carcinoma of the Ovary and Breast. In: Kavanaugh, J. J., Singletary, S. E., Eoinhorn, N. and DePetriello, A. D. (eds), Cancer in Women, Blackwell Science, 1998: 30–53
16. Evans, A. C. Jr. and Berchuck, A. Tumor Markers. In: Hoskins, W. J., Parez, C. A. and Young, R. C. (eds), Principles and Practice of Gynecologic Oncology, 2nd edn, Lippincott-Raven, Philadelphia, 1997: 177–95
17. Alessandro, R., Bicher, A. and Kohn, E. Tumor Invasion and Metastases. In: Hoskins, W. J., Parez, C. A. and Young, R. C. (eds), Principles and Practice of Gynecologic Oncology, 2nd edn, Lippincott-Raven, Philadelphia, 1997: 87–106
18. Williams, P. L. (ed.) Gray's Anatomy, Volume 3. Embryology and Development. Churchill Livingstone, New York,1995: 166–73
19. Benirscke, K. and Kaufman, P. Pathology of Human Placenta, 2nd edn, Springer-Verlag, New York, 1990
20. Jones, C. J. P. and Fox, H. Ultrastructure of the normal human placenta. Electron. Microscop. Rev. 1991; 4:120–78
21. Teasdale, F. Gestational changes in the functional structure of the human placenta in relation to fetal growth: a morphometric study. Am. J. Obstet. Gynec. 1980; 137:560–8
22. Teasdale, F. and Jean-Jacques, G. Morphometric evaluation of the microvillous surface enlargement factor in the human placenta from mid-gestation to term. Placenta. 1985; 6:375–81
23. Van der Velde, W. J., Peereboom-Stegeman, J. H. J., Treffers P. E. and James, J. Basal lamina thickening in the placentae of smoking mothers. Placenta 1983; 6:329–40
24. Cantle, S. J., Kaufman, P., Luckhadt, M. and Schweikart, G. Interpretation of syncytial sprout and bridges in the human placenta. Placenta 1987; 8:221–34
25. Kaufman, P., Luckhardt, M., Schweikhart, G. and Cantle, S. J. Cross-sectional feature and three dimensional structure of human placental villi. Placenta 1987; 8:235–47
26. Morriss, F. H., Boyd, R. D. H. and Mahendran, D. Placental Transport. In: Knobil, E. and Neill, J.D. (eds), The Physiology of Reproduction, 2nd edn, Volume 2, Raven Press, New York, 1994: 813–861
27. Sibley, C. P. and Boyd, R. D. H. Mechanism of Transfer Across the Human Placenta. In: Polin, R. A. and Fox. H. (eds), Fetal and Maternal Physiology, W. B. Saunders, Philadelphia, 1992: 62–74
28. Mihaly, G. W. and Morgan, D. J. Placental drug transfer: effect of gestational age and species. Pharmacol. Therap. 1984; 23:253–66
29. Patten, B. M. Human Embryology, 3rd edn, McGraw-Hill, New York, 1968: 500–83
30. Heymann, M. A. Fetal Cardiovascular Physiology. In: Creasy, R. K. and Resnik, R. (eds) Maternal-Fetal Medicine, W. B. Saunders, Philadelphia,1984: 276–87
31. Benet, L. Z., Koetz, D. L. and Sheiner, L. B. Pharmacokinetics. In: Hardman, J. G. and Limbird, L. E. (eds), Goodman and Gilman's The Pharmacological Basis of Therapeutics, 9th edn, McGraw-Hill, New York, 1996: 3–27
32. Ross, E. M. Pharmacodynamics. In: Hardman, J. G. and Limbird, L. E. (eds), Goodman and Gilman's The Pharmacological Basis of Therapeutics, 9th edn, McGraw-Hill, New York, 1996: 29–41
33. Ratain, M. J. Pharmacokinetics and Pharmacodynamics. In: DeVita, V. T. Jr., Hellman, S. and Rosenberg, S. A. (eds) Cancer Principles and Practice of Oncology, 5th edn, Lippincott-Raven, Philadelphia, 1997; 375–85
34. Reynolds, F. Pharmacokinetics. In: Chamberlain, G. and Pipkin, F. B. (eds), Clinical Physiology in Obstetrics, 3rd edn, Blackwell Science, Oxford, 1998: 239–260
35. Riddick, D. S. Drug Biotranformation. In: Kalant, H. and Roschlau, W. H. E. (eds) Principles of Medical Pharmacology, 6th edn, Oxford University Press, New York, 1998: 38–54

36. Wong, L. L. Cytochrome P450 monoxygenases. Curr. Opinion in Chem. Biol. 1998; 2:263–8
37. Hinson, J. A. and Forkert, P. G. Phase II enzymes and bioactivation. Can. J. Physiol. Pharmacol. 1995; 73:1407–13
38. Nebert, D. W., Nelson, D. R., Adesnik, M. et al. The P450 gene superfamily. Update on the naming of new genes and nomenclature of chromosomal loci. DNA 1989; 8:1–13
39. Nelson, D. R., Kamataki, T., Waxman, D. J. et. al. The P450 superfamily: update on new sequence, gene mapping, accession numbers, early trivial names of enzymes and nomenclature. DNA Cell Biol. 1993; 12:1–51
40. Black, S. D. Cytochrome P450 Structure and Function. In: Schenkman, J. B. and Greim, H. (eds), Handbook of Experimental Pharmacology, Springer, Berlin, 1993: 155–68
41. Shimada, T., Mimura, M., Inoue, K. et al. Cytochrome P450 dependent drug oxidation activities in liver microsomes of various animal species including rats, guinea pigs, dogs, monkeys and humans. Arch. Toxicol. 1997; 71:401–8
42. Kivisto, K. T., Kroemer, H. K. and Eichelbaum, H. The role of human cytochrome P450 enzymes in the metabolism of anticancer agents: implications in drug interactions. Br. J. Clin. Pharmacol. 1995; 40:523–30
43. Guengerich, F. P. Role of cytochrome P450 enzymes in drug-drug interactions. Adv. Pharmacol. 1997; 43:7–35
44. Clarke, L. and Waxman, D. J. Oxidative metabolism of cyclophosphamide: identification of hepatic monoxygenase catalysis of drug activation. Cancer Res. 1989; 49:2344–50
45. Chang, T. K., Weber, G. F., Crespi, C. L. and Waxman, D. J. Differential activation of cyclophosphamide and ifosfamide by cytochrome P450 2B and 3A in human liver microsomes. Cancer Res. 1993; 53:5629–37
46. Bohnenstengel, F., Hofmann, U., Eichelbaum, M. and Kroemer, H. K. Characterization of the cytochrome P450 involved in side chain oxidation of cyclophosphamide in humans. Eur. J. Clin. Pharmacol. 1996; 51:297–301
47. Chang, T. K., Yu, L., Goldstein, J. A. and Waxman, D. J. Identification of polymorphically expressed CYP 2C19 and the wild type CYP269-ILE359 allele as low Km catalysis of cyclophosphamide and ifosfamide activation. Pharmacogenetics 1997; 7:211–21
48. Ren, S., Yang, J. S., Kalhorn, T. F. and Slattery, J. T. Oxidation of cyclophosphamide to 4-hydroxycyclophosphamide and deschlooethylcyclophosphamide in human liver microsomes. Cancer Res. 1997; 57:4229–35
49. Hengstker, J. G., Hengst, A., Fuchs, A. et al. Induction of crosslinking and DNA strand lesion by cyclophosphamide after activation by cytochrome P450 2B1. Mut. Res. 1997; 373:215–23
50. Pariani, S., Buscaglia, M., Piantanide, M., and Simoni, G. Cyclophosphamide increases frequency of sister chromatid exchanges in direct preparations of human chorionic villi in the absence of supplementary enzymatic activation systems. J. Med. Genetics 1992; 29:109–11
51. Cuisido, L., Pujol, R. Egocue, J. and Garcia, M. Cyclophosphamide-induced synaptonemal complex damage during meiotic prophase of female *Rattus norvgicus*. Mut. Res. 1995; 329:131–41
52. Cutts, S. M., Persons, P.G., Saturn,R. A. and Phillips, D. R. Adriamycin-induced DNA adducts inhibits the DNA interaction of transcription factors and RNA polymerase. J. Biol. Chem. 1996; 271:5422–9
53. Boyer, M. J. Bioreductive agents: a clinical update. Oncology Res. 1997; 9:391–5
54. Tomaz, M. and Palom, Y. The mitomycin bioreductive antitumor agents: crossl-inking and alkylation of DNA as the molecular basis of their activity. Pharmacol. Ther. 1997; 76:73–87
55. Masters, J. R., Know, R. J., Hartley, J. A., et al. KW-2149 (7-N-[2-[gamma-L-gluta-amyl amino] ethyl dithioethyl] mitomycin C) a new mitomycin C analogue activated by serum. Biochem. Pharmacol. 1997; 53:279–85
56. Haffty, B. G., Son, Y. H., Papac, R. et al. Chemotherapy as an adjunct to radiation in the treatment of squamous cell carcinoma of the head and neck: results of Yale mitomycin randomized trial. J. Clin. Oncol. 1997; 15: 268–76
57. Raymond, E., Favivre, S., Woynarowski, J. M. and Chaney, G. G. Oxiplatin: mechanism of action and antineoplastic activity. Semin.Oncol. 1998; 25: (2 suppl. 5):4–12
58. Nagani, N., Okuda, R. Kinoshita, M. and Ogata, H. Decomposition kinetics of cisplatin in human biological fluids. J. Pharmacy Pharmacol. 1994; 48:918–24
59. Saris, C. P., Van der Vaart, P. J., Rietbroek, R. C. and Blommaerrt, F. A. In vitro formation of DNA adducts by cisplatin, loboplatin, and oxoplatin in calf thymus DNA in solution and in cultured human cells. Carcinogenesis 1996; 17:2763–9
60. Mani, C., Gelboin, H. V., Park, S. S. et al. Metabolism of the antimammary cancer antiestrogenic agent tamoxifen. I. Cytochrome P 450 catalysed N-demethylation and 4-hydroxylation. Drug Metab. Dispos. 1993; 21:645–56

61. Jordan, V. C. Tamoxifen: Toxicities and drug resistance during the treatment and prevention of breast cancer. Ann. Rev. Pharmacol. Toxicol. 1995; 35:195–211
62. Crewe, H. K., Ellis, S. W., Lennard, M. S. and Tucker, G. T. Variable contribution of cytochrome P 450 2D6, 2C9 and 3A4 to the 4-hydroxylation of tamoxifen by human liver microsomes. Biochem. Pharmacol. 1997; 53:171–8
63. Dorr, R. T. Pharmacology of Taxanes. Pharmacotherapy. 1997; 17 (5 pt 2): S96–104
64. Harris, J. W., Rahman, A., Kim, B. et al. Metabolism of taxol by human hepatic microsomes and liver slices: participation of cytochrome P450 3A4 and an unknown P450 enzymes. Cancer Res. 1994; 54:4026–35
65. Walle, T. Assays of CYP2C8 and CYP3A4 mediated metabolism of taxol in vivo and vitro. Methods in Enzymology 1996; 272:145–51
66. Kumar, G. N., Oatis, J. E. Jr., Thornberg, K. R. et al. 6-alpha-hydroxytaxol: isolation and identification of the major metabolite of taxol by human liver microsomes. Drug Metab. Dispos. 1994; 22:177–9
67. Kumar, G. N., Walle, U. K. and Walle, T. Cytochrome P450 3A-mediated human liver microsomal taxol 6 alpha-hydroxylation. J. Pharmacol. Exp. Ther. 1994; 268:1160–65
68. Royer, I., Monsarrat, B., Sonnier, M., et al. Metabolism of docetaxel by human cytochrome P450: interactions with paclitaxel and other neoplastic drugs. Cancer Res. 1996; 56:58–65
69. Gidding, C. E., Kellie, S. J., Kamps, W. A. and Graff, S. S. Vincristine revisited. Crit. Rev. Oncol. 1999; 29:267–87
70. Zhou-Pan, X., R., Serree, E., Zhou, X. J. et al. Involvement of human liver cytochrome P4503A in vinblastin metabolism: drug interactions. Cancer Res. 1993; 53:5121–6
71. Lobert, S., Vulevic, B. and Correica, J. J. Interaction of vinca alkaloids with tubulin: a comparison of vinblastin, vincristin and vinorelbine. Biochemistry 1996; 35:6808–14
72. Panda, D., Miller, H. P., Islam, K. and Wilson, L. Stabilization of microtubule dynamics by estramustine by binding to a novel site in tubulin: a possible mechanistic basis for its antitumor action. Proc. Natl. Acad. Sci. USA 1997; 94:10560–4
73. Hagen, B., Walseth, P., Walstad, P. et. al. Single and repeated dose pharmacokinetics of thio-TEPA in patients treated for ovarian cancinoma. Cancer Chemotherap. Phamocol. 1987; 19:143–8
74. Ng, S. and Waxman, D. J. Activation of thio-TEPA cytotoxicity toward human breast cancer cells by hepatic cytochrome P450. Int. J. Oncol. 1993; 2:731–8
75. Chang, T. K. H., Chen, G. and Waxman, D. J. Modulation of thiotepa antitumor activity in vivo by alteration of liver cytochrome P450 catalyzed drug metabolism. J. Pharmacol. Exp. Therap. 1995; 274:270–5
76. Raha, A. and Tew, K. D. Glutathione S-transferase. Cancer Treat. and Res. 1996; 87:83–122
77. Ferrandina, G., Scambia, G., Damia, G. et al. Glutathione S-transferase activity in epithelial ovarian cancer: association with response to chemotherapy and disease outcome. Ann. Oncol. 1997; 8:343–50
78. Tanner, B., Hengstler, J. G. Dietrich, B. et al. Glutathione, glutathione S-transferase alpha and pi, and aldehyde dehydrogenase content in relationship to drug resistance in ovarian cancer. Gynec. Oncol. 1997; 65:54–62
79. Renes, J., deVries, E. G., Nienhuis, E. F et al. ATP and glutathione-dependent transport of chemotherapeutic drugs by multidrug resistant protein MRPI. Br. J. Pharmacol. 1999; 126:681–8
80. Aran, J. M., Pastan, I. and Gottesman, M. M. Therapeutic strategies involving the multidrug resistance phenotype: the MDR1 gene as target, chemoprotectant, and selectable marker in gene therapy. Adv. Phamacol. 1999; 46:1–42
81. Deeley, R. G. and Cole, S. P. C. Function, evolution and structure of multidrug resistance protein (MRP). Semin. Cancer Biol. 1997; 8:193–204
82. Sancar, A. DNA excision repair. Ann. Rev. Biochem. 1996; 65:43–81
83. Crul, M., Schellans, J. H. M, Beijnen, J. H.and Maliepaard, M. Cisplatin resistance and DNA repair. Cancer Treat. Reviews 1997; 23:341–66
84. Filler, R. and Lew, K. J. Developmental onset of mixed function oxidase activity in preimplantation mouse embryos. Proc. Natl. Acad. Sci. USA 1981; 78:6991–5
85. Pedersen, R. A., Meneses, J., Spindle, A. et al. Cyotchrome P450 metabolic acivity in embryonic and extraembryonic tissue lineage of mouse embryos. Proc. Natl. Acad. Sci. USA 1985; 82:3311–15
86. Dey, A., Westphal, H. and Nebert, D. W. Cell specific induction of mouse cyp1a1 mRNA during development. Proc. Natl. Acad. Sci. USA 1989; 86:7446–50
87. Berry, D. L., Zachariah, P. K., Namkung, M. J. and Juchau, M. R. Transplacenal induction of carcinogen by hydroxylation system with 2,3,7,8-tetrachlorodibenzo-p-dioxin (TCDD). Toxicol. Appl. Pharmacol. 1976; 36:569–84
88. Wu, D. and Cederbaum, A. I. Expression of P4502E1 in rat fetal hepatocyte culture. Mol. Pharmacol. 1996; 49:802–807

89. Borlakoglu, J. T., Scott, A., Henderson, C. J. and Wolf, C. R. Expression of P450 isoenzymes during rat liver organogenesis. Int. J. Biochem. 1993; 25:1659–68
90. Juchau, M. R., Harris, C., Stark, K. L. et al. Cytochrome P450-dependent bioactivation of prodysmorphogens in cultured conceptuses. Reprod. Toxicol. 1991; 5:259–64
91. Juchau, M. R., Lee, Q. P. and Fantel, A. G. Xenobiotic biotransformation/bioactivation in organogenesis-stage conceptal tissues: implication for embryotoxicity and teratogenesis. Drug Metab. Rev. 1992; 24:195–234
92. Sanyal, M. K. and Naftolin, F. In vitro development of mammalian embryo. J. Exp. Zool. 1983; 228:235–51
93. Sanyal, M. K., Kitchin, K. T. and Dixon, R. L. Rat conceptus development in vitro: Comparative effects of alkylating agents. Toxicol. Appl. Pharmacol. 1981; 57:14–19
94. Kitchin, K. T., Schmid, B. P. and Sanyal, M. K. Teratogenicity of cyclophosphamide in a coupled microsomal activating/embryo culture system. Biochem. Pharmacol. 1981; 30:59–64
95. Schmid, B. P., Goulding, E., Kitchin, K. T. and Sanyal, M. K. Assessment of the teratogenic potential of acrolein and cyclophosphamide in a rat embryo culture system. Toxicology 1981; 22:235–4
96. Satish, J., Pratt, B. M., and Sanyal, M. K. Differential dysmorphogenesis induced by microinjection of an alkylating agent into rat conceptuses cultured in vitro. Teratology 1985; 31:61–72
97. Biggers, W. J., Barnea, E. T. and Sanyal, M. K. Anomalous neural differentiation induced by 5-bromo-2deoxy-uridine during organogenesis in the rat. Teratology 1987; 35:63–75
98. Lee, Q. P., Fantel, A. G. and Juchau, M. R. Human embryonic cytochrome P450s: phenoxazone ethers as probes for expression of functional isoforms during organogenesis. Biochem. Pharmacol. 1991; 42:2377–86
99. Juchau, M. R. and Yang, H. L. Cytochrome P450-dependent monooxygenase of embryonic/teratogenic chemicals in human embryonic tissues. Fundment. Appl. Toxicol. 1996; 34:166–8
100. Naftolin, F., Diamond, M. P., Pinter, E., Reece, A. and Sanyal, M. K. A hypothesis concerning the general basis of organogenetic congenital anomalies. Am J. Obstet. Gynecol. 1987; 157:1–4
101. Juchau, M. R. Chemical teratogenesis in humans: biochemical and molecular mechanisms. Prog. Drug Res. 1997; 49:25–92
102. Juchau, M. R., Boutelet-Bochan, H. and Huang, Y. Cytochrome P450 dependent biotransformation of xenobiotics in human and rodent embryonic tissues. Drug Metab. Rev. 1998; 30:541–68
103. Wells, P. G. Chemical Teratogenesis. In: Kalant, H. and Roschlau, W. H. E. (eds), Principles of Medical Pharmacology, 6th edn, Oxford University Press, New York, 1998: 873–90
104. Hakkola, J., Pelkonen, O., Pasanen, M. and Raunio, H. Xenobiotic-metabolizing cytochrome P450 enzymes in human feto-placental unit: role in intrauterine toxicity. Crit. Rev.Toxicol. 1998; 28:35–72
105. Yaffe, S. J., Rane, A., Sjoqvist, F. et al. The presence of monooxygenase system in human fetal liver microsomes. Life Sci. 1970; 9:1189–200
106. Farrar, H. C. and Blumer, J. L. Fetal effects of maternal drug exposure. Ann. Rev. Pharmacol. Toxicol. 1991; 31:525–47
107. Krauer, B. and Dayer, P. Fetal drug metabolism and its possible clinical implication. Clin. Pharmacokinet. 1991; 21:70–80
108. Kitada, M. and Kamataki, T. C. Cytochrome P450 in human fetal liver: significance and fetal specific expression. Drug Metab. Rev. 1994; 26:305–23
109. Raucy, J. L. and Carpenter, S. J. The expression of xenobiotic metabolizing cytochrome P450 in fetal tissues. J. Pharmacol. Toxicol. Methods 1993; 29:121–8
110. Jones, A. H., Fantel, A. G., Kocan, R. M. and Juchau, M. R. Bioactivation of procarcinogens to mutagens in human fetal and placental tissues. Life Sci. 1997; 21:1831–7
111. Hakkola, J., Pasanen, M. Purkunen, R. et al. Expression of xenobiotic-metabolizing cytochrome P450 forms in human adult and fetal liver. Biochem. Pharmacol. 1994; 48:59–64
112. Murray, G. I., Foster, C. O., Barnes, T. S. et al. Cytochrome P450 1A expression in adult and fetal human liver. Carcinogenesis 1992; 13:165–9
113. McKinnon, R. A., Burgess, W. M., Gonzales, F. J. et al. Species specific expression of CYP4B1 in rabbit and human gastrointestinal tissues. Pharmacogenetics 1994; 4:260–70
114. Shimada, T., Yamazaki, H. , Mimura, M., et al. Characterization of microsomal cytochrome P450 enzymes involved in the oxidation of xenobiotic chemicals in human fetal livers and adult lungs. Drug Metab. Dispos. 1996; 24:515–22
115. Guengerich, F. P., Shimada, T., Yamazaki, H. and Mimura, M. Comparison of cytochrome P450 enzymes and their activities in human fetal and adult liver. Fund. Appl. Toxicol. 1996; 34:168–72
116. Yang, H. L., Namkung, M. J. and Juchau, M. R. Expression of functional cytochrome P4501A1 in human embryonic hepatic tissues during organognesis. Biochem. Pharmacol. 1995; 49:717–26

117. Treluyer, J. M., Jacqz-Aigrain, E., Alvarez, F. and Cresteil, T. Expression of CYP 2D6 in developing human liver. Eur. J Biochem. 1991; 202: 583–8
118. Gilham, D. E., Cairns, W., Paine, M. J. I. et al. Metabolism of MTPT by cytochrome P450 2D6 and demonstration of 2D6 mRNA in human fetal and adult brain by in situ hybridization. Xenobiotica 1997; 27:111–25
119. Carpenter, S. P., Lasker, J. M. and Raucy, J. L. Expression, induction and catalytic activity of the ethanol induced cytochrome P450 (CYP 2E1) in human fetal liver. Molec. Pharmacol. 1996; 49:260–8
120. Jones, S. M., Boobis, A. R., Moore, G. E. and Stanier, P. M. Expression of CYP2E1 during human fetal development: methylation of the CYP2E1 gene in human fetal and adult liver samples. Biochem. Pharmacol. 1992; 43:1876–80
121. Boutelet-Bochan, H., Huang, Y. and Juchau, M. R. Expression of CYP 2E1 during embryogenesis and fetogenesis in human cephalic tissues: implication for the fetal alcohol syndrome. Biochem. Biophysis. Res. Commun. 1997; 238:443–7
122. Vieira, I., Sonnier, M. and Cresteil, T. Developmental expression of CYP 2E1 in the human liver. Hypermethylation control of gene expression during the neonatal period. Eur. J. Biochem. 1996; 238:476–83
123. Yang, H. L., Lee, Q. P., Rettie, A. E. and Juchau, M. R. Functional CYP3A isoform in human embryonic tissues: expression during organogenesis. Molec. Phamacol. 1994; 46:922–9
124. Schuetz, J. D., Beach, D. L. and Guzelian, P. S. Selective expression of cytochrome P4503A mRNAs in embryonic and adult human liver. Pharmacogenetics 1994; 4:11–20
125. Greuet, J., Pichard, L., Bonfils, C. et al. The fetal specific gene CYP 3A7 is inducible by rifampcin in adult human hepatocytes in primary culture. Biochem. Biophys. Res. Commun. 1996; 225:689–94
126. Schuetz, J. D., Schuetz, E. G., Thottassery, J. V. et al. Identification of novel dexamethasone responsive enhancer in the CYP 3A5 gene and its activation in human and rat liver cells. Mol. Pharmacol. 1996; 49: 63–72
127. LaCroix, D., Sonnier, M., Moncion, A., Cheron, G. and Cresteil, T. Expression of CYP 3A in the human liver. Evidence that the shift between CYP3A7 and CYP3A4 occurs immediately after birth. Eur. J. Biochem. 1997; 247:625–34
128. Juchau, M. R. Drug biotransformation in the placenta. Pharmacol. Ther. 1980; 8:501–24
129. Pasanen, M. and Pelkonen, O. Human placental xenobiotic and steroid biotransformations catalyzed by cytochrome P450, epoxide hydrolase and glutathione S-transferase activities and their relationships to maternal cigarette smoking. Drug Metab. Rev. 1989; 21:427–61
130. Pasanen, M. and Pelkonen, O. The expression and environmental regulation of P450 enzymes in human placenta. Crit. Rev. Toxicol. 1994; 24:211–29
131. Juchau, M. R. Human placental hydroxylation of 3,4-benzo(a)pyrene during early gestation and at term. Toxicol. Appl. Pharmacol. 1971; 18:665–75
132. Juchau, M. R. and Smuckler, E. A. Subcellular localization of human placental aryl hydrocarbon hydroxylase. Toxicol. Appl. Pharmacol. 1973; 26:163–79
133. Manchester, D. K. and Jacoby, E. H. Sensitivity of human placental monooxygenase activity to maternal smoking. Clin. Pharmacol. Ther. 1081; 30:687–92
134. Manchester, D. K. and Jacoby, E. H. Decreased placental monooxygenase activities associated with birth defects. Teratology 1984; 30:31–3
135. Gurtoo, H. L., Williams, C. J., Gottlieb, K. et al. Population distribution of placental benz(a)pyrene metabolism in smokers. Int. J. Cancer 1983; 31:29–37
136. Fujino, T., Gottlieb, K, Manchester, D. K. et al. Monoclonal antibody phenotyping of interindividual differences in cytochrome P450-dependent reactions of single and twin placenta. Cancer Res. 1984; 44:3916–23
137. Huel, G., Girard, F., Nessmann, C. et al. Placental aryl hydrocarbon hydroxylase activity and placental calcification. Toxicology 1992; 71:257–66
138. Pasanen, M., Haaparanta, T., Sundin, M. et al. Immunochemical and molecular biological studies on human placental cigarette smoke inducible cytochrome P450 dependent monooxygenase activities. Toxicology 1990; 62:175–87
139. Hakkola, J., Raunio, H., Purkunen, R. et al. Detection of cytochrome P450 gene expression in human placenta in first trimester pregnancy. Biochem. Pharmacol. 1996; 52:379–83
140. Hakkola, J., Pasanen, M., Hukkanen, J. et al. Expression of xenobiotic-metabolizing cytochrome P450 forms in human full term placenta. Biochem. Pharmacol. 1996; 51:403–11
141. Hakkola, J., Pasanen, M., Pelkonen, O., et al. Expression of CYP1B1 in human adult and fetal tissues and differential ineducability of CYP1B1 and CYP1A1 by Ah receptor ligands in human placenta and cultured cells. Carcinogenesis 1997; 18:391–7

142. Sanyal, M. K., Li, Y. L., Biggers, W. J., Satish, J. and Barnea, E. R. Augmentation of polynuclear aromatic hydrocarbon metabolite of human first trimester pregnancy by cigarette smoke exposure. Am. J. Obstet. Gynecol. 1993; 168:1587–97
143. Sanyal, M. K., Li, Y. L. and Belanger, K. Metabolism of polynuclear aromatic hydrocarbon in human term placenta influenced by cigarette smoke exposure. Reprod. Toxicol. 1994; 8:411–18
144. Sanyal, M. K. and Barnea, E. R. Expression of aryl hydrocarbon hydroxylase (CYP1A1) in human placentas. In: Barnea, E. R. Check, J. H., et al. (eds), Implantation and Early Pregnancy, Parthenon Publishing Group, London, 1994:379–86
145. Howie, A. F., Hayes, J. D. and Beckett, G. J. Purification of acidic glutathion S-transferase from human lungs, placenta and erthythrocyte and development of specific radioimmunoassay for their measurement. Clin. Chem. Acta. 1988; 177:65–75
146. Aiso, S., Yasuda, K., Shiozawa, M., et al. Preparation of monoclonal antibodies to glutathione S-transferase pi application to immunohistochemical study. J. Histochem. Cytochem. 1989; 37:1247–52
147. Manchester, D. K. and Jacoby, E. H. Glutathione S-transferase activities in placentas from smoking and nonsmoking women. Xenobiotica 1982; 12:543–47
148. Pasanen, M and Pelkonen, O. Xenobiotic and steroid metabolizing monoxygenase catalysed by cytochrome P450 and glutathione S-transferase conjugations in the human placenta and their relationship to maternal cigarette smoking. Placenta 1990; 11:75–85
149. Wixtrom, R. N., Silva, M. H. and Hammock, B. D. Cytosolic epoxide hydrolase in human placenta. Placenta 1988; 9:559–63
150. Farin, F. M., Pohlman, T. H. and Omiecinski, C. J. Expression of cytochrome P450s and microsomal epoxide hydrolase in primary cultures of human umblical vein endothelial cells. Toxicol. Appl. Pharmacol. 1994; 124:1–9
151. Manchester, D. K., Gordon, S. K., Golas, C. L. et al. Ah receptor in human placenta: solubilization by molybdate and characterization by binding of 2,3,7,8- tetrachlorobenzo-p-dioxin, 3-methylcholanthrene and benzo(a)pyrene. Cancer Res. 1987; 47:4861–8
152. Sogowa, K., Nakano, R., Kobayashi, A. et al. Possible function of Ah receptor nuclear translocator (Arnt) homodimer in transcriptional regulation. Proc. Natl. Acad. Sci. USA 1995; 92:1936–40
153. Botto, F., Seree, E., Khyari, S. E., et al. Tissue-specific expression and methylation of the human CYP2E1 gene. Biochem. Pharmacol. 1994; 48:1095–103
154. Rasheed, A., Hines, R. N. and McCarver-May, D. G. Variation in induction of placental ^{3}CYP2E1: possible role is susceptibility to fetal alcohol syndrome. Toxicol. Appl. Pharmacol. 1997; 144:396–400
155. Schuetz, J. D., Kauma, S. and Guzelian, P. S. Identification of the fetal liver cytochrome CYP3A7 in human endometrium and placenta. J. Clin. Invest. 1993; 92:1018–24
156. Cummingham, F. G., McDonald, P. C., Gant, N. et al. (eds) Williams Obstetrics, 20th edn, Appleton & Lange, Stamford, CT, 1997:125–190
157. Ryan, K. J. Biological aromatization of steroids. J. Biol. Chem. 1959; 234:268–72
158. Diczfalusy, E. and Toren, P. Endocrine functions of human placenta. Vit. Horm. 1961; 19:229–311
159. Siiteri, P. K. and MacDonald, P. C. Placental estrogen biosynthesis during human pregnancy. J. Clin. Endocrinol. 1966; 26:751–61
160. Baulieu, E. E.and Dray, F. Conversion of ^{3}H-dehydroepiandrosterone (3ß-hydroxysteroid Δ^{5}-androstene-17-one) sulfate to ^{3}H-estrogens in normal pregnant women. J. Clin. Endocrinol. 1963; 23:1298–301
161. Canick, J. A. and Ryan, K. J. Cytochrome P450 and aromatization of 16-hydroxytestosterone and androstenedione by human placental microsomes. Mol. Cell. Endocrinol. 1976; 6:105–15
162. Mason, J. I. and Rainey, W. E. Steroidogenesis in the human fetal adrenal: a role for cholesterol synthesized de novo. J. Clin. Endocrinol. Metab. 1987; 64:140–7
163. Simpson, E. R., Mahendroo, M. S., Means, G. D. et al. Aromatase cytochrome P450, the enzyme responsible for estrogen biosynthesis. Endocrn. Rev. 1994; 15:342–55
164. Means, G. D., Kilgore, M. W., Mahendroo, M. S. et al. Tissue specific promoters regulate aromatase cytochrome P450 gene expression in human ovary and fetal tissues. Mol. Endocrinol. 1991; 5: 2005–13
165. Kilgore, M. W., Means, G. D., Mendelson, C. R. and Simpson, E. R. Alternate promotion of aromatase P-450 expression in the human placenta. Mol. Cell Endocrinol. 1992; 83:R9–16
166. Kalow, W. and Grant, D. M. Human Pharmacogenetics. In: Kalant, H. and Roschlau, W. H. E. (eds), Principles of Medical Pharmacology, 6th edn, Oxford University Press, New York, 1998:120–31
167. May, D. G. Genetic differences in drug disposition. J. Clin. Pharmacol. 1994; 34:881–97
168. Shimada, T., Yamazaki, H., Mimura, M., et al. Interindividual variation in human liver cytochrome P450 enzymes involved in oxidation of drugs, carcinogens and toxic chemicals: studies with liver microsomes of 30 Japanese and 30 Caucasians, J. Pharmacol. Exp. Ther. 1994; 270:414–23
169. Spielberg, S. Pharmacogenetics: from scientific curiosity to a central theme in drug development and therapeutics. Can. J. Pharmacol. 1995; 2:54–6

170. Gonzalez, F. J., Skoda, R. C., Dimura, S. et al. Characterization of the common genetic defects in humans deficient in debisquin metabolism. Nature 1988; 331:442-6
171. Lennard, L., Lilleyman, J. S., Van-Loon, J. and Weinshilboum, R. M. Genetic variation in response to 6-mercaptopurine for childhood acute lymphoblastic leukemia. Lancet 1990; 336:225–29
172. Krynetski, E., Tai, H. L. and Yates, C. R. Genetic polymorphism of thiopurina S-methyltransferase: Clincal importance and molecular mechanisms. Pharmacogenetics 1996; 6:279–90
173. Meyers, U. A. Pharmacogenetics: the slow, the rapid and ultrarapid. Proc. Natl. Acad. Sci. USA 1994; 91:1983–4
174. Nebert, D. W., McKinnon, R. A. and Puga, A. Human drug-metabolizing enzyme polymorphism: effects on risk of toxicity and cancer. DNA Cell Biol. 1996; 15:273–80
175. Eaton, D. L., Gallagher, E. P., Bammler, T. K. and Kunze, K. L. Role of cytochrome P4501A2 in chemical carcinogenesis: implication for human variability in expression and enzyme activity. Pharmacogenetics 1995; 5: 259–74
176. Kawajiri, K., Nakachi, K. Imai, K. et al. Identification of genetically high risk individuals to lung cancer by DNA polymorphism on cytochrome P4501A1 gene. Letter, FEBS 1990; 263:131–3
177. Peterson, D. D., Mckinney, C. E., Ikeya, K. et al. Human CYP1A1 gene: cosegregation of the enzyme inducibility phenotype and an RFLP. Am J. Hum. Genet. 1991; 48:720–25
178. Raunio, H., Husgafvel-Pursiainen, K., Antilla, S. et al. Diagnosis of polymorphism in carcinogen-activating and inactivating enzymes and cancer susceptibility – review. Gene 1995; 159:113–21
179. Flaws, J. A. and Bush, T. L. Racial differences in drug metabolism: an explanation for higher breast cancer mortality in blacks? Medical Hypoth. 1998; 50:327–9
180. Nebert, D. W. Polymorphism in drug-metabolizing enzymes: what is their clinical relevance and why do they exist? Am. J. Hum. Genet. 1997; 60:265–71
181. Linder, M. W., Prough, R. A. and Valdes, R. Jr. Pharmacogenetics: a laboratory tool for optimizing therapeutic efficiency. Clin. Chem. 1997; 43:254–66
182. Kelsey, K. T., Ross, D., Traver, R. D. et al. Ethnic variation in the prevalence of a common NAD (P) H quinone oxidoreductase polymorphism and its implication for anticancer chemotherapy. Brit. J. Cancer 1997; 76:852–4
183. Vermes, A., Guchelaar, H. J. and Koopmans, R. P. Individualization of cancer chemotherapy based on cytochrome P450 polymorphism: a pharmacogenetic approach. Cancer Treat. Rev. 1997; 23:321–39
184. Gonzalez, F. J. and Idle, J. R. Pharmacogenetic phenotyping and genotyping. Present status and future potential. Clin. Pharmacokinet. 1994; 26:56–70
185. Seidegard, T., Voracheck, W. R., Pero, R. W. and Pearson, W. R. Hereditary differences in the expression of human glutathione transferase active on transstilbane oxide are due to gene deletion. Proc. Natl. Acad. Sci. USA 1988; 85:7293–7
186. Beard, P. Genetic Polymorphism of Glutathione Transferase in Men. In: Pickett, C. B. and Mantle, T. J. (eds), GlutathioneTransferase and Drug Resistance (eds:) Taylor and Francis, 1990:232–41
187. Norris, K. K., DeAngelo, T. M. and Vessell, S. E. G. Genetic and environmental factors that regulate cytosolic epoxide hydrolase acivity in human lymphocytes. J. Clin. Invest. 1989; 84:1749–56

15 Adverse Reproductive Outcome Potential of Cancer Therapies During Pregnancy

Mrinal K. Sanyal

Introduction

A vast majority of chemotherapeutic drugs and radiation treatments for cancer are deleterious to the developing conceptus (placenta and embryo-fetus). Developing conceptuses and cancer tissues exhibit close similarities in biological characteristics, and both are exposed to treatment agents given through the maternal system during cancer therapy of pregnant women (Table 15.1). At present, a wide variety of chemotherapeutic drugs are used for cancer treatment.[1] Chemotherapeutic drugs are genotoxic, damaging the genome, thereby affecting the expression of genes, preventing cell division and destroying cancer cells. These drugs are of different types and molecular processes, for killing of cancer cells may involve affecting DNA synthesis and its replication (antimetabolites), breaking and unwinding of the DNA strands (antibiotics) and cross-linking with DNA or other macromolecules (alkylating agents). Inhibiting functions of the mitotic apparatus associated with cell division (plant alkaloids) and influencing hormonal effects (antihormonal agents) are also important mechanisms of chemotherapeutic drugs. (See also chapters 11, 13.)

The growing chorionic villi of the placenta invade the maternal uterine tissues and progressively immerse themselves in the maternal blood, exposing the conceptus to deleterious effects of drugs and radiation.[2] Such exposure may lead to anomalous fetal development and adverse reproductive outcome (Table 15.2).[3] However, pregnancy is a specialized condition and has adaptations for a selective transport of substances from the maternal compartments to the fetus (Fig. 15.1).[4] The pregnancy state is associated with changes in cardiac, hematological, renal, immunological, nutritional and metabolic processes in the mother.[5] Drug metabolism and phamacokinetics during pregnancy are different from that in the non-pregnant state, and these processes change progressively with growth and development of the conceptus. The drug metabolizing enzymes (phase 1 and phase 2) are expressed in both maternal and conceptus tissues.[6-9] Expression of these enzymes varies widely and is determined by specific genetic characteristics. A more effective, personalized cancer therapy, based on the drug metabolism potential of the individual (pharmacogenetics), is emerging.[10-12] These physiological, metabolic, and genetic factors influence reproductive outcomes related to cancer treatment of pregnant women.

Table 15.1. Similarities and differences between conceptus and cancer tissues

Conceptus (placenta–embryo/fetus)	Cancer tissue
Originates from one cell (fertilized ovum) with progressive differentiation into normal cell types and organs	Originate as a clone of a few mutated cells that progressively become heterogenous abnormal cancer (tumor) cells
Differentiating cells may migrate to form functioning organs	Cancer cells may migrate and colonize to destroy host tissues
Placenta tissue (fetal genotype) invades into genetically different maternal tissues	Cancer tissue, modified by mutation and other genetic changes, invades host organs
Generates immunosuppressive substances to survive within maternal body	Creates immunosuppressive mechanisms for invasion and destruction of host cells
Produces numerous growth and cytokine factors independent of the mother and also by simultaneous maternal influences	Produces numerous growth and cytokine factors different from the host (tumor markers); few resemble conceptus factors
Fast cell cycle rate compared to maternal cells	Fast cell cycle rate compared to host tissues
Placental trophoblast villi with proliferating cells are bathed in maternal blood and derive nutrients from the maternal system	Tumor with dividing cells is infiltrated by the capillary system of the host for supply of nutrients
Active and selective transport system for systemic drugs from the maternal to fetal compartment, trophoblast cell layer is a barrier for drug transport	Reduced barrier for the availability of systemic drugs from the host to tumor tissues
Drug activation and detoxification systems are present in maternal, placental and fetal compartments	High activation and reduced detoxification systems for drugs in tumor tissues

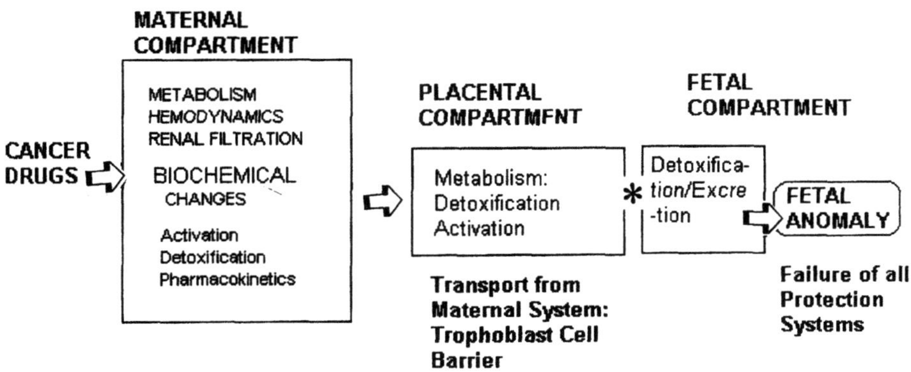

Fig. 15.1. A brief outline of the various biological processes occurring during pregnancy. The three basic compartments (maternal, placental and fetal) are active in protecting fetal development, and failure of all protection systems results in fetal anomalies. The human placenta is hemochorial and trophoblastic villi with fetal blood capillaries are bathed within the maternal blood. The villi are exposed directly to systemic maternal drugs. The interface between the maternal and the fetal compartments are the layers of trophoblast cells (cytotrophoblast and syncytiotrophoblast) of the villi. Although these cells have potent metabolic systems for drug metabolism, cytotoxic drugs still can damage them and affect the drug transport processes into the fetus.

Table 15.2. Mechanisms of adverse effects of cytotoxic drugs and radiation cancer therapies during early pregnancy influencing pregnancy outcome and maternal reproduction potential

Target of effects		Cytotoxic drugs	Radiation exposure
Birth defects in offspring:	(i)	Cell processes for organogenesis: Cell cycle (most important), cell-migration, interaction, and death; gene expression and differentiation of somatic and germ cells	Same processes for organogenesis are affected as with cyto-toxic drugs, but by a different mechanism
	(ii)	Genotoxic mechanisms: molecular adduct formation leading to gene mutation, chromosome breaks and reorganization	Genotoxic mechanisms: energy transfer leading to gene mutation, chromsome breaks and reorganization
Maternal reproduction:	(i)	Germ cell death, genotoxic changes, hormone imbalance, and damaged accessory reproductive organs	Germ cell death and genotoxic changes

Since the treatment procedures for cancer during pregnancy can be hazardous to fetal development and the offspring born, a register of exposures is in place for collection of data at the University of Oklahoma Medical Center[13] (Dr John Mulvihill, Director). Assessment of specific teratogenic and mutagenic effects of different chemotherapeutic drugs have been extremely difficult as the samples are relatively rare, and therapeutic procedures are rapidly evolving. Also the cases are to a great extent unreported. Most of the present knowledge of deleterious effects of cancer treatment during pregnancy is based on experimental studies with animal species and observation of abnormal outcomes in clinical case reports. This review will describe these adverse reproductive outcomes associated with cancer therapy and the influences of newer drugs and protocols on this process.

Animal and Historical Early Human Exposure Studies

Exposure to Chemotherapeutic Drugs

Birth defects are dysmorphogenesis of fetal organs induced during pregnancy. The malformation in the fetus may be due to inherent genetic causes, or to involuntary environmental toxic exposure, or to treatment procedures such as cancer chemotherapy and radiation during pregnancy. Abnormal development may be structural, or functional, or both. The malformations are highly variable in animal species and in humans, and depend on the period of exposure during development.[3] Although there are significant differences in dysmorphology between experimental studies of animals and reports on human exposures,[14] animal studies remain the basic foundation for drug effect analysis. Recognition of the absence of reliable human data is an important consideration in cancer therapy counseling and in prevention of unnecessary termination of pregnancy.[15]

Chemotherapeutic agents for cancer treatment are teratogenic and they induce different types of anomalies in the fetus and ultimately in the offspring.[16] Among the chemotherapeutic drugs, cyclophosphamide, an alkylating agent, has been studied extensively. It induces teratogenic effects by maternal treatment in common laboratory animal species, and a biochemical activation process produces the specific teratogenic agent.[16-19] Exposure to this agent has produced major congenital anomalies in humans. On the basis of few case reports, cyclophosphamide induces structural deformities of the limbs, cleft palate, and cardiac and eye abnormalities.[20-21] Methotrexate, a widely used antimetabolite drug, induces malformations in various animal species, including humans. The adverse effect is mostly embryo lethality and fetal growth retardation.[22] The drug is also known to produce craniofacial and limb anomalies.[23-26] Similar examples of multiple congenital anomalies have been observed in animal species and humans exposed to fluorouracil derivatives.[27]

The initial studies of vinca alkaloids in different animal species, including monkeys, indicated that the agent was teratogenic; however, human exposure studies have failed to substantiate such deleterious effects.[28-31] Retinoic acids are potent and emerging new drugs for cancer therapy.[32] They are known to be teratogenic in various animal test systems and in monkeys.[33-35] The teratogenic effect of retinoic acid in humans remains controversial.[35] Among anticancer agents, doxorubicin and other antibiotics are known to be less toxic to fetal development in spite of the fact that these drugs cross the placental barrier and enter the fetal compartment.[36-39] During the 1980s, cancer therapy advanced to a more effective multimodal chemotherapy (combination of several drugs) and radiation.[40] Effects of cancer treatments with more than one chemotherapeutic drug in combination with radiation on fetal development and reproductive outcomes are being assessed in recent case reports. The sequence of administration and relative doses of the therapeutic agents may influence the reproductive outcomes.

Exposure to Radiation

At present, irradiation in combination with chemotherapy is a major modality of cancer treatment, and often a high dose of radiation is applied for a rapid remission and cure.[41-42] The radiation from such treatment to a pregnant patient may impact embryo-fetal development in utero and postnatal life significantly. Experimental animal studies and observation of human exposure have revealed that prenatal radiation produces embryo-fetal death, a spectrum of congenital anomalies, growth retardation, developmental delays and various functional deficits depending upon the dose and gestational phase of the exposure.[43-44] It is known from animal studies that maternal radiosensitivity is markedly increased during pregnancy. There is also induction of major genomic and carcinogenic alterations in embryonic primordial cells by in utero radiation exposure.[45-47]

Significant human anomalies are produced by in utero radiation exposure during the period of organogenesis (8–15 weeks of pregnancy). Deleterious effects on the brain and other neurological damage are dramatic during 16–25 weeks of gestation. Anomalies include microcephaly, eye abnormalities (cataracts and retinal degeneration), skeletal and genital dysmorphology.[48-49] Abnormal gray matter suggesting abnormal neural cell migration has also been reported in humans. In addition, functional neurological deficits of mental retardation and reduced scholastic skills during postnatal life have been shown to be important deleterious effects caused by in utero radiation exposure.[50-52] The recent studies showing the positive relationship of intrauterine radiation exposure to childhood cancer have also been of great concern.[53-55]

Deleterious effects of prenatal radiation exposure on human diseases have been studied in atomic bomb survivors[56-61] and those of the Chernobyl reactor accident.[62-67] The observed effects include various types of congenital anomalies, fetal growth retardation, increase of cancer incidence, and brain damage, reduced intelligence quotient and reduced scholastic skills. Since the mathematical models of radiation exposure predict the possibility of human cancer even at very low levels of exposure, and public health studies support this possibility, re-evaluation of the threshold regulation for radiation therapy during pregnancy has been urged.[68-71] Thus, scattered radiation during radiation therapy has the potential for inducing damage to the fetus. Strategies for the management of pregnant cancer patients and reduction of fetal exposure by measuring fetal dose with anthropomorphic phantoms and by using different types of radioprotective shields are being developed for specific cancers.[72-77]

Analysis of Birth Defects' Potential Based on Clinical Cases

Background Estimates

The Birth Defects Monitoring Program of the Centers for Disease Control and Prevention estimates an overall rate of 3–4% of infants diagnosed with birth defects in the first year of life based on the surveillance of more than 17 million births in the USA.[78] This estimate does not consider environmental exposure information. The prevalence of types of birth defect varies year to year, and among subgroups of the population, maternal age groups, geographic regions and socioeconomic statuses. At present, the 3–4% rate is generally considered to be the baseline value. The background rate for spontaneous abortion of recognized pregnancy is approximately 15%, premature delivery 6–8%, and full term delivery 80%.[79]

Pregnancy Outcomes Related to Cancer Treatment During Pregnancy

Comprehensive surveys of human exposure cases such as that by Nicholson in 1968[80], established that treatment of cancer during pregnancy may produce adverse reproductive outcomes. Cancer care procedures for pregnant patients changed significantly during the 1970s and 1980s based on advances in drug discovery. In 1987, Mulvihill et al. showed in a large cooperative study on pregnancy outcomes that, in spite of improvements in cancer therapy, cancer treatment procedures during pregnancy still produced adverse outcomes.[81] This clinical report contained data from 133 pregnancies comprised of 3 groups: 43 ending before therapy commenced, 32 receiving therapy at conception or during pregnancy, and 58 after therapy had been completed. The risk of teratogenic outcome by cancer treatment during the first treatment of pregnancy was greater; among 10 live born infants, 8 were normal and 2 abnormal. In the group of women who received chemotherapy after pregnancy, 40% of next pregnancies showed low birth weight or premature termination of pregnancy. These adverse effects were presumably due to inadequate functioning of the uterus and hormonal secretion related to reproduction. Subsequent clinical series established further that chemotherapy during the first trimester increased the likelihood of spontaneous abortions and birth defects, and with treatment after this period of pregnancy, these risks were reduced.[82-83]

Recently, Ebert et al. reviewed pregnancies in which of cytotoxic therapy was used, published between 1983 and 1995.[84] The information on drug type, dose and gestational age during exposure were analyzed with respect to teratogenicity, stillbirth, spontaneous abortion, and premature birth. Available data in this regard for leukemia, lymphoma and gynecological and/or breast cancer are outlined in Table 15.3, and graphically shown in Fig. 15.2. These data showed that there is a trend of increased congenital anomalies (6–17 %) among live-born infants. In addition, there is a marked increase of preterm births ranging from 30–50% in patients treated for cancer during pregnancy. These rates are well above background levels and appear to be significantly different from untreated controls.

Among 96 cases recorded for perigestational treatment of leukemia, 2 women died, and therapeutic abortion was performed on 2 cases, and 2 children were stillborn.[84] These pregnant cancer patients received a combination therapy with chemotherapeutic drugs: 6-mercaptopurine, cytarabine, vincristine, daunorubicin, doxorubicin and prednisone. There were also cases treated with cyclophosphamide, busulfan, aminopterine, methotrexate and mitoxantrone. Nine children were born with congenital anomalies of varying degree, and 9 other newborns without apparent morphological anomalies had bone marrow hypoplasia or other hematological abnormalities. In lymphoma cases, the drug exposure was also combination chemo-

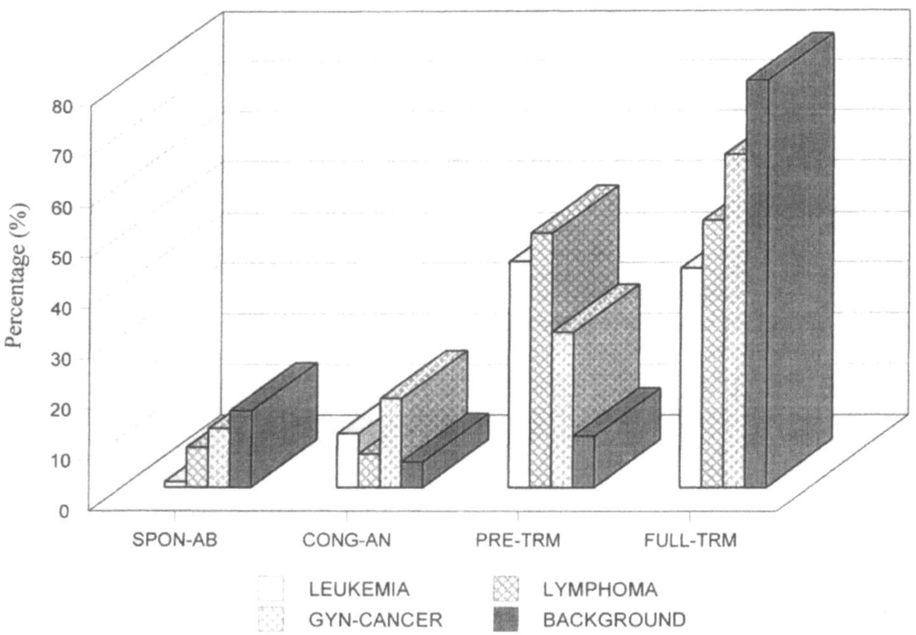

Fig. 15.2. Graphic representation of data available from the review by Ebert et al. and Table 15.3 (ref. 84) showing comparative effects on the reproductive outcome of treatment of leukemia, lymphoma and gynecological cancer during pregnancy. There is a trend of increased congenital anomalies (CONG-AN) in the fetus for all the three treatment groups. However, there is a substantial increase in the preterm birth (PRE-TRM) presumably induced by treatment of the cancer with chemotherapeutic drugs during pregnancy. This may be due to toxicity of the drugs on the placental tissues. The values for spontaneous abortion (SPON-AB) during the first trimester are low for all the groups. A statistical significance of the difference between groups cannot be ascertained, as the data collection conditions were variable without simultaneous controls.

Table 15.3. Estimates of deleterious effects on birth outcomes associated with cancer therapy during pregnancy*

Disease	No. of cases	Spontaneous abortion	Congenital anomalies (live-born infants)	Pre-term birth (normal and abnormal)	Full-term birth 35+ wks
Leukemia	92	1.1** (1/92)++	10.5 (9/89)	44.3 (39/88)	42.9 (33/77)
Lymphoma	51	7.8 (4/51)	6.5 (3/46)	50 (Approx.)	52.4 (22/42)
Gynecologic cancer	26	11.5 (3/26)	17.4 (4/23)	30.4 (7/23)	65.2 (15/23)

* Based on data available from References 82–84
** Percentage
++ Number of cases/total examined

therapy. In this group of patients, therapeutic abortions were performed in 5 of 57 patients, 4 pregnancies spontaneously aborted, 1 fetus was stillborn, and 3 of 46 live-born children exhibited anomalies. It is noteworthy that approximately one half of pregnancies resulted in preterm deliveries. Similarly, the gynecological and/or breast cancer group showed 3 cases of spontaneous abortion, 4 of 23 live-born infants with congenital anomalies, and more than 30% (15 of 23) of births were from preterm deliveries.

Some Recent Cases of Treatment and the Pregnancy Outcome

Recent progress in cancer treatment procedures during pregnancy is summarized in a number of reviews.[85-89] A general recommendation for cancer treatment is to avoid the first trimester, as it is the most sensitive period for birth defects. In addition, antimetabolite and alkylating drugs and radiation treatments are also not to be used whenever possible. At present, cancer treatment during pregnancy may include a number of new drugs (e.g.; carboplatin, paclitaxel, docetaxel, interferons, all-*trans* retinoic acid (ATRA), etoposide, teniposide, bleomycin, idarubicin, tamoxifen and GnRH agonists) along with established drugs for chemotherapy. Limiting treatment to the second and third trimesters of pregnancy, and being cautious in the use of radiation, seem to have reduced apparent birth defects in the progeny. Another basic strategy has been Cesarean section delivery, as soon as competency of the fetus for postnatal survival is ascertained, to allow for aggressive treatment of the mother.

The details of current management for specific cancers have been outlined in several recent reviews. The treatment procedures during pregnancy for blood cancers,[90-93] gynecological cancers[94-104] and melanoma[105-107] include considerations of risk to the fetus and a comparative assessment of the drugs used. A number of studies also show that surgical removal of solid tumors is highly beneficial for some cancers during pregnancy with variable results for reproductive outcome.[108-114] Delay in therapy to the second and third trimester of pregnancy is an option also frequently considered at the expense of the maternal cure.

Table 15.4. Some examples of current therapeutic procedures and pregnancy outcomes

Disease	No. of patients	Treatment drugs	Trimester treatment	Fetal outcome	References
Breast	24	Fluorourocil Doxorubicin Cyclophosphamide	2nd, 3rd	All normal Av .38 wk delivery	Berry et al.[115]
Ovary	1	Bleomycin Cisplatin Etoposide	2nd	Abnormal (cerebral atrophy) 28 wk; C-sec	Elit et al.[116]
Cervix	1	Cisplatin	2nd	Normal 32 wk; C-sec	Giacalone et al.[117]
same	2	Vincristin Cisplatin	1st 2nd	Normal 34 wk; C-sec Normal 32 wk; C-sec	Tewari et al.[118]
Multiple myeloma	1	Interferon-alpha	1st	Normal 38 wk	Sakata et al.[119]
Acute promyelocytic leukemia	1	ATRA	2nd, 3rd	Normal 30 wk; C-sec	Harrison et al.[120]
same	3	ATRA	2nd, 3rd	Normal Premature	Hoffman et al.[121]
same	1	ATRA	1st	Normal; 38 wk	Simone et al.[122]
same	1	ATRA	3rd	Normal; 38 wk	Watanabe et al.[123]
same	1	ATRA	3rd	Normal; 38 wk	Lipovsky et al.[124]
same	1	ATRA: CSF EPO	1st	Normal; 40 wk	Lin et al.[125]
same	1	ATRA	3rd	Normal; 33 wk	Terada et al.[126]
Acute leukemia	1	Cytarabine Daunorubin Mitoxantrone	2nd	Stillborn; 40 wk	Reynoso et al.[127]
same	1	C-Arabinoside Daunorubicine Etoposide	2nd	Normal; C-sec 32 wk	Murray et al.[128]
same	1	Idarubicin C-Arabinoside	2nd	Normal; premature; 33 wk	Claahsen et al.[129]
Lymphoblastic leukemia	1	Vincristine Prednisone	3rd	Normal; 35 wk	Tewari et al.[130]

Table 15.4 (cont.)

Disease	No. of patients	Treatment drugs	Trimester treat-ment	Fetal outcome	References
same		6-mercaptopurine	1st	Spontaneous abortion	Bergstrom et al.[131]
		Vincristine,			
		Methotrexate	2nd	Normal; 34 wk	
		Prednisone			
Rhabdosarcoma	1	Vincristine	3rd	Normal; 36 wk C-sec	Martin et al.[132]
		Actinomycin D			
		Cyclophosphamide			
Melanoma	1	Tamoxifen	2nd	Normal; 30 wk C-sec	DiPaola et al.[133]
		Carmustine			
		Dacarbazine			
		Cisplatin			
Lung	2	Cisplatin	2nd	Normal; Full term	Chen et al.[134]
		Radiation			
			3rd	Normal; Full term	

Some examples of current therapeutic procedures and pregnancy outcomes are shown in Table 15.4. Among these, management of breast cancer during pregnancy has been encouraging. A standardized treatment protocol for breast cancer with fluorouracil (1,000 mg/m^2), doxorubicin (50 mg/m^2) and cyclophosphamide (500 mg/m^2) administered every 3–4 weeks after first trimester pregnancy for 4 cycles, developed at the M. D. Anderson Hospital, University of Texas, resulted in normal pregnancy outcomes in 24 patients.[115] Ovarian and cervical cancer treatment procedures mostly relied on cisplatin and had variable reproductive outcomes.[116-118]

New therapeutic protocols for multiple myeloma using interferon-alpha[119] and for promyelocytic leukemia using all-*trans* retinoic acid (ATRA),[120-126] appear to be extremely promising in a number of case reports. Although retinoic acids are known to be teratogenic agents in animal experiments,[32-35] thus far, treatment of pregnant patients with these drugs has resulted in complete remission of leukemia and normal live births with minimal delivery complications. The current therapies for leukemia and other blood cancers with antibiotic drugs, bone marrow transplantation and activation of stem cells by interleukin and other cytokines are successful therapeutic procedures with a reduced possibility of adverse outcomes.[127-131] Attempts at therapy for cancers of other organs during pregnancy with favorable reproductive outcomes are also being made.[132-134]

Maternal Cancer Survival and Ethical Aspects of Fetal Wellbeing

The conceptus generates high levels of specific proteins, hormones, growth factors and cytokines, and also induces an immunosuppressive process for maintenance of the pregnancy in the face of a fetus genetically different from the mother.[135-138] Any of these factors may significantly influence the development and progression of cancer during pregnancy, especially in cancers of endocrine responsive tissues. Whether a current pregnancy or variables related to previous pregnancies increase or decrease the risk of cancer in humans still remains unclear.[139-143] However, estrogen and progesterone, major hormones of pregnancy, have been shown to regulate some cancer conditions.[144-145] Cancer therapy during pregnancy is not comparable to that in the non-pregnant state.

There is a growing concern that antenatal exposure to drugs may be a source of cancer in the future progeny.[146-148] Cancer treatment during pregnancy also influences future maternal reproductive processes significantly as both chemotherapeutic drugs and radiation may cause injuries to germ cells and uterine tissues.[149-152] The long-term effects of maternal cancer treatment during pregnancy on the overall growth and development of children seem minimal,[153-154] but the risks of cancer and other diseases are significant. In addition, there are cases of maternal malignancy that metastasizes to placenta or fetus and thereby inflicts maternal disease on the progeny.[155-158]

Fetal development is highly sensitive to cancer therapy (drugs and radiation) during the first trimester of pregnancy, the period of organogenesis. Progressively the fetus becomes more resistant during the second and third trimesters. Delay in therapy benefits the fetus, but this can markedly compromise maternal survival and the chances of her cancer cure. Nettleton et al. have developed a mathematical model that recognizes primary breast tumor size and lymph node pathology as the most important prognostic indicators of survival.[159] Delay in therapy progressively increases the risks of axillary node involvement and maternal survival. At present, maintenance of pregnancy without treatment of cancer has a cost to maternal life, whereas early treatment may lead to numerous short-term and long-term deleterious effects to the progeny.

Thus, treatment of cancer during pregnancy is an extremely complex process. It involves consideration of various ethical issues, including abortion and loss of life, risks of cancer in the progeny, infertility of the offspring and mother, and expenses of the disabilities associated with congenital anomalies.[160] Clinical management and treatment procedures for cancer during pregnancy require evaluation of both the benefits of therapy to the mother and the safety of the embryo-fetus. Our present knowledge is insufficient in this area.

Conclusion

The rapidly growing and differentiating conceptus during pregnancy resembles in many ways a cancerous condition. The invading placental trophoblastic tissues are bathed in maternal blood and are exposed to the maternal cancer chemotherapeutic drugs and effects of radiation. Cancer cell eradication is based on inflicting genotoxic effects on the molecular processes of gene expression and cell division in the neoplastic cells. In spite of maternal physiological processes and the placental barriers and mechanisms for detoxification provided by the placenta and fetus, these drugs may produce deleterious effects on both placental and fetal tissues resulting in adverse reproductive outcomes. Animal studies and historical observations of human exposures have established that a vast majority of chemotherapeutic drugs and radiation, even at a low level, may be hazardous to fetal wellbeing. They may also be a source of major diseases, including cancer and mental retardation, in postnatal life. In addition, these studies have shown that fetal development is affected at all stages of development. The first trimester of pregnancy is highly sensitive to drug effects and fetal morphological anomalies generally appear during this period. The most significant deleterious effect of current chemotherapy is induction of preterm delivery. Treatment protocols should consider the risks to the fetus and benefits to the mother, as delay in therapy until the second and third trimester of pregnancy may benefit the fetus at the cost of maternal life and cure of her cancer. At present, information is not available on the handling of numerous cancer chemotherapeutic drugs during pregnancy and their transfer potential across the placenta. An aggressive research effort in this direction will benefit pregnant patients and their progeny.

Acknowledgments

The author is grateful to Dr. Maurice J. Mahoney, Professor of Genetics and Obstetrics and Gynecology, Yale University, for the numerous constructive suggestions and extensive editorial help in preparation of the manuscript. He is also thankful to Dr. F. Naftolin, Chairman, Department of Obstetrics & Gynecology, for generous support of author's research in this area, and to Dr. Albert B. Deisseroth, Ensign Professor of Oncology and Medicine, Yale University, for discussions regarding the manuscript. Research support of the author was from the National Institutes of Health.

References

1. Moore, M. J. and Goldenberg, G. J. Antineoplastic Drugs. In: Kalant, H. and Roschlau, W. H. E. (eds), Principles of Medical Pharmacology, Oxford University Press, New York, 1998:759–74
2. Patten, B. M., Human Embryology. VI. Fetal Membranes and Placenta. McGraw-Hill, New York, 1968:102–38
3. Moore, K. The Developing Human (Clinically Oriented Embryology) 8. The causes of Human Congenital Malformations, 4th edn, W. B. Saunders, Philadelphia, 1988:131–58
4. Morriss, F. H., Boyd, R. D. H. and Mahendran, D. Placental Transport. In: Knobil, E. and Neill, J. D. (eds), The Physiology of Reproduction, 2nd edn, pp. Raven Press, New York, 1994:813–816
5. Chamberlain, G. and Pipkin, F. B. (eds), Clinical Physiology in Obstetrics, 3rd edn, Blackwell Science, Malden, MA, 1998
6. Juchau, M. R., Boutelet-Bochan, H. and Huang, Y. Cytochrome-P450-dependent biotransformation of xenobiotics in human and rodent embryonic tissues. Drug Metab. Rev. 1998; 30:541–68
7. Hakkola, J., Pelkonen, O. Pasanen, O. and Raunio, H. Xenobiotic-metabolizing cytochrome P450 enzymes in human feto-placental unit: role in intrauterine toxicity. Crit. Rev. Toxicol. 1998; 28:35–72
8. Sanyal, M. K., Li, Y. L, Biggers, W. J. et al. Augmentation of polynuclear aromatic hydrocarbon metabolism of human placental tissues of first trimester pregnancy by cigarette smoke exposure. Am. J. Obstet. Gynecol. 1993; 168:1587–97
9. Sanyal, M. K., Li, Y. L. and Belanger, K. Metabolism of polynuclear aromatic hydrocarbon in human term placenta influenced by cigarette smoke exposure. Reprod. Toxicol. 1994; 8:411–18
10. Krynetsky, E. Y. and Evans, W. E. Pharmacogenetics of cancer therapy: getting personal. Am. J. Human Genet. 1998; 63:11–6
11. Vermes, A., Guchelaar, H. J. and Koopmans, R. P. Individualization of cancer chemotherapy based on cytochrome P450 polymorphism: pharmcogenetic approach. Cancer Treat. and Rev. 1997; 23:321–39

12. Flaws, J. A. and Bush, T. L. Racial differences in drug metabolism: an explanation for higher breast cancer mortality in blacks? Med. Hypothesis 1998; 50:327–9
13. Randall, T. National registry seeks scarce data on pregnancy outcomes during chemotherapy. JAMA 1993; 269:323
14. Holmes, L. B. Exposures in pregnancy that are harmful to the fetus i.e., human teratogen. Pediatr. Res. 1999; 45:286–7
15. Koren, G. and Pastuszak, A. Prevention of unnecessary pregnancy termination by counseling women on drug, chemical and radiation exposure during first trimester. Teratology 1990; 41:657–61
16. Shepard, T. H. Catalog of Teratogenic Agents, 8th edn, The Johns Hopkins University Press, Baltimore, 1995
17. Sanyal, M. K., Kitchin, K. T. and Dixon, R. L. Rat conceptus development in vitro: comparative effects of alkylating agents. Toxicol. Appl. Pharmacol. 1981; 57:14–19
18. Kitchin, K. T., Schimid, B. P. and Sanyal, M. K. Teratogenicity of cyclophosphamide in a coupled microsomal activating/embryo culture system. Biochem. Phamacol. 1981; 30:59–64
19. Satish, J., Pratt, B. M. and Sanyal, M. K. Differential dysmorphogenesis induced by microinjection of an alkylating agent into rat conceptuses cultured in vitro. Teratology 1985; 31:61–72
20. Greenberg, L. H., Palos, V. and Tanaka, K. R. Congenital anomalies probably induced by cyclophosphamide . JAMA 1964; 188:423–26
21. Toledo, T. M., Harper, R. C. and Moser, R. H. Fetal effects during cyclophosphamide and irradiation therapy. Ann. Intern. Med. 71971; 4:87–91
22. Wilson, J. G., Scott, W. J., Ritter, E. J. and Fradkin, R. C. Comparative distribution and embryotoxicity of methotrexate in pregnant rats and in monkeys. Teratology 1979; 19:71–80
23. Kirshon, B., Wasserstrum, N., Willis, R. et al. Teratogenic effects of first trimester cyclophosphamide therapy. Ostet. Gynecol. 1988; 72:462–6
24. Milunsky, A., Graef, J. W. and Gaynor, M. F. Methotrexate-induced congenital malformation with review of the literature. J. Pediatr. 1968; 72:790–95
25. Powell, H. R. and Ekert, H. Methotrexate-induced congenital malformation. Med. J. Aust. 1971; 2:1076–7
26. Bawle, E. V., Conrad, J. V. and Weiss, L. Adult and two children with fetal methotrexate syndrome. Teratology 1998; 57:51–5
27. Stephens, T. D., Golbus, M., Miller, J. R. et al. Multiple congenital anomalies in a fetus exposed to 5-fluorouracil during the first trimester. Am. J. Obstet. Gynecol. 1980; 137:747–9
28. Courtney, K. D. and Valerio, D. A. Teratology in the *Macaca mulatta*. Teratology 1968; 1:163–72
29. Lacher, M. J. Use of vinblastin sulfate to treat Hodgkin's disease during pregnancy. Ann. Intern. Med. 1964; 61:113–15
30. Armstrong, J. G., Dyke, R. W., Fouts, P. J. and Jansen, C.J. Delivery of a normal infant during the course of oral vincristine sulfate therapy for Hodgkin's disease. Ann. Intern. Med. 1964; 61:106–7
31. Rosenberg, A. L., Crews, Q. E. and Hopwood, H. G. Vinblastine sulfate in Hodgkin's disease in pregnancy. Ann. Intern. Med. 1964; 61:108–12
32. Miller, W. H. The emerging role of retinoids and retinoic acid metabolism blocking agents in the treatment of cancer. Cancer 1998; 83:1471–82
33. Fantel, A. G., Shepard, T. G., Neuell-Morris, L. L. and Moffett, B. C. Teratogenic effects of retinoic acid in pigtail monkey (*Macaca nemestrina*). Teratology 1977; 15: 65–71
34. Collins, M. D. and Mao, G. E. Teratology of retinoids. Ann. Rev. Pharmacol. Toxicol. 1999; 39:399–430
35. Lammer, E. J., Chen, D. T., Hoar, R. M. et al. Retinoic acid embryopathy. New Engl. J. Med. 1985; 313:837–41
36. Newcomb, M., Balducci, L., Thigpen, J. T and Morrison, F. S. Acute leukemia in pregnancy: successful delivery after cytarabine and doxorubicin. JAMA 1978; 239:2691–2
37. Garcia, V., San Miguel, J. and Bourasca, A. L. Doxorubicin in the first trimester pregnancy. Ann. Intern. Med. 1981; 94:547
38. Catanazarite, A. V. and Ferguson, J. E. Acute leukemia and pregnancy: a review of management and outcome 1972–1982. Obstet. Gynecol. Survey 1984; 39:663–78
39. Karp, G. I., von Oeyen, P., Valone, F. et al. Doxorubicin in pregnancy: possible transplacental passage. Cancer Treat. Report 1983; 67:773–7
40. Murray, C. L., Reicheert, J. A., Anderson, J. and Twiggs, L. B. Multimodal cancer therapy for breast cancer in the first trimester of pregnancy. JAMA 1984; 252:2607–8
41. Chao, H. T., Wang, P. H., Yuan, C. C. et al. Successful pregnancy in a woman with acute myeloid leukemia treated with high dose whole body irradiation. J. Reprod. Med. 1998; 43:703–6
42. Wang, W. S., Tzeng, C. H., Hsieh, R. K. et al. Successful pregnancy following very high dose total body irradiation (1575 cGy) and bone marrow transplantation in a woman with myeloid leukemia. Bone Marrow Transpl. 1998; 21:415–7

43. Brent, R. L. The effect of embryonic and fetal exposure to X-ray, microwaves, and ultrasound: counseling the pregnant and non-pregnant patient about their risks. Semin. Oncol. 1989; 16:347–68
44. Streffer, G. Health impacts of large releases of radionucleotides: Biological effects of prenatal irradiation. CIBA Foundation Symp. 1997; 203:155–66
45. Ricoul, M., Sabatier, L., and Dutrillaux, B. Increased chromosomal radiosensitivity during pregnancy. Mut. Res. 1997; 374:73–8
46. You, K., Bergstrom, R., Klemm, M. et al. Chromosome deletion comlexes in mice by radiation of embryonic stem cells. Nature Genetics 1997; 15:285–8
47. Lumniczky, K., Antal, S., Unger, E. et al. Carcinogenic alteration in murine liver, lung, and uterine tumors induced by in utero exposure to ionizing radiation. Mol. Carcinogenesis 1998; 21:100–10
48. Nakagawa, K., Aoki, Y., Kusama, T. et al. Radiotherapy during pregnancy: effects on fetus and neonates. Clin. Therap. 1997; 19:770–7
49. Mayr, N. A., Wen, B. C. and Saw, C. B. Radiation therapy during pregnancy. Obstet. Gynecol. Clinics in N. America 1998; 25:301–21
50. Miller, R. W. Intrauterine radiation exposure and mental retardation. Health Phys. 1988; 55:295–98
51. Kimler, B. F. Prenatal irradiation: a major concern for the developing brain. Int. J. Radiation Biol. 1998; 73:423–34
52. Nyagu, A. I., Loganovsky, K. and Loganvoskaja, T. K.. Psychophysiologic effects of prenatal irradiation. Int. J. Psychophysiology 1998; 30:303–11
53. Doll, R. and Wakeford, R. Risk of childhood cancer from fetal irradiation. Br. J. Radiol. 1997; 70:130–9
54. Bolande, R. P. Prenatal exposure and childhood cancer. Pediatr. Develop. Pathol. 1999; 2:208–14
55. Mangano, J. J. A rise in the incidence of childhood cancer in the United States. Int. J. Health Services 1999; 29:393–408
56. Neel, J. O. Genetic studies of the atomic bomb casualty commission – radiation effects research foundation: 1946–1997. Proc. Natl. Acad. Sci. USA. 1998; 95:5432–6
57. Delongchamp, R. R., Mabuchi, K. Yoshimoto, Y. and Preston, D. L. Cancer mortality among atomic bomb survivors exposed in utero or as young children, October 1950–May 1997. Radiation Res. 1997; 147:385–95
58. Miller, R. W. and Boice, J. D. Cancer after intrauterine exposure to the atomic bomb. Radiation Res. 1997; 147:396–7
59. Little, M. P. and Muirhead, C. R. Curvilinearity in the dose–response curve for cancer in Japanese atomic bomb survivors. Env. Health Perspectives 1997; 105 (Suppl. 6):1505–9
60. Otake, M. and Schull, W. J. Radiation related brain damage and growth retardation among the prenatally exposed atomic bomb survivors. Int. J. Radiation Biol. 1998; 74:159–71
61. Schull, W. J. Brain damage among individuals exposed prenatally to ionizing radiation: a 1993 review. Stem Cells 1997; 15 (Suppl. 2):129–33
62. Raytomaa, T. Ten years after Chernobyl. Ann. Med. 1996; 28:83–7
63. Kruslin, B., Jukic, S., Kos, M., Simic, G. and Cviko, A. Congenital anomalies of the central nervous system at autopsy in Croatia in the period before and after the Chernobyl accident. Acta Med. Croatia 1998; 52:103–7
64. Schwenn, M. R. and Brill, A. B. Childhood cancer 10 years after the Chernobyl accident. Curr. Opinions in Pediatr. 1997; 9:51–4
65. Petrova, A., Gnedko, T., Maistrova, I. et al. Morbidity in a large cohort study of children born to mothers exposed to radiation from Chernobyl. Stem Cells 1997; (Suppl. 2):141–50
66. Lazjuk, G. I., Nikolaev, D. L. and Novikova, I. V. Changes in registered congenital anomalies in the Republic of Belarus after Chernobyl accident. Stem Cells 1997; 15 (Suppl. 2):225–60
67. Kolominsky, Y., Igumnov, S. and Drozdovitch, V. The psychological development of children from Belarus exposed in the prenatal period to radiation from the Chernobyl atomic power plant. J. Child. Psychol. Psychiat Allied Discipl. 1999; 40:299–305
68. Doll, R. Effects of small doses of ionizing radiation. J. Radiol. Protec. 1998; 18:163–74
69. Hoel, D. G. and Li, P. Threshold models in radiation carcinogenesis. Health Phys. 1999; 75:241–50
70. Nussbaum, R. H. The linear no-threshold dose-effect relation: is it relevant to radiation protection regulation? Med. Phys. 1998; 25:291–9
71. Mangano, J. J. Low-level Radiation and Immune System Damage – an Atomic Age Legacy. Lewis Publication, CRC Press, Boca Rotan, 1999
72. Stabin, M. G., Tagesson, M., Thomas, S. R. et al. Radiation dosimetry in nuclear medicine. Appl. Rad. Isotopes 1999; 50:73–87
73. Mazonakis, M., Damilakis, J., Theoharopoulos, N. et al. Brain radiotherapy during pregnancy: an analysis of conceptus dose using anthropomorphic phantoms. Br. J. Radiol. 1999; 72:274–8

74. Podgorsak, M., Meiler, R. J., Kowal, H. et al. Technical management of a pregnant patient undergoing radiation therapy to the head and neck. Med. Dosimetry 1999; 24:121–8
75. Antypas, C., Sandilos, P., Kouvaris, J. et al. Fetal dose evaluation during breast cancer radiotherapy. Int. J. Radiat. Oncol. Biol. Phys. 1998; 40:995–9
76. Van der Giessen, P. H. Measurement of the peripheral dose of the tangential breast treatment technique with Co-60 gamma radiation and high energy X-rays. Radiother. Oncol. 1997; 42:257–64
77. Cygler, J., Ding, G. X., Kendal, W. and Cross, P. Fetal dose for a patient undergoing mantle field irradiation for Hodgkin's disease. Med. Dosimetry 1997; 22:135–7
78. CDC's Reproductive Health Surveillance – Prevalence of Birth Defects; State use of Birth Defects Surveillance, January 1999; *http://www.cdc.gov/nccdphp/drh/datoact/birout.htm*
79. Review Guidance (Evaluation of Human Pregnancy Outcome Data). US Department of Health and Human Services, June *1999. http://www.fda.gov/cder/guidance/index.htm*
80. Nicholson, H. O. Cytotoxic drugs in pregnancy. J. Obstet. Gynaecol. Brit. Comwlth. 1968; 75:307–12
81. Mulvihill, J. J., Mckeen, E. A., Rosner, F. and Zarrabi, M. H. Pregnancy outcome in cancer patients. Experience in a large cooperative group. Cancer 1987; 60:1143–50
82. Zemlicks, D., Lishner, M., Degendorf, P. et al. Fetal outcome after in utero exposure to cancer chemotherapy. Arch. Intern. Med. 1992; 152:573
83. Wiebe, V. J. and Sipila, P. E. H. Pharmacology of antineoplastic agents in pregnancy. Crit. Rev. Oncol. Hematol. 1994; 16:75–112
84. Ebert, U., Loffler, H., and Kirch, W. Cytotoxic therapy and pregnancy. Pharmacol. Therap. 1997; 74:207–20
85. Antonelli, N. M., Dotters, D. J., Katz, V. L. and Kuller, J. A. Cancer in pregnancy: review of the literature. Part I. Obstet. Gynecol. Survey 1996; 5:125–34
86. Antonelli, N. M., Dotters, D. J., Katz, V. L. and Kuller, J. A. Cancer in pregnancy: review of the literature. Part II. Obstet. Gynecol. Survey 5:135–42
87. Sorosky, J. I., Sood, A. K. and Buekers, T. E. The use of chemotherapeutic agents during pregnancy. Obstet. Gynecol. Clinics of N. America 1997; 24:591–9
88. Buekers, T. E. and Lallas, T. A. Chemotherapy in pregnancy. Obstet. Gynecol. Clinics of N. America 1998; 25:323–9
89. Falkenbury, S. S. Cancer in pregnancy. Surg. Oncol. Clinics of N. America 1998; 7:373–97
90. Peleg, D. and Ben-Ami, M. Lymphoma and leukemia complicating pregnancy. Obstet. Gynecol. Clinics of N. America 1998; 25:365–83
91. Barnes, M. N., Barrett, J. C., Kimberlin, D. F. and Kilgore, L. C. Burkitt's lymphoma in pregnancy. Obstet. Gynecol. 1998; 92:675–8
92. Stiles, G. M., Stance, L. M., Saven, A. and Hoffman, K. D. Splenectomy for hairy cell leukemia in pregnancy. J. Perinatology 1998; 18:200–201
93. Silva, P. T., de Almeida, H. M. N., Principe, F. and Pereira-Leite, L. Non-Hodgkin's lymphoma during pregnancy. Eur. J. Obstet. Gynecol. Reprod. Biol. 1998; 77:249–51
94. Merkel, D. E. Pregnancy and breast cancer. Semin. Surg. Oncol. 1996; 12:370–5
95. Kuerer, H. M., Cunnigham, J. D. Brower, S. T. and Tartter, P. I. Breast carcinoma associated with pregnancy and lactation. Surg. Oncol. 1997; 6:93–8
96. Espie, M. and Cuvier, C. Treating breast cancer during pregnancy. What can be taken safely? Drug Safety 1998; 18:135–42
97. Sorosky, J. I. and Scott-Conner, C. E. Breast disease complicating pregnancy. Obstet. Gynecol. Clinics of N. America 1998; 25:535–63
98. Shivvers, S. A. and Miller, D. S. Preinvasive and invasive breast and cervical cancer prior to or during pregnancy. Clin. In Perinatol. 1997; 24:369–89
99. Grendys, E. Jr. and Barnes, W. A. Ovarian cancer in pregnancy. Surg. Clinic of N. America. 71995; 5:1–14
100. Bouley, R. and Podczaski, E. Ovarian cancer complicating pregnancy. Obstet. Gynecol. Clinic of N. America 1998; 25:385–99
101. Sood, A. K. and Sorosky, J. I. Invasive cervical cancer complicating pregnancy. How to manage the dilemma. Obstet. Gynecol. Clinic of N. America 1998; 25:343–52
102. Connor, J. P. Non-invasive cervical cancer complicating pregnancy. Obstet. Gynecol. Clinic of N. America 1998; 25:331–42
103. Orr, J. W. Cervical cancer. Obstet. Gynecol. Clinic of N. America 1998; 25:299–316
104. Method, M. W. and Brost, B. C. Management of cervical cancer in pregnancy. Sem. Surg. Oncol. 1999; 16:251–60
105. Squatrito, R. C. and Harlow, S. P. Melanoma complicating pregnancy. Obstet. Gynecol. Clinic of N. America 1998; 25:407–16
106. Grein, C. M., Driscoll, M. S. and Grant-Kels, J. M. The relationship of pregnancy, hormones and melanoma. Sem. Cut. Med. Surg. 1998; 17:167–71

107. Mackie, R. M. Pregnancy and exogenous hormones in patients with cutaneous malignant melanoma. Curr. Open. Oncol. 1999; 11:129–31
108. Skilling, J. S. Colorectal cancer complicating pregnancy. Obstet. Gynecol. Clinic of N. America 1998; 25:417–21
109. Walsh, C. and Fazio, V. W. Cancer of the colon, rectum and anus during pregnancy. The surgeon's perspective. Gastroentrology Clinics of N. America 1998; 27:257–67
110. Cappell, M. S. Colon cancer during pregnancy. The gastroenterologist's perspective. Gastroentrology Clinics of N. America 1998; 27:225–56
111. Anthanassiou, A. M. and Craigo, S. D. Liver mass in pregnancy. Sem. Perinatol. 1998; 22:166–77
112. Sciscione, A. C., Villeneuve, J. B., Pitt, H. A. and Johnson, T. R. Surgery for pancreatic tumor during pregnancy: a case report and review of literature. Am. J. Perinatol. 1996; 13:21–5
113. Gross, A. J., Zoller, G., Hermanns, M. and Ringert, R. H. Renal cell carcinoma during pregnancy. Br. J. Urology 1995; 75:254–5
114. Hendry, W. F. Management of urological tumors in pregnancy. Br. J. Urology 1997; 80 (Suppl. 1):24–8
115. Berry, D. L., Theriault, R. L., Holmes, F. N. et al. Management of breast cancer during pregnancy using a standardized protocol. J. Clin. Oncol. 1999; 17:855–61
116. Elit, L., Bocking A., Kenyon, C. and Natale, R. An endometrial sinus tumor diagnosed in pregnancy: case report and review of literature. Gynec. Oncol. 1999; 72:123–7
117. Giacalone, P. L., Laffargue, F., Benos, R., Rpousseau, O. and Hedon, B. Cis-platinum neoadjuvant chemotherapy in pregnant women with invasive carcinoma of the uterine cervix. Br. J. Obstet. Gynecol. 1996; 103:932–4
118. Tewari, K., Cappuccini, F., Gambino, A. et al. Neoadjuvant chemotherapy in the treatment of locally advanced cervical carcinoma in pregnancy: a report of two cases and review of issues specific to the management of cervical carcinoma in pregnancy including planned delay of therapy. Cancer 1998; 82:1529–34
119. Sakata, H.., Karamitsos, J., Kundaria, B. and Disaia, P. J. Case report of interferon alfa therapy for multiple myeloma during pregnancy. Am J. Obstet. Gynecol. 1995; 172:217–9
120. Harrison, P., Chipping, P. and Fothergill, G. A. Successful use of all-trans retinoic acid in acute promyelocytic leukemia presenting during second trimester of pregnancy. Br. J. Haematol. 1994; 86:681–2
121. Hoffman, M. A., Wiernik, P. H. and Kleiner, G. J. Acute promyelocytic leukemia and pregnancy. A case report. Cancer 1995; 76:2237–41
122. Simone, M. D., Stasi, R., Venditt, A. et al. All-trans retinoic acid (ATRA) administration during pregnancy in relapsed acute promyelocytic leukemia. Leukemia 1995; 9:1412–3
123. Watanabe, R., Okamoto, S., Morki, T. et al. Treatment of acute promyelocytic leukemia with all-trans retinoic acid during the third trimester of pregnancy. Am J. Hematol. 1995; 48:210–1
124. Lipovsky, M. M., Biesma, D. H., Christiaens, G. C. and Petersen, E. J. Successful treatment of acute promyelocytic leukemia with all-trans retinoic acid during late pregnancy. Br. J. Haematol. 1996; 94:699–701
125. Lin, C. P., Huang, M. J., Liu, H. J., et al. Successful treatment of acute promyelocytic leukemia in pregnant Jehovah's Witness with all-trans retinoic acid, rhG-CSF and erythropoietin. Am J. Hematol. 1996; 51:251–2
126. Terada, Y., Shindo, T., Endoh, A. et al. Fetal arrhythmia during treatment of pregnancy-associated acute promyelocytic leukemia with all-trans retinoic acid and favorable outcome. Leukemia 1997; 11:454–5
127. Reynoso, E. E. and Huerta, F. Acute leukemia and pregnancy – fetal outcome after exposure to idarubicin during the second trimester. Acta Oncol. 1994; 33:709–12
128. Murray, N. A., Acolet, D., Deave, M. et al. Fetal marrow suppression after maternal chemotherapy for leukemia. Arch. Dis. Child. 1994; 71:F209–10
129. Claahsen, H. L., Semmekrat, B. A., Van Donegan, P. W. and Mattijssen, V. Successful fetal outcome after exposure to idarubicin and cytosine arabinoside during the second trimester of pregnancy – a case report. Am J. Perinatol. 1998; 15:295–7
130. Tewari, K., Cappuccini, F., Rosen, R. B. et al. Relapse of acute lymphoblastic leukemia in pregnancy: survival following chemoirradiation and autologous transfer of interleukin-2- activated stem cells. Gynecol. Oncol. 1999; 74:143–6
131. Bergstrom, S. K. and Altman, A. J. Pregnancy during therapy for childhood acute lymphoblastic leukemia: two case reports and review of literature. J. Ped. Hematol. Oncol. 1998; 20:154–9
132. Martin, D., Winter, S. S., Gardner, M. O. and Nicklause, P. Rhabdomyosarcoma treated with chemotherapy during the third trimester. Obstet. Gynecol. 1997; 89:828–31
133. DiPaola, R. S., Goodin, S. Ratzelle, M. et al. Chemotherapy for metastatic melanoma during pregnancy. Gynecol. Oncol. 1997; 66:526–30

134. Chen, K. Y., Wang, H. C., Shih, J. Y. and Yang, P. C. Lung cancer in pregnancy: report of two cases. J. Formosa Med. Assoc. 1998; 97:573-6
135. Ogren, L. and Talamantes, F. The placenta as an endocrine organ: polypeptides. In: Knobil, E. and Neill, J. D. (eds), The Physiology of Reproduction, 2nd edn, pp. Raven Press, New York, 1994: 875–945
136. Chard, T. Placental Metabolism. In: Chamberlain, G. and Pipkin, F. B. (eds), Clinical Physiology in Obstetrics, 3rd edn, Blackwell Science, Oxford, 1998: 419–35
137. Manyonda, I. T. The Immune System. In: Chamberlain, G. and Pipkin, F. B. (eds), Clinical Physiology in Obstetrics, 3rd edn, Blackwell Science, Oxford, 1998:129–62
138. Sanyal, M. K., Brami, C. J. Bischof, P. et al. Immunoregulatory activity in the supernatant from cultures of normal human trophoblast cells of the first trimester. Am. J. Obstet. Gynecol. 1989; 161:446–53
139. Holmes, F. N. Pregnancy, hormone replacement, and reproductive factors. In: Kavanaugh, J. J., Singletary, S. E., Einhorn, N. and DePetrillo, A. D. (eds), Cancer in Women, Blackwell Science, Malden, MA, 1998:215–37
140. Bonnier, P., Romain, S., Dilhuydy, M. et al. Influence of pregnancy on the outcome of breast cancer: a case-control study. Int. J. Cancer 1997; 72:720–7
141. Wohlfahrt, J. and Melbye, M. Maternal risk of breast cancer and birth characteristics of offspring by time since birth. Epidemiology 1999; 10:441–4
142. Sanderson, M., Williams, M. A., Daling, J. R. et al. Maternal factors and breast cancer among young women. Ped. Perinatal Epidemiol. 1998; 12:397–407
143. Troisi, R., Weiss, H. A., Hoover, R. N. et al. Pregnancy characteristics and maternal risk of breast cancer. Epidemiology 1998; 9:641–7
144. Gusman, R. C., Yang, J. Rajkumar, L. et al. Hormonal prevention of breast cancer: mimicking the protective effect of pregnancy. Proc. Natl. Acad. Sci. USA; 1999:96:2520–5
145. Schneider, H. P. and Jackisch, C. Potential benefits of oestrogens and progesterone on breast cancer. Int. J. Fertil. Womens Med. 1998; 43:278–85
146. Satge, D., Sasco, A. J. and Little, J. Antenatal therapeutic drug exposure and fetal/neonatal tumors: review of 89 cases. Pediatr. Perinat. Epidemiol. 1998; 12:84–117
147. Hemninke, E., Gissler, M. and Toukomaa, H. Exposure to female hormone drugs during pregnancy: effect on malformation and cancer. Br. J. Cancer 1999; 80:1092–7
148. Ekbom, A. Growing evidence that several human cancers may originate in utero. Sem. Cancer Biol. 1998; 8:237–44
149. Reichman, B. S. and Green, K. B. Breast cancer in young women: effect of chemotherapy on ovarian function, fertility, and birth defects. J. Natl. Cancer Inst. Monograph 1994; 16:125–9
150. Surbone, A. and Petrek, J. A. Childbearing issues in breast carcinoma survivors. Cancer 1997; 79:1271–8
151. Hensley, M. L. and Reichman, B. S. Fertility and pregnancy after adjuvant chemotherapy for breast cancer. Crit. Rev. Oncol-Hematol. 1998; 28:121–8
152. Averette, H. E., Mirhashemi, R. and Moffat, F. L. Pregnancy after breast carcinoma: the ultimate medical challenge. Cancer 1999; 85:2301–4
153. Reynoso, E. E., Shepard, F. A., Messner, H. A. Acute leukemia during pregnancy: The Toronto leukemia study group experience with long-term follow-up of children exposed in utero to chemotherapeutic agents. J. Clin. Oncol. 1987; 5:1098–106
154. Aviles, A., Diaz-Maqueo, J. C., Talavera, A. et al. Growth and development of children of mothers treated with chemotherapy during pregnancy: current status of 43 children. Am. J. Hematol. 1991; 36:243–8
155. Didley, G. Y. III, Moise, K. J. Carpenter, R. J. et al. Maternal malignancy metastatic to the products of conception: a review. Obstet. Gynec. Survey 1989; 44:535–40
156. Osada, S., Horibe, K., Oiwa, K. et al. A case of infantile acute monocytic leukemia caused by vertical transmission of mother's leukemia cells. 1990; Cancer 65:1146–9
157. Catlin, E. A., Roberts, J. D., Erana, R. et al. Transplacental transmission of natural killer cell lymphoma. New Engl. J. Med. 1999; 341:85–91
158. Resnick, R. Cancer during pregnancy. New Engl. J. Med. 1999; 341:120–21
159. Nettleton, J., Long, J. and Kuban, D. et al. Breast cancer during pregnancy: quantifying the risk of treatment delay. Obstet. Gynecol. 1996; 87:414–18
160. Iseminger, K. A. and Lewis, M. A. Ethical challenges in treating mother and fetus when cancer complicates pregnancy. Obstet. Gynec. Clinics of N. America 1998; 25:273–85

16 Immunomodulatory Analogies Between Trophoblastic and Cancer Cells and Their Hosts

Carolyn Coulam and Daniel Rukavina

Introduction

All living organisms have a defense mechanism, the immune system, that protects them from potentially harmful invaders. It has become apparent that in humans the defense mechanisms of the immunologic system against microorganisms is but a part of a broader reactivity concerned with the recognition of self and non-self. Using this mechanism of recognition, the human immune system provides for the surveillance and elimination of native cells "gone wild" or that undergo malignant transformation. Malignant transformation of normal cells poses an inherent danger to the survival of the organism and, therefore, raises a threat to the species. The immune system acts in response to antigens present on the surface of transformed or neoplastic cells, but not on normal cells. As a result, the aberrant cells are destroyed before they can proliferate. Cancer results when an immune response fails to perform appropriately or adequately. Thus, immunity has come to mean a specific protective response with which the host maintains the constancy of its internal environment when confronted with substances that are recognized as foreign, be they generated from within the host or introduced from the external environment.

The immune response is mediated by a variety of cells and soluble factors, broadly divided according to whether they mediate innate (natural) or adaptive (acquired) immunity. Innate immunity is dependent on a variety of mechanisms which are neither specific to a particular agent nor improved by repeated encounters with the same agent. Adaptive immunity is specific to the inducing agent and is marked by an enhanced response on repeated encounters with that agent, thus displaying memory. The mechanisms capable of exhibiting immune responses have an evolutionary history of some 400 million years. The forms taken by the response during this period have maintained a remarkable consistency both at the molecular and functional levels. Memory, specificity, and the recognition of non-self are central and preserved mechanisms of the adaptive immune response. As nature evolved these mechanisms that dictated survival of the species, a remarkable adaptation to this system was an essential prerequisite for embarking on the evolution of mammals. A response was evolved that protected the fetus and the mother from immunologic hazards during pregnancy and the lack of response allowed development of cancers in respective hosts.

The immune system recognizes self and responds to non-self antigens, yet pregnancy and cancer seem to represent exceptions to this rule. The mechanisms by which these two conditions are able to affect survival in the face of an immune response are the topics presented in this chapter. A discussion of the role of the cellular immune response will be followed by discussion on the role of the cellular products or cytokine immune response.

Cellular Immune Response

The Trophoblast: Frontier to the Maternal Immune System

Peter Medawar[1] first recognized the paradox that the fetus in mammals, in spite of its position of being semi-allogenic to an immunologically competent mother, is well tolerated. Very soon it was recognized that what is transplanted is not the fetus itself, but the trophoblast cells which are a real semiallogenic transplant.

The trophoblast is the only cell population of fetal origin which forms the ultimate interface with the maternal tissues, including maternal immunocompetent cells and antibodies. Owing to its unique properties, trophoblast serves not only as a physical barrier but also to prevent fetoplacental damage by maternal immune responses.

Syncytiotrophoblast and mononuclear cytotrophoblast, two main classes of fetal trophoblast, come into contact with maternal decidua. Extravillous cytotrophoblastic cells infiltrate deeply through the maternal decidua as far as the inner myometrium, and in the first trimester of pregnancy display many of the characteristics of tumor cells in their proliferative and invasive properties.[2] These distinct subpopulations of trophoblast cells contain different levels of HLA class I mRNA and express the protein antigen differently from one another. This regulated expression of MHC genes by placental trophoblast cells represents one of the key factors in preventing maternal rejection of the fetoplacental unit allograft.

Generally, first trimester trophoblast cells transcribe more HLA class I mRNA[3] and contain more HLA class I protein[4] than term trophoblast cells. On the basis of MHC antigen expression, trophoblastic cells can be divided into three subpopulations:

1 There is no class I or class II MHC antigen expression on the syncytiotrophoblastic cells (neither mRNA nor protein).

2 Villous cytotrophoblast cells express MHC class I mRNA, but not protein.

3 Invasive extravillous cytotrophoblast cells express mRNA and protein for nonclassical HLA-G class I antigens, and additionally the classical HLA-C molecule.[3,5-8]

Thus, villous trophoblastic cells represent an HLA-negative fetal cell layer that continuously separates HLA-positive fetal cells (e.g. Hofbauer macrophages) from maternal immunocompetent cells. HLA-G, which is expressed on invasive extravillous cytotrophoblast,[9] like classical class I MHC molecules,[5] is non-covalently associated with b2 microglobulin, but has a truncated cytoplasmic tail, and a molecular weight of 39 kDa rather than 44 kDa. It has been clearly demonstrated that HLA-G is polymorphic. HLA-G can be transcribed in four different "membrane bound" and two soluble isoforms[9-12] which are present in various trophoblast cell subpopulations from first trimester and term human placentas.[13] NK cells largely recognize and lyse target cells which are deficient in class I HLA expression. However, selective HLA-G expression (in the absence of classical class I MHC) may render extravillous cytotrophoblast resistant to NK cells. This raises the question of how trophoblast cells expressing HLA-G and HLA-C escape recognition and subsequent destruction by alloreactive and HLA-C specific T cells. Possible explanation is the suppressive function of soluble forms of HLA-G suppressing maternal CTL. Soluble HLA-G could bind either directly to the TCR or alternatively to CD8 molecules on the T cells and thereby inhibit the interaction between T cells and class I antigens on the target cells. The lack of expression of the most of classical polymorphic class I HLA antigens on trophoblast cells would also hinder CTL-mediated lysis, thus making this vital fetal tissue interface resistant to both the innate and the adaptive arms of the cell-mediated cytotoxic response.[14]

A lot of experimental work has been done recently to identify HLA-G recognizing cells and their putative HLA-G receptors. Uterine NK cells (see later) that predominate during the first trimester of pregnancy come into direct contact with trophoblast cells and many express receptors for HLA-G on their surfaces. HLA-G decreases the susceptibility of target cells to lysis by fresh peripheral blood NK cells. Blocking trophoblast cell expression of HLA class I molecules (including HLA-G) with the monomorphic anti-HLA class I W6/32 monoclonal antibody prevents cell lysis by fresh decidual effector cells.[15] Both soluble and membrane-bound full length HLA-G isoforms are able to bind intracellularly processed peptides[16,17] and thus capable of presenting them to CD8+ T cells. This means that virally infected cytotrophoblast cells expressing HLA-G may present viral peptides to the T cells, and so would contribute to limiting the spread of infection in the placenta.[18]

It has been hypothesized that HLA-G restricted CTL either survey the trophoblast for viral infections or malignancy through the presented peptide pool or that HLA-G has an inhibitory effect on those NK cells that would normally recognize the absence of the classical MHC class I molecules, therefore destroying the fetal cytotrophoblast.[17,19] For reproductive immunologists the second hypothesis looks more attractive, since the cells of NK phenotype are the most abundant cell population in decidual tissue and are in close contact with trophoblast. It is believed that regulation of NK cell activity occurs which is mediated by signals that are transmitted through killer inhibitory receptors (KIR) and killer activatory receptors (KAR) on NK cells on contact with their ligands: HLA class I molecules on trophoblast.[15,19] KIRs are also expressed on a small number of T cells and can mediate inhibition of lysis of target cells expressing the specific HLA ligands.[20] This would be a potential mechanism for preventing lysis of trophoblast by decidual T cells.[21] There are also mechanisms to protect fetal trophoblast against damage mediated by maternal humoral immunity with both maternal antibodies and complement. Members of the family of complement regulatory proteins expressed by trophoblast cells may be responsible for the survival of these cells in contact with maternal antibodies and complement. There are three cell surface complement regulatory proteins which are selectively expressed at high levels by all trophoblastic populations and are able to prevent complement mediated damage of trophoblast cells by both classical or alternative pathways. Trophoblast cells express extraordinarily high levels of these proteins that interfere with the complement cascade such as CD46 (membrane cofactor protein, or MCP), CD55 (decay accelerating factor, or DAF) and membrane attack complex (C5b-C9) inhibitory protein (CD59). CD46 enhances inactivation of C3b, whereas CD55 prevents formation of C3 convertases and accelerates their decay.[22-24]

Bone Marrow-Derived Cells Infiltrating the Decidua of Pregnancy

Decidual Large Granulated Lymphocytes

Prior to and during pregnancy the uterine epithelium and stroma undergo changes known as the decidual reaction. This involves the appearance of highly specialized cell classes which are end products of proliferation and differentiation of fibroblast-like stromal cell precursors. The non-pregnant midsecretory endometrium, as well as first and third trimester basal decidua, is heavily infiltrated by cells of bone marrow origin.[25,26] Three principal populations of decidual leukocytes can be recognized by immunohistological techniques. The most prominent populations are decidual macrophages and decidual granulated lymphocytes (dGL) most of which are CD2+ and CD56bright+, but are negative for CD3, CD4, CD5, CD8 and CD16 markers.[27]

The phenotype of the dGL strongly resembles that of PBL NK cells, but they are CD16 negative and have lower cytotoxic activity, in spite of the fact that they are full of perforin (perforin bright+).[28] In non-pregnant endometrium CD56+ cells increase in their number from the proliferative to midsecretory phase of the menstrual cycle.[29] We have found CD56+ cells in midsecretory endometrium at more than three times the number of mature T lymphocytes (CD3+ cells). Moreover, the number of CD56+ cells showed a discernible increase in the first trimester basal decidua, causing an increase in the CD56/CD3 cell ratio to more than five.[30] Numbers of these cells have decreased greatly by term indicating that their primary function is during implantation and early pregnancy.

Because large granulated lymphocytes (LGL) with NK activity are so abundant in the first trimester of pregnancy, an important question concerns their role in pregnancy. Although there are some hypotheses about their function, such as limitation of the trophoblast invasion, prevention of the vertical transmission of viral infection, or production of lymphokines which may influence locally other cells,[27,28] their precise role still remains unknown.

Macrophages

Macrophages are abundantly represented in both non-pregnant endometrium and basal decidua, and their number does not change significantly during pregnancy which could suggest that their function(s) is not likely to be related to normal pregnancy.[30] All possible functions of macrophages in endometrium and/or decidua are far from being clear but there is no doubt about their immunological role and phagocytic potential. Macrophages have a unique ability to produce a wide range of substances on demand and it has been postulated that they play a pivotal role in the success of pregnancy.[31] Macrophages are the site of prostaglandin E2 (PGE2) production and it is known that PGE2 suppresses lymphocyte functions, such as blastic proliferation and generation of cytotoxic T lymphocytes (CTL),[32] and this could contribute to the suppression of maternal rejection of the fetal allograft. On the other hand, uterine macrophages may also have detrimental effects, particularly in cases of infection.[31] Activated macrophages may produce many potent effector molecules like interleukin-1 (IL-1), tumor necrosis factor-alpha (TNFα), IL-6, nitric oxides (NO) and transforming growth factor-beta (TGF-β)[31,33] which can be associated with pregnancy termination in case of infection. Nitric oxide is the smallest, lightest molecule known to act as a biological second messenger in mammals. NO is essential for a very broad range of activities from digestion and blood pressure regulation to antimicrobial and antitumor defense.[34] Nitric oxides decline dramatically during gestation,[35] and this is an indication that macrophage-derived NO could be important in myometrial relaxation and subsequent contraction.

Lymphocytes

CD3+ T lymphocytes and their subpopulations CD4+ and CD8+ cells are represented in much higher percentages at the end of the pregnancy than in the first trimester.[30] Nevertheless, it is obvious that cytolytic lymphocytes with the potential of both antigen-specific and MHC-restricted killing and MHC-nonrestricted killing are present in the vicinity of the fetoplacental unit from the early beginning of pregnancy.

We have shown that decidual lymphocytes are functionally distinct from PBL. Spontaneous proliferation of DL is significantly higher than the proliferation of PBL from the same patients.[36] This higher level of activity may be the result of either the presence of more growth promoting cytokines produced by LGLs within decidua,[37] or greater proliferative capacity of decidual LGLs which share the same phenotype as a subpopulation of PBL showing high proliferative capacity.[38] However, induced proliferation of DL to polyclonal mitogens is many times lower than the proliferation of PBL.[36] This lower level of blastic transformation can be explained rather as a result of the lower number of responsive cells than the lower capacity to respond to polyclonal mitogens. Namely, we repeatedly have found that the relative numbers of CD3 positive DL in suspensions of DL preparations are regularly three to four times lower than in the corresponding PBL suspensions (unpublished). Accordingly, lower proliferation probably does not represent suppression on the level of the cell reactivity to polyclonal mitogens, in agreement with the conclusion of others.[39] Investigating the role of decidua-trophoblast interactions, we have found that human decidual lymphocytes, both adherent (predominantly macrophages) and nonadherent (predominantly lymphocytes) cells from normal pregnancy and anembryonic pregnancy (viable trophoblast), have very strong immunosuppressive potential. However, adherent and nonadherent cells from missed abortion patients (dead trophoblast) had the opposite effect, i.e. the facilitation of immune reactivity.[36,40]

Molecular Mechanisms of Cell Mediated Cytotoxicity at the Maternal–Fetal Interface

Perforin (pore forming protein)

Cytotoxic lymphocytes, both CTL and NK cells, contain in their granules a pore forming protein, perforin (P), a cytolytic molecule which is a mediator in cell-mediated cytotoxicity reactions.[41-43] In unstimulated peripheral blood lymphocytes, perforin is constitutively expressed in NK and γ/δ T cells (high level of expression) and in the subpopulation of CD8+ cells expressing the CD11b antigen (moderate expression). However, perforin can be induced in the CD8+CD11b-subpopulation and in some of CD4+ T cells.[44] In the cytotoxic pathway mediated by regulated secretion of granules the formation of membrane pores by P is a prerequisite for apoptosis of the target cell.[45,46] Besides P the main protein component of granules is a group of serine proteases known as granzymes.[47] Their main function is to mediate target DNA degradation upon gaining entry into the target cell through the presence of P pores.[48,49]

There are very few data showing P expression in human decidua. By immunohistochemistry and flow cytometric analyses we have found P-containing cells in both decidua basalis and decidua parietalis, the number of P+ cells in decidua parietalis being even higher then in decidual basalis.[28] The percentage of P+ cells in the suspension of decidual lymphocytes is twice that of PBL from the same women (55% vs 27%); however, NK activity of these CD56+ cells is much lower than NK activity of PBL[28,50] in spite of the fact that they are full of perforin.[28] The question could be raised as to when and how these cells can be activated. The answer seems especially important in light of the data that in the same granules of decidual NK cells perforin, granzymes and TIA-1 colocalize.[51] Decidual NK cells are nonclassical NK cells, since only 2% of CD56+ cells are CD16+ (77% in PBL). Furthermore, decidual NK are almost all (91%) perforin positive, and their phenotype is CD3-CD16-CD56bright+Pbright+ 28). In the first trimester decidua CD8+ cells are either CD3+CD8bright+CD56-P- or CD3- CD8dim+CD56+P+. There are very few classical CTL (CD3+CD8+P+) and the question remains how can they be induced.[28] The CD16 molecule is the IgGFcRIII that is exclusively responsible for lymphocyte-mediated antibody-dependent cellular cytotoxicity (ADCC) reactions[38,52] which may be important for some types of rejection of allogenic grafts. Early pregnancy could be the period when the fetoplacental unit allograft needs to be protected against ADCC, which is a combination of both natural (innate) and adaptive immunity. It is important to emphasize that this protection (the downregulation of CD16+P+ cells) in the first trimester of pregnancy is realized at both local (decidua)[28] and systemic (peripheral blood) levels. Namely, we have found profound changes in the CD16+ subpopulation (a drastic decrease of CD16+P+ cells; CD16+ cells among P+ cells; P+ cells among CD16+ cells).[53] In contrast, at the time of parturition we have found a many-fold increase of CD16+P+ cells.[53] An increase of CD16+P+ cells was found in the PBL of kidney allograft recipients in the early post-transplantation period and at the time of acute rejection reaction as well,[54] and the parturition can be viewed also as a maternal rejection reaction of the fetoplacental allograft. Investigation of the perforin expression in both decidual lymphocytes and peripheral blood lymphocytes in the first trimester of pathological pregnancies (anembryonic pregnancy and missed abortion) showed that significant decreases in the prevalence of perforin positive lymphoid cells, their subpopulations, and mean fluorescence intensity for perforin are associated with pregnancy failure.[55] We are still far from understanding basic mechanisms regulating P expression in decidual lymphocytes. There is an almost complete absence of IL-2 at the maternofetal tissue interface[56] and IL-2 is one of the most powerful stimulators of P induction and upregulation of expression.[57] Recently, attention has been focused on the expression of IL-15 in the placenta. In spite of many similarities there are some essential differences between IL-2 and IL-15. Even though it does not share sequence homology with IL-2, both cytokines bind to the same receptor with the noted exception of a cytokine specific alpha chain.[58] Despite the fact that IL-2 and IL-15 apparently use shared receptor components, resting T cells do not respond to IL-15 unless exogenous IL-2 is added, and then only poorly, compared with their response to IL-2.[59] While IL-2 is produced predominantly by activated T lymphocytes, IL-15 appears to be produced by a variety of cell types and tissues, but not by T cells.[60] The mRNA coding for IL-15 has been detected in monocyte-macrophages, fibroblasts and epithelial cell lines, as well as tissues and organs including placenta.[60] Experiments in mice have shown that IL-15 can enhance the expression of P in pregnant uterine tissues maintained in short-term in vitro culture.[61] Preliminary results of experiments in our laboratory with human first trimester pregnancy decidual lymphocytes clearly showed that P expression in cultured decidual lymphocytes and PBL can be upregulated by coculture with decidual adherent cells and their supernatants. However, these effects can be blocked completely by the addition of monoclonal antibodies against IL-15.[62]

FasL- Fas Pathway

The non-secretory pathway of cell-mediated cytotoxicity is mediated by the Fas ligand molecule on the effector cell which induces apoptosis in the susceptible target cell upon the interaction with the Fas receptor.[24,25] Immunohistochemical staining of first trimester human placental tissue sections revealed the presence of Fas ligand in cytotrophoblasts in the free floating villi, anchoring villi and cytotrophoblastic island,[63] while the Fas was detected in amnion, chorion, decidua and placenta,[64] suggesting that apoptosis and Fas signaling may play a role in remodeling of fetal membrane architecture during gestation.[64]

The Potential Role of Perforin Mediated Cytotoxicity in Tumor Control.

There are numerous data accumulated demonstrating tumor specific immune responses and supporting the possibility of immune surveillance against the formation and growth of tumors. Cell-mediated cytotoxicity is an important mechanism of tumor control in vivo. Cytolytic cells, both CTL and NK cells, are a crucial component in the immune response to tumors. Tumor antigens are recognized as peptides presented to the T cell receptor via class I or class II major histocompatibility complex molecules.[65,66] For elimination of tumor cells by CD8+CTL it is necessary that tumor specific peptides are presented in the context of MHC class I molecules.[67,68] Further, a perforin mediated cytolytic pathway is essential for tumor rejection, since approximately 83% perforin deficient mice with IL-2 producing Lewis lung carcinoma injected subcutaneously develop tumor.[69] CD8+ CTL and NK cells expressing perforin and granzyme B were found in tissue sections of follicular lymphomas[70] and it was hypothesized that these cells are present as a part of the host immune response against malignant B lymphocytes. Perforin positive lymphocytes were found in stroma of the colorectal cancer, and they were more numerous in the vicinity of tumor infiltration than in the normal mucosa. Perforin positive cells were more numerous in CD8+ cells than in CD16+ cells, and decreased according to the progression of tumors.[71] As has been discussed previously, at the maternal-fetal interface there is very few CD8+ CTL[30] and it has been found that most of these cells have predominantly noncytolytic phenotype CD3+CD8bright P negative.[28]

The question is, how are these cells converted to classical cytolytic cells (CD3+CD8+P+) able to eliminate cells expressing tumor specific peptides in the context of MHC class I molecules? It is well known that some tumors downregulate MHC class I expression[72-74] and escape immune surveillance by CTL. However, these tumors could be eliminated by NK-like Pbright+ decidual large granulated lymphocytes, which are abundantly represented at the maternal-fetal interface in quantities much higher than in any other tissue either in physiological or pathological conditions. Therefore, one important message of extremely high cytolytic potential expressed at the maternal-fetal interface could be the surveillance of tumors, or virus infected cells, expressing low or no MHC class I. It is well known that NK cells use predominantly the perforin-dependent pathway in cytolytic action.[75,76]

Cytokine Immune Response

Cytokines are a broad, heterogeneous group of proteins that regulate intercellular communication. Intercellular signaling can result in a wide range of biochemical and behavioral changes in a cell. The existence of such a system of cell-to-cell communication is critical to governing the behavior of cells. Normal embryonic development and tissue homeostasis depend upon cell-to-cell communication mediated through cytokines. As the molecular basis for malignant transformation has been documented,[77] it is apparent that a common means by which a tumor becomes autonomous of external control is by becoming independent of the need for external growth factor stimulation. One of the central problems in the understanding of embryogenesis is to account for how the cell-to-cell communication results in the influence of sequential development. An important trend in embryogenesis has been to study the role of cytokines in development. Cytokines involved in trophoblastic development and malignant transformation include growth factors, colony stimulating factors, interferons, interleukins and tumor necrosis factor.

Growth Factors

Growth factors represent a diverse group of proteins that are produced by a variety of cells and were originally defined by their capacity to affect growth and differentiation of cells. The growth factors generally are directed toward specific cell types. In the process of cell-to-cell interactions, growth factors produced by one cell can act at a cell surface receptor or on the target cell. Intercellular signaling that results from the receptor–ligand complex can result in a wide range of biochemical and behavioral changes in a cell. This diversity is the result of a complex array of signal transduction pathways mediated by the intracellular portion of the receptor protein and includes protein phosphorylation, calcium channel effects and C AMP formation. A number of clinical conditions may reflect an abnormal response to growth factors including cancer and recurrent pregnancy loss. Examples of such factors include platelet-derived growth factor (PDGF), fibroblast growth factors (FGF), transforming growth factors (TGF) and vascular endothelial growth factor (VEGF).

Platelet Derived Growth Factor

PDGF can affect the growth of a variety of cells including trophoblastic and endothelial cells as well as enhancing angiogenesis and prostaglandin metabolism – both necessary for normal placentation.[78,79]

A common means by which normal cells undergo malignant change is by becoming independent of the need for external growth factor stimulation. This event can occur through the cell producing the growth factors needed for its own growth. One example of this mechanism is malignant transformation of fibroblasts by the simian sarcoma virus.[80] This virus carries the cis oncogene that is the cause of this transformation. This oncogene codes for a protein closely homologous with platelet derived growth factor (PDGF), an important growth stimulus for fibroblasts. It has been shown that fibroblasts transformed by the cis oncogene express PDGF, that PDGF appears in the media, and that this peptide binds to its cell surface receptor. Anti-PDGF antibodies bind to and inactivate PDGF present in the media and slow the rate of cell proliferation.

Fibroblast Growth Factors

FGFs are examples of analogues between malignant transformation and early embryogenesis.[81,82] FGFs have a range of important biological effects. First, they are an important growth signal for many cells, especially those of mesenchymal origin. Thus, they stimulate fibroblast growth as expected. In addition, they stimulate the growth of osteoblasts and cause these cells to deposit amorphous calcium phosphate in vitro. They are the major growth factor for capillary endothelial cells in culture and have been implicated as the major mechanism for neovascularization in inflammation, tumor growth and in the chick allantoic membrane. At present, there are six clearly documented members of this family. Only three have a signal sequence that allows for transmembrane movement and can therefore be expected to be transported extracellularly with any efficiency. These same three, hst/k-FGF, FGF-5 and int-2, are also the only ones clearly documented as acting as transforming oncogenes and act by establishing an autocrine loop for FGF. Hst/k-FGF has been implicated in Kaposi's sarcoma. Int-2 and hst/k-FGF are both located at 11q13 and tend to be coamplified. This has been documented in 50% of primary esophageal carcinoma lesions and in 100% of metastatic esophageal carcinoma lesions. Similarly, 40–50% of head and neck carcinomas show int-2 amplification.

It also is these three FGFs that have been implicated in embryogenesis. One aspect of these oncogenes is that their expression during embryogenesis exhibits a striking temporal and spatial restriction. Fgf-5 has been implicated as the endodermal signal that triggers mesoderm differentiation. Int-2 appears to be important in mesoderm migration. Hst/k-FGF is expressed in the periimplantation stage and, given the ability of FGFs to cause neovascularization, may play an important role in the process of implantation.

Transforming Growth Factors

TGFs are mitogenic proteins that confer on normal cells a transformed phenotype and control the growth and differentiation of a variety of cell types including trophoblastic and endothelial cells.[83.84] In mammals, TGF-β1, -β2, and -β3 have been identified in various cells and tissues that are normal and/or transformed.[85] The biologic activities of the TGF-βs are mediated through specific cell-surface receptors found in all of their target cells.[86/87] Three cell surface proteins, designated types I, II and II, have been identified as TGF-β receptors.[88-91] The heromeric complex of type I (TβR-I) and type II (TβR-II) receptors is thought to be an important element that mediates the multiple actions of TGF-βs, whereas the type III receptor binds and presents TGF-βs to the type II receptor.[87,89]

TGF-β has been shown to be implicated in implantation.[92] TGF-β mRNAs and immunoreactive proteins have been demonstrated in both pre-and postimplantation tissues.[92-94] In addition, their receptors have been detected immunohistologically at periimplantation sites.[95] The predominant expression of TGF-β1 in the villous tissues and of TGF-β2 in the decidual tissues indicated that they are likely to be an important factor controlling the invasion, growth and activities of the placenta as an invasive graft. Because TGF-β2-like molecules are released by CD56+ natural killer cells, are detected in human first-trimester pregnancy decidua, and act as an immunosuppressive factor,[96] high levels of TGF-β2 mRNA expression in the endometrium and decidua might represent a local immune reaction preventing rejection of the fetal allograft. TGF-β3 protein is localized in the myometrium, vascular smooth muscle and epithelium of the uterus,[94] suggesting that TGF-β3 regulates myometrial differentiation and cyclic changes during menstruation.[97]

TGF-β inhibits the proliferation of both normal and malignant cells. TGF-β1 has been shown to inhibit the growth of different ovarian cancer cell lines as well as some human leukemic cell lines.[98,99] Resistance to TGF-β mediated growth inhibition is frequently observed in cancers derived from epithelial and lymphohematopoietic cells.[100]

In the process of malignant transformation of normal cells, the transformed cell becomes independent of external growth regulation. One mechanism employed by the transformed cell to obviate the need for external growth signals is the production of the growth factor that stimulates its own growth. An example of this mechanism is TGF-∝ which has manifest as an autocrine loop that has been implicated in breast cancer. In addition to inappropriate growth factor production, there are a series of growth factor receptor mutants that can result in transformation. In the case of breast cancer, the TGF-∝ receptor external portion acts to inhibit the intracellular signal transduction machinery unless the appropriate ligand is bound. The erb-b oncogene represents a TGF-∝ receptor mutant in which the external portion of the receptor is missing. Thus, the receptor is always on independent of the presence of TGF-∝ and transformation results. In a similar fashion, the her-2/neu oncogene represents a mutant in a TGF-∝ related cell surface receptor in which the receptor linked tyrosine kinase has experienced a mutation which results in a dramatic increase in activity. This alteration has been shown to correlate with a much worse prognosis in patients with breast cancer.[77]

Vascular Endothelial Growth Factor

VEGF is a potent angiogenic growth factor. Intense vascular growth and remodeling are associated with development of a competent placenta. Trophoblast expression of VEGF and its homolog placental growth factor (PlGF) suggest that these factors play a pivotal role in implantation and placental function.[101] The potential role for these factors to influence both vascular endothelial cells and trophoblasts suggests that aberrant trophoblastic production could compromise cellular function during gestation and contribute to vascular and placental pathologies noted in many obstetrical complications including pre-eclampsia.[102] As a promoter of angiogenesis, VEGF is believed to play a role in tumor growth and metastasis.[103] Tumor angiogenesis is essential for solid tumor growth. Patients with early stage ovarian carcinoma with increased VEGF expression had a poorer prognosis.[104] In ovarian cancer, tumor derived VEGF is obligatory for ascites formation.[105]

Colony Stimulating Factors

Hematopoiesis, or formation of blood cells, is unique in that all blood cells arise from a small common set of pluripotent stem cells that reside mainly in the bone marrow. These stem cells, which have an extensive capacity for self-renewal, can differentiate to various types of progenitor cells, which in turn give rise to circulating erythrocytes, granulocytes, monocytes, platelets and lymphocytes. In the mid-1960s semi-solid culture systems were developed for the in vitro clonal growth of progenitor cells, which generated mature progeny cells (e.g. granulocytes and macrophages) of the various hematopoietic lineages. A study of these semi-solid cultures indicated that hematopoietic precursor cells cannot survive or proliferate unless specifically stimulated. It was discovered that cellular proliferation of hematopoietic progenitor cells was dependent on continuous stimulation by a set of glycoproteins, which were later shown to affect some of the functional properties of the various hematopoietic lineages. Based on the fact that colony formation was employed to identify and characterize these factors, these cytokines were referred to as colony stimulating factors. These factors are granulocyte–macrophage colony stimulating factor (GM-CSF), granulocyte colony stimulating factor (G-CSF), and IL-3 (multi-CSF).

Receptors for GM-CSF, G-CSF, and IL-3 have been shown to be present on cell membranes of trophoblastic and cancer cells. Their ligands have also been shown to be present at the sites of implantation and invasion.[77,106,107] The sources of the growth factors are from the activated immune cells surrounding the invading cells as well as from the invaders (trophoblastic and cancer cells) themselves.[77,106,107] In response to the ligand engaging their receptor, the trophoblastic and cancer cells are stimulated to proliferate. Cellular proliferation and growth are also stimulated by transferrin engaging its receptor.[108,109] Transferrin receptors are present in high concentrations on the cell surfaces of trophoblastic and cancer cells.[110,111]

Interestingly, CSF induces and enhances interferon production.[112]

Interferons

In 1957 Isaacs and Lindenmann[113] discovered that the supernatant obtained from cells incubated with heat-inactivated influenza virus contained a substance capable of preventing the growth of active virus. This substance, named interferon (IFN), was later shown to be composed of a family of structurally related proteins that act directly on the target cells, not on the virus. Many types of animal cells produce these proteins in response to various external stimuli (e.g. viruses, certain types of double-stranded RNA, antigens or mitogens). Three classes of IFNs have been described that differ in their amino acid sequences, as well as immunochemical and physicochemical properties: alpha (leukocyte), beta (fibroblast), and gamma (immune) IFN. Alpha and beta IFNs have also been designated as type I (acid-stable) and gamma IFN as type II (acid-labile). The alpha IFNs, which are produced by various cells including macrophages and B cell lines, are a family of at least 14 species that share a 75% or greater amino acid sequence homology. Beta IFN is produced mainly by fibroblasts and epithelial cells. Gamma IFN is predominantly a product of T cells and natural killer (NK) cells and shares little homology with type IFNs. More recently, five classes of IFN have been identified, namely α, β, γ, ω, and τ, based primarily on divergence in amino acid sequence and antigenicity.[112]

In humans, IFN have been detected in the placenta.[112] Human trophoblast populations produce different levels of IFN at different stages of pregnancy.

During embryonic development, some trophoblast populations exhibit invasive behavior as a normal part of the differentiation program. It is noteworthy that the period of high trophoblast IFN production is also the period of invasive behavior of the trophoblast. However, several in vitro and in vivo studies show that IFNs enhance the invasive and metastatic potential of a number of different tumor cells.[114-117] The three events that occur during trophoblast or tumor invasion are cell attachment, proteolysis and migration. All these three events are regulated by IFNs.

Interleukins

The name "interleukin" (IL) was chosen to describe a group of proteins produced by either monocytes and tissue macrophages or lymphocytes that served to mediate communication between leukocytes. The first interleukin to be discovered was IL-1, which was described as a factor that could enhance the response of T cells to mitogens or antigens.[118] IL-1 at this time was referred to as lymphokine activating factor (LAF) and was later shown to be identical to endogenous pyrogen, a heat-labile protein that could produce fever in animals. It was shown by molecular cloning that two forms of IL-1 existed: IL-1α and IL-1β. Both species are synthesized as precursors and show only about 20% homology at the amino acid level. IL-1 is required for maximal induction of another interleukin, IL-2, from T cells. IL-2 can enhance the proliferation of T and B lymphocytes and thymocytes. Importantly, IL-2 can activate killer cells that subsequently become cytotoxic to tumor cells.

IL-3 is a member of a group of proteins referred to as colony stimulating factors (see above) and can stimulate hematopoietic precursors to differentiate into a variety of lymphoid and myelomonocytic cells. Although IL-4 was originally discovered as a mouse factor that could stimulate the proliferation of anti-IgM activated B cells (i.e. B cell stimulating factor-1), it has also been observed to interact with T cells and myelomonocytic cells. IL-5 and IL-6 can influence the growth and differentiation of B cells and hence are also referred to as B cell growth factor-II and B cell stimulating factor-2, respectively. IL-7 is a hemopoietic factor that induces the proliferation of early B cell lineages. IL-8 is a neutrophil chemotactic factor. IL-9 is p40, which supports the growth of helper T cells and IL-10 is the cytokine synthesis inhibition factor. IL-11 is a pleiotropic cytokine that inhibits anti-inflammatory and mucosal protective effects. IL-12 stimulates the production of IFNγ, by NK and T cells as well as GMCSF and IFNα by granulocytes and macrophages.[119,120] Plasma IL-12 has been reported to be elevated in women with pre-eclampsia.[121] IL-13 has 25% sequence homology to IL-4 and mirrors many of IL-4 actions. IL-14 is a high molecular weight B cell growth factor. IL 15 binds to and induces signaling through the IL-2 receptor. Like IL-2, IL-15 activates T cell proliferation, B cell antibody production and promotes NK cell cytotoxicity.

A number of interleukins have been shown to play a role in trophoblastic and cancer cell functions. IL-1 may serve as an important regulator of implantation and trophoblastic as well as cancer cell invasion.[122] IL-1 is present in trophoblasts as well as macrophages within the chorionic villi and maternal decidua.[123] The type I IL receptor has also been localized to the trophoblast. IL-1 has been implicated as a paracrine–autocrine regulator by hCG[124] and estrogen[125] biosynthesis by human trophoblasts.

IL-2 is weakly expressed at the implantation site. Because deciduae NK cells exhibit enhanced killing activity when stimulated with IL-2,[126] the tight regulation of IL-2 expression at the maternal–fetal interface may be a key feature in the establishment and maintenance of pregnancy immunotolerance. Furthermore, peripheral blood mononuclear cells from pregnant women produce less IL-2 when stimulated with antigen or mitogen than non-pregnant women.[127] IL-2 can enhance the growth of tumor infiltrating lymphocytes specific for autologous melanoma[128] and can induce the generation of cytotoxic T cell clones specific for transformed stimulator cells.[129]

IL-4 is a TH-2 cytokine that can enhance the proliferation of preactivated B cells and decrease the production of TH-1 cytokines by T cells. These properties of IL-4 suggest a role of IL-4 in the success of pregnancy and tumor growth. IL-4 production is enhanced in stimulated peripheral blood monocytes among pregnant women[130] and individuals with colorectal cancer[100] compared with normal controls.

IL-6 is expressed by first trimester trophoblasts.[131] The IL-6 –IL-6 receptor system induces hCG secretion by activating a tyrosine kinase and may play a role as an autocrine–paracrine mediator of trophoblast endocrine function.[132] IL-6 is also produced by ovarian carcinoma cells as well as IL-6 receptors.[133] Some patients with ovarian carcinoma have been shown to have elevated levels of IL-6 in the serum and peritoneal cavity in comparison to patients with benign ovarian tumors.[134] Furthermore, patients with advanced ovarian cancer according to Figo stages III / IV demonstrated higher IL-6 levels in serum and ascites than patients with Figo stages I / II, reflecting low tumor burden.[135] These observations suggest that IL-6 plays a key role in tumor–host interaction, particularly in the possible facilitated spread of ovarian cancer cells.

The expression of IL-10 by first trimester human trophoblasts has important implications for pregnancy immunotolerance, because IL-10 suppresses the production of TH-1 cytokines including IL-2, IFNγ and TNFα – all of which are detrimental to pregnancy.[136] Preliminary studies have shown that GM-SCF enhances in vitro production of IL-10 by cancer cells, suggesting a possible paracrine regulation of neoplastic IL-10 production by host growth factors.[137]

Tumor Necrosis Factor (TNFα)

TNFα is a TH-1 cytokine that is detrimental to early embryos and is elevated in the serum of women with carcinomas.[135,136] TNFα has been reported to have a number of effects within the placenta including regulation of trophoblastic apoptosis.[138] TNFα and soluble TNFα receptors are altered in plasma, amniotic fluid and placentae of patients with pre-eclampsia.[139]

Summary

Cytokines control cell growth. The mechanisms by which trophoblastic cells proliferate and invade the endometrium at the time of implantation are analogous to the processes involved in cancer invasion and metastasis. This analogy seems appropriate in that the biologic phenomenon of trophoblastic invasiveness is a reflection of two traits common to cancer cell growth: high cell proliferation and lack of cell contact inhibition. Other analogies between cancer and pregnancy include the ability of both to evade immune rejection as well as cytokine production and usage. Successful mammalian pregnancy is dependent upon maternal immunologic recognition and upon the release and actions of an array of cytokines. The trophoblast seems to be a key cell in the development and maintenance of this complex interplay between fetal and maternal systems.[140]

A major conceptual advance in cancer research was made when it was demonstrated that cancers do provoke a specific immune response in the organism within which they appear.[77] More recent data have documented similar immunologic responses of the mother toward her pregnancy.[141] Thus, trophoblastic and cancer cells employ the same protective mechanisms from their host to allow their survival.

In spite of these analogies, there is a fundamental difference between cancer and pregnancy. The process of implantation and placentation consists of trophoblastic cell proliferation and invasion that is rigidly controlled by cytokines. In contrast, cancer represents a state in which normal cell growth patterns become altered such that the cells can replicate continuously. Thus the preeminent biologic difference between placentation and cancer is the loss of growth regulation in the latter. This loss of regulation can occur through the cell losing its need for external growth factor stimulation by producing its own growth factors, or by mutating growth factor receptors so that these receptors give a positive signal even when no growth factor is bound to the receptor. Thus all growth is under cytokine control. Control of cellular proliferation is demonstrated at the time of implantation. Understanding the cytokines responsible for control of proliferation and invasion will offer new approaches to cancer therapy and treatment of recurrent pregnancy loss.

References

1. Medawar PB. Some immunological and endocrinological problems raised by the evolution of viviparity in vertebrates. Symp Soc Exp Biol 1953; 44:320–38
2. Johnson PM. Reproductive and maternofetal relations. In: Lachmann, PJ, Peters DK, Rosen FS, Walport MJ (eds), Clinical aspects of immunology, 5th edn, Oxford: Blackwell Scientific Publications, 1993: 755–67
3. Chumbley G, King A, Gardner L, Howlett S, Holmes N, Lokoe YW. Generation of an antibody to HLA-G in transgenic mice and demonstration of the tissue reactivity of this antibody. J Reprod Immunol 1994; 27:173–86
4. Koller BH, Geraghty DE, Shimizu Y, DeMars R, Orr HT. HLA-E: a novel HLA class I gene expressed in resting T lymphocytes. J Immunol 1988; 141:897–904
5. King A, Boocock C, Sharkey AM, Gardner L, Beretta A, Siccardi AG, Loke YW. Evidence for the expression of HLAA-C class I mRNA and protein by human first trimester trophoblast. J Immunol 1996; 156:2068–76
6. Hutter H, Hammer A, Blaschitz A, Hartmann M, Ebbesen P, Dohr G, Ziegler A, Uchanska-Ziegler B. Expression of HLA class I molecules in human first trimester and term placenta trophoblast. Cell Tissue Res 1996; 286:439–47
7. Hunt JS, Orr HT. HLA and maternal-fetal recognition. FASEB J 1992; 6:2344–8
8. Hunt JS. Immunobiology of pregnancy. Curr Opin Immunol 1992; 4:591–6
9. Ober C, Aldrich CL. HLA-G polymorphisms: neutral evolution or novel function? J Reprod Immunol 1997; 36:1–21
10. Ishitani A, Geraghty DE. Alternative splicing of HLA-G transcripts yields proteins with primary structures resembling both class I and class II antigens. Proc Natl Acad Sci USA 1992; 89:3947–51
11. Fujii T, Ishitani A, Gerghty DE. A soluble form of the HLA-G antigen is encoded by a messenger ribonucleic acid containing intron 4. J Immunol 1994; 153:5516–24
12. Kirszenbaum M, Moreau P, Gluckman E, Dausset J, Carosella E. An alternatively spliced form of HLA-G mRNA in human trophoblasts and evidence for the presence of HLA-G transcript in adult lymphocytes. Proc Natl Acad Sci USA 1994; 91:4209–13
13. Le Bouteiller P, Lenfant F. Antigen-presenting function(s) of the non-classical HLA-E, -F and -G class I molecules: the beginning of a story. Res Immunol 1996; 147:301–13
14. Le Bouteiller P. GLA-G: what's new? Am J Reprod Immunol 1997; 38:146–9
15. King A, Jokhi PP, Burrows TD, Gardner L, Sharkey AM, Loke YW. Functions of human decidual NK cells. Am J Reprod Immunol 1996; 35:258–60
16. Lee N, Malacko AR, Ishitani A, Chen MC, Bajorath J, Marquardt H, Geraghty DE. The membrane-bound and soluble forms of HLA-G bind identical sets of endogenous peptides but differ with respect to TAP association. Immunity 1995; 3:591–600
17. Diehl M, Munz C, Keilholz W, Stevanovic S, Holmes N, Loke YW, Rammensee HG. Nonclassical HLA-molecules are classical peptide presenters. Curr Biol 1996; 6:305–14
18. Parham P. Antigen presentation by class I major histocompatability complex molecules: a context for thinking about HLA-G. Am J Reprod Immunol 1995; 34:10–19
19. Loke YW, King A. Human Implantation: Cell Biology and Immunology. Cambridge: Cambridge Univ Press, 1995, pp83-90

20. Lanier LL, Phillips JH. Inhibitory MHC class I receptors on NK cells and T cells. Immunol Today 1996; 17:86–91
21. Jones RK, Vince GS, Christmas SE. Human endometrial granulated lymphocytes: phenotype and function. Current Trends in Immunology 1999: 60:871-878.
22. Johnson PM. Immunological characterization of the trophoblast-decidual interface in human pregnancy. In Hunt, JS (ed), Immunology of reproduction, New York: Springer-Verlag, 1994: 3–13
23. Holmes CH, Simpson KL, Okada H, Okada N, Wainwright SD, Purcell DF, Houlihan JM. Complement regulatory proteins at the feto-maternal interface during human placental development: distribution of CD59 by comparison with membrane cofactor protein (CD46) and decay accelerating factor (CD55). Eur J Immunol 1992; 22:1579–85
24. Holmes CH, Simpson KL. Complement and pregnancy: new insights into the immunobiology of the fetomaternal relationship. Baillieres Clin Obstet Gynaecol 1992; 6:439–60
25. Bulmer JN. Decidual cellular responses. Curr Opin Immunol 1989; 1:1141–7
26. Dietl J, Ruck P, Horny HP, Handgretinger R, Marzusch K, Ruck M, Kaiserling E, Griesser H, Kabelitz D. The decidua of early human pregnancy: immunohistochemistry and function of immunocompetent cells. Gynecol Obstet Invest 1992; 33:197–204
27. King A, Loke YW. On the nature and function of human uterine granular lymphocytes. Immunol Today 1991; 12:432–5
28. Rukavina D, Rubesa G, Gudelj L, Haller H, Podack ER. Characteristics of perforin expressing lymphocytes within the first trimester decidua of human pregnancy. Am J Reprod Immunol 1995; 33:394–404
29. King A, Welllings V, Gardner L, Loke YW. Immunocytochemical characterization of the unusual large granular lymphocytes in human endometrium throughout the menstrual cycle. Hum Immunol 1989; 24:195–205
30. Haller H, Radillo O, Rukavina D, Tedesco F, Candussi G, Petrovic O, Randic L. An immunohistochemical study of leukocytes in human endometrium, first and third trimester basal decidua. J Reprod Immunol 1993; 23:41–9
31. Hunt JS, Robertson SA. Uterine macrophages and environmental programming for pregnancy success. J Reprod Immunol 1996; 32:1–25
32. Parhar RS, Yagel S, Lala PK. PGE2-mediated immunosuppression by first trimester human decidual cells blocks activation of maternal leukocytes in the decidua with potential anti-trophoblast activity. Cell Immunol 1989; 120:61–74
33. Silver RM, Lohner WS, Daynes RA, Mitchell MD, Branch DW. Lipopolysaccharide-induced fetal death; the role of tumor necrosis factor alpha. Biol Reprod 1994; 50:1108–12
34. Nathan C. Nitric oxide as a secretory product of mammalian cells. FASEB J 1992; 6:3051–64
35. Natuzzi ES, Ursell PC, Harrison M, Buscher C, Riemer RK: Nitric oxide synthase activity in the pregnant uterus decreases at parturition. Biochem Biophys Res Commun 1993; 194:1–8
36. Petrovice O, Gudelj L, Rubesa G, Haller H, Beer AE, Rukavina D. Decidual-trophoblast interactions: decidual lymphoid cell function in normal anembryonic, missed abortion and ectopic human pregnancy. J Reprod Immunol 1994; 26:217–31
37. Johnson PM, Deniz G, McLaughlin PJ. Functional properties of cloned CD3-decidual leukocytes and low-affinity cytokine receptor expression on human trophoblast. In: Dondero F and Johnson PM (eds), Reproductive Immunology, New York: Raven Press 1993: 141–4
38. Nagler L, Lanier LL, Curila S, Philips JH. Comparative studies of human FcR III-positive and negative natural killer cells. J Immunol 1989; 143:3183–91
39. Mincheva-Nilsson L, Hammarstrom S, Hammarstrom ML. Human decidual leukocytes from early pregnancy contain high numbers of g/d+ cells and show selective downregulation of alloreactivity. J Immunol 1992; 149:2203–11
40. Haller H, Gudelj L, Rubesa G, Petrovic O, Rukavina D. Suppressive effect of decidual leukocytes. Period Biol 1993; 95:327–33
41. Podack ER, Hengartner H, Lichtenheld MG. A central role of perforin in cytolysis? Ann Rev Immunol 1991; 9:129–57
42. Podack ER, Lichtenheld MG. Perforin and the mechanisms of lymphocyte mediated cytolysis. Curr Topics Membrane Transport 1990; 36:161–75
43. Podack ER. Perforin: structure, function and regulation. Curr Topics Microbiol Immunol 1992; 178:175–84
44. Yagita H, Nakata M, Kawaswaki A, Shinkai Y, Okumura K. Role of perforin in lymphocyte-mediated cytolysis. Adv Immunol 1992; 51:215–41
45. Shi L, Kam CM, Powers JC, Aebersold R, Greenberg AH. Purification of three cytotoxic lymphocyte granule serine proteases that induce apoptosis through distinct substrate and target cell interactions. J Exp Med 1992; 175:1521–9

46. Shiver JW, Su L, Henkart PA. Cytotoxicity with target DNA breakdown by rat basophilic leukemia cells expressing both cytolysin and granzyme A. Cell 1992; 71:315–22
47. Hameed A, Lowrey DM, Lichtenheld M, Podack ER. Characterization of three serine esterases isolated from human interleukin-2 activated killer cells. J Immunol 1988; 141:3142–7
48. Podack ER. Functional significance of two cytolytic pathways of cytotoxic T lymphocytes. J Leukoc Biol 1995; 57:548–52
49. Podack ER. Execution and suicide: cytotoxic lymphocytes enforce Draconian laws through separate molecular pathways. Curr Opin Immunol 1995; 7:11–16
50. King A, Birkby C, Loke YW. Early human decidual cells exhibit NK activity against the K562 cell line but not against first trimester trophoblast. Cell Immunol 1989; 118:337–44
51. King A, Wooding P, Gardner L, Loke YW. Expression of perforin, granzyme A and TIA-1 by human uterine CD56+ NK cells implies they are activated and capable of effector functions. Human Reprod 1993; 8:2061–7
52. Abrams SI, Brahmi Z. Target cell directed NK inactivation – concomitant loss of NK and antibody-dependent cellular cytotoxicity activities. J Immunol 1988; 140:2090–95
53. Rukavina D, Podack ER, Rubesa G, Spanjol-Pandelo S, Randic L. Downregulated expression of perforin-positive/CD16+ cells in the peripheral blood lymphocytes in the first trimester of pregnancy and upregulation at the end of pregnancy. Am J Reprod Immunol 1997; 38:189–96
54. Rukavina D, Balen-Marunic S, Rubesa G, Orlic P, Vujaklija K, Podack ER. Perforin expression in peripheral blood lymphocytes in rejecting and tolerant kidney transplant recipients. Transplantation 1996; 61:285–91
55. Gulan G, Podack ER, Rukavina D, Gudelj L, Rubesa G, Petrovic O, Johnson PM, Christmas SE. Perforin-expressing lymphocytes in peripheral blood and decidua of human first trimester pathological pregnancies. Am J Reprod Immunol 1997; 38:9–18
56. Jokhi PP, King A, Sharkey AM, Smith SK, Loke YW. Screening for cytokine messenger ribonucleic acids in purified human decidual lymphocyte populations by the reverse-transcriptase polymerase chain reaction. J Immunol 1994; 153:4427–35
57. Smyth MJ, Ortaldo JR, Bere W, Yagita H, Okumura K, Young HA. IL-2 and IL-6 synergize to augment the pore-forming protein gene expression and cytotoxic potential of human peripheral blood T cells. J Immunol 1990; 145:1159–66
58. Lorenz HM, Hieronymus T, Grunke M, Manger B, Kalden JR. Differential role of IL-2 and IL-15 in the inhibition of apoptosis in short-term activated human lymphocytes. Scand J Immunol 1997; 45:660–69
59. Doherty TM, Seder RA, Sher A. Induction and regulation of IL-15 expression in murine macrophages. J Immunol 1996; 156:735–41
60. Grabstein KH, Eisenman J, Shanebeck K, Rauch C, Srinivasan S, Fung V, Beers C, Richardson J, Schoenborn MA, Ahdieh M, et al. Cloning of a T cell growth factor that interacts with the beta chain of the interleukin-2 receptor. Science 1994; 264:965–8
61. Ye W, Zheng LM, Young JD, Liu CC. The involvement of interleukin-15 in regulating the differentiation of granulated metrial gland cells in mouse pregnant uterus. J Exp Med 1996; 184:2405–10
62. Strbo N, Laskarin G, Randiae LJ, Rukavina D. The role of IL-15 on the maintaining of perforin protein in decidual and peripheral blood lymphocytes. Per Biol 1997; 99 (Suppl. 2):23
63. Runic R, Lockwood CJ, Ma Y, Dispasquale B, Guller S. Expression of fas ligand by human cytotrophoblasts: implications in placentation and fetal survival. J Clin Endocrinol Metab 1998; 81:3119–22
64. Runic R, Lockwood CJ, LaChapelle L, DiPasquale B, Demopoulos RI, Kumar A, Guller S. Apoptosis and fas expression in human fetal membranes. J Clin Endocrinol Metab 1998; 83:660–66
65. Van der Bruggen P, Traversari C, Chomez P, Lurquin C, De Plaen E, Van den Eynde B, Knuth A, Boon T. A gene encoding an antigen recognized by cytolytic T lymphocytes on a human melanoma. Science 1991; 254:1643
66. Mandelbolm O, Berke G, Fridkin M, Feldman M, Einstein M, Eisenbach L. CTL induction by a tumor-associated antigen octapeptide derived from a murine lung carcinoma. Nature 1994; 369:67–71
67. Melief CJ. Tumor eradication by adoptive transfer of cytotoxic T lymphocytes. Adv Cancer Res 1992; 58:143–75
68. Boon T, Cerottini JC, Van den Eynde B, Van der Bruggen P, Van Pel A. Tumor antigens recognized by T lymphocytes. Ann Rev Immunol 1994; 12:337–65
69. Podack ER, Zhao D, Ohe Y, Nishio M, Cassileth PA, Roderick JF, Spielman J, Savaraj N. Gene therapy for small cell lung carcinoma and demonstration of tumor specific CTL restricted by HLA A2. Proc Intl Cancer Congress, Monduzzi Editore 1994:1261–4

70. Leger-Ravet MB, Devergne O, Peuchmaur M, Solal-Celigny P, Brousse N, Gaulard P, Galanaud P, Emilie D. In situ detection of activated cytotoxic cells in follicular lymphomas. Am J Pathol 1994; 144(3):492–9
71. Nakanishi H, Monden T, Morimot H, Kobayashi T, Shimano T, Mori T. Perforin expression in lymphocytes infiltrated to human colorectal cancer. Br J Cancer 1991; 64(2):239–42
72. Doherty PC, Knowled BB, Wettstein PJ. Immunological surveillance of tumors in the context of major histocompatibility complex restriction of T cell function. Adv Cancer Res 1984; 42:1–65
73. Hill A, Jugovic P, York I, Russ G, Bennink J, Yewdell J, Ploegh H, Johnson D. Herpes simplex virus turns off the TAP to evade host immunity. Nature 1995; 375(6430):411–5
74. Fruh K, Ahn K, Djaballah H, Sempe P, Van Endert PM, Tampe R, Peterson PA, Yang Y. A viral inhibitor of peptide transporters for antigen presentation. Nature 1995; 375(6530):415–8
75. Kagi D, Ledermann B, Burki K, Seiler P, Odermatt B, Olsen KJ, Podack ER, Zinkernagel RM, Hengartner H. Cytotoxicity mediated by T cells and natural killer cells is greatly impaired in perforin-deficient mice. Nature 1994; 369(6475):31–7
76. Henkart PA. Mechanism of lymphocyte-mediated cytotoxicity. Ann Rev Immunol 1985; 3:31–58
77. Meyers C. Peptide growth factors: the parallel between fetal development and malignant transformation. Am J Reprod Immunol 1991; 25:133–6
78. Torry DS, Torry RJ. Angiogenesis and the expression of vascular endothelial growth factor in endometrium and placenta. Am J Reprod Immunol 1997; 37:21–9
79. Sananes N, Baulieu EE, Le Goascogne C. Prostaglandins as inductive factor of decidualization in the rat uterus. Mol Cell Endocrinol 1976; 6:153–8
80. Deuel TF, Silverman NJ, Kawahara RS. Platelet-derived growth factor: a multifunctional regulator of normal and abnormal cell growth. Biofactors 1988; 1(3):213–7
81. Liu LM, Nicoll CS. Evidence for a role of basic fibroblast growth factor in rat embryonic growth and differentiation. Endocrinology 1988; 123(4):2027–31
82. Wilkinson DG, Bhatt S, McMahon AP. Expression pattern of the FGF-related proto-oncogene int-2 suggests multiple roles in fetal development. Development 1989; 105(1):131–6
83. Pelton RW, Hpgan BLM, Miller DA, Moses HL. Differential expression of genes encoding TGFs β1, β2 and β3 during murine palate formation. Dev Biol 1990; 141:456–60
84. Sporn MB, Roberts AB. The transforming growth factor betas: past, present, and future. Ann NY Acad Sci 1990; 593:1–6
85. Gupta A, Bazer FW, Jaeger LA. Differential expression of beta transforming growth factors (TGFβ1, TGFβ2, and TBFβ3) and their receptors (type I and type II) in peri-implantation porcine conceptuses. Biol Reprod 1996; 55:796–802
86. Segarini PR, Rosen DM, Seyedin SM. Binding of transforming growth factor-β to cell surface proteins varies with cell type. Mol Endocrinol 1989; 3:261–72
87. Lyons RM, Miller DA, Graycar JL, Moses HL, Derynck R. Differential binding of transforming growth factor-β1, -β2 and -β3 by fibroblasts and epithelial cells measured by affinity cross-linking of cell surface receptor. Mol Endocrinol 1991; 5:1887–96
88. Lin HY, Wang X-F, Ng-Eaton E, Weinberg RA, Lodish HF. Expression cloning of the TGF-β type II receptor, a functional transmembrane serine/threonine kinase. Cell 1992; 68:775–85
89. Massagu J. Receptors for the TGF-β family. Cell 1992; 69:1067–70
90. Ebner R, Chen R-H, Shum L, Lawler S, Zioncheck TF, Lee A, Lopez AR, Derynck R. Cloning of a type I TGF-β receptor and its effect of TGF-β binding to the type II receptor. Science 1993; 260:1344–8
91. Bassing CH, Yingling JM, Howe DJ, Wang T, He WW, Gustafson ML, Shah P, Donahoe PK, Wang X-F. A transforming growth factor β type I receptor that signals to activate gene expression. Science 1994; 263:87–9
92. Lea RG, Flanders KC, Harley CB, Manuel J, Banwatt D, Clark DA. Release of a transforming growth factor (TGF)-β2 related suppressor factor from post-implantation murine decidual tissue can be correlated with the detection of a subpopulation of cells containing RNA for TGF-β2. J Immunol 1992; 148:778–87
93. Altman DJ, Schneider SL, Thompson DA, Cheng H-L, Tomasi TB. Transforming growth factor-β2 (TGF-β2)-like immunosuppressive factor in amniotic fluid and localization of TGF-β2 mRNA in the pregnant uterus. J Exp Med 1990; 172:1391–401
94. Das SK, Flanders KC, Andrews GK, Dey SK. Expression of transforming growth factor-β isoforms (β2 and β3) in the mouse uterus: analysis of the peri-implantation period and effects of ovarian steroids. Endocrinology 1992; 130:3459–66
95. Tang X-M, Zhao Y, Rossi MJ, Abu-Rustum RS, Ksander GA, Chegini N. Expression of transforming growth factor-β (TGFβ) isoforms and TGFβ type II receptor messenger ribonucleic acid and protein, and the effect of TGFβs on endometrial stromal cell growth and protein degradation in vitro. Endocrinology 1994; 135:450–59

96. Clark DA, Vince G, Flander KC, Hirte H, Starkey P. CD56+ lymphoid cells in human first trimester pregnancy decidua as a source of novel transforming growth factor beta 2 related immunosuppressive factors. Hum Reprod 1994; 9:2270–77
97. Arici A, MacDonald PC, Casey ML. Modulation of the levels of transforming growth factor β messenger ribonucleic acids in human endometrial stromal cells. Biol Reprod 1996; 54:463–9
98. De Benedetti #, Falk LA, Ellingsworth LR, Ruscetti FW, Faltynek CR. Synergy between transforming growth factor beta and tumor necrosis factor alpha in the induction of monocytic differentiation of human leukemic cell lines. Blood 1990; 75:626–32
99. Berchuck A, Olt GJ, Everitt L, Soisson AP, Bast RC, Boyer CM. The role of peptide growth factors in epithelial ovarian cancer. Obstet Gynecol 1990; 75:255–62
100. Massague J. The transforming growth factor beta family. Ann Rev Cell Biol 1990; 6:597–641
101. Torry PS, Ahn H, Barnes EL, Torry RJ. Placental growth factor; potential role in pregnancy. Am J Reprod Immunol 1999; 41: 79-85
102. Roberts JM, Taylor RN, Musci TJ, Rodgers GM, Hubel CA, McLaughlin MK. Pre-eclampsia: an endothelial cell disorder. Am J Obstet Gynecol 1989:161:1200–04
103. Torry RJ, Rongish BJ. Angiogensis in the uterus: potential regulation and relation to tumor angiogenesis. Am J Reprod Immunol 1992; 27:171–9
104. Paley PJ, Staskus KA, Gebbard K, Mohanraj D, Twiggs LB, Carson LF, Ramakrishnan S. Vascular endothelial growth factor expression in early stage ovarian carcinoma. Cancer 1997; 80:98–106
105. Mesiano S, Ferrara N, Jaffe RB. Role of vascular endothelial factor in ovarian cancer: inhibition of ascites formation by immunoneutralization. Am J Path 1998; 153:1249–56
106. Trotta PP. Cytokines: an overview. Am J Reprod Immunol 1991; 25:137–41
107. Clark DA, Chaouat G. What do we know about spontaneous abortion mechanisms? Am J Reprod Immunol 1980; 19:28–35
108. Laskey J, Webb J, Schulman HM, Ponka P. Evidence that transferrin supports cell proliferation by supplying iron for DNA synthesis. Exp Cell Res 1988; 88:205–209
109. May WS, Cuatrecacas P. Transferrin receptor: its biological significance. J Member Biol 1988; 88:205–209
110. Faulk WP and Galbraith GMP. Trophoblast transferrin and transferrin receptors in the host-parasite relationship of human pregnancy. Proc R Soc Lond B 1979; 204:83–97
111. Faulk WP, Hsi BL, Stevens PJ. Transferrin and transferrin receptors in carcinoma of the breast. Lancet 1980; 2:390–92
112. Ababgye-Matthiesen G, Toth FD, Zdravkovic H, Ebbesen P. Human trophoblast interferons: production and possible roles in early pregnancy. Early Preg. Biol Med 1995; 1:41–53
113. Isaacs A, Lindenmann J. Virus interferences: The Interferon. Proc R Soc B 1957; 147: 258–67
114. Siegal GP, Thorgursson UP, Russo RG, Wallace DH, Liotta LA, Berger SL. Interferon enhancement of the invasive capacity of living sarcoma cells in vitro. Proc Natl Acad Sci USA 1982; 79:4064–8
115. Brunda MG, Rosenbaum D, Steen L. Inhibition of experimentally induced metastasis by interferon alpha: correlation between the modulatory effect of interferon treatment on natural killer cell activity and inhibition of metastasis. Int J Cancer 1984; 34:421–26
116. Lollini PL, Giovanni C, Del Re B, Nicoletti G, Prodi G, Nanni P. Inteferon-mediated enhancement of metastasis: are MHC antigens involved? Clin Exp Metast 1987; 5:277–87
117. Ramani P, Balkwill FR. Enhanced metastasis of mouse carcinoma after in vitro treatment with murine interferon gamma. Int J Cancer 1987; 40:830–34
118. Gery I, Waksman B. Potentiation of the T lymphocyte response to mitogens II: the cellular source of potentiating mediator(s). J Exp Med 1972; 136:143–55
119. Chan SH, Perussia B, Gupta JW, Kobayashi M, Pospisil M, Young HA Wolf SF, Young D, Clark SC, Trinchieri G. Induction of interferon gamma production by natural killer cell stimulatory factor: characterization of the receptor cells and synergy with other inducers. J Exp Med 1991; 173:869–79
120. Kubin M, Kambun M, Trinchieri G. Interleukin 12 synergized with B7/CD28 interaction in inducing efficient proliferation and cytokine production in human T cells. J Exp Med 1994; 180:211–22
121. Daniel Y, Kupferminc J, Baram A, Jaffa AJ, Fait G, Wolsman I, Lessing JB. Plasma interleukin 12 is elevated in patients with pre-eclampsia. Am J Reprod Immunol 1998; 38:376–80
122. Librach CL, Feigenbaum SL, Bass KE, Cui TY, Verastas N, Sadorvsky Y et al. Interleukin-1 beta regulates human cytotrophoblast metalloproteinase activity and invasion in vitro. J Biol Chem 1994; 269:17125–131
123. Simon C, Frances A, Piquette G, Hendrickson M, Milki A, Polan ML. Interleukin-1 system in the materno-trophoblast unit in human implantation: immunohistochemical evidence for autocrine–paracrine function. J Clin Endocrinol Metab 1994; 78:847–54

124. Steele GL, Currie WD, Leung EH, Yen BH, Lueng PCK. Rapid stimulation of human chorionic gonadotropin secretion by interleukin-1 beta from perfused first trimester trophoblast. J Clin Endocrinol Metab 1992; 75:783–8
125. Nestler JE. Interleukin-1 stimulates the aromatase activity of human placental cytotrophoblasts. Endocrinol 1993; 132:566–70
126. Saito S, Morii T, Enomoto M, Sakakura S, Nishikawa K, Narita N, et al. The effect of interleukin-2 and transforming growth factor-beta 2 (TGF-beta 2) on the proliferation and natural killer activity of decidual CD16-CD56 bright natural killer cells. Cell Immunol 1993; 152:605–13
127. Marzi M, Vigano A, Trabattoni D, Villa ML, Salvaggio A, Clerici E, et al. Characterization of type 1 and type 2 cytokine production profile in physiologic and pathologic human pregnancy. Clin Exp Immunol 1996; 106:127–33
128. Kawakami Y, Eister MC, Roseberg SH, Lotze MT. IL-4 regulates IL-2 induction of lymphokine-activated killer activity from human lymphocytes. J Immunol 1989; 142:3452–561
129. Paliard X, Yssel H, Blanchard D, Waitz JA, de Vires JE, Spits H. Antigen specific and MNC nonrestricted cytotoxicity of T cell receptor $\alpha\beta^+$ and $\gamma\alpha\delta^+$ human T cell clones isolated in IL-4. Immunol 1989; 143:452–7
130. Matthiesen L, Ekerfelt C, Berg G, Ernerudh J. Increased numbers of circulating interferon γ and interleukin 4 secreting cells during normal pregnancy. Am J Reprod Immunol 1998; 39:362–7
131. Bennett WA, Lagro-Deenadayalan S, Stopple JA, Barber WH, Hale E, Brackin MN, Cawan BD. Cytokine expression by first trimester human chorionic villi. Am J Reprod Immunol 1998; 40:309–18
132. Neki R, Matsuzaki N, Yamanaka K, Shimoya K, Okada T, Saji F, et al. The interleukin-6 (IL-6) /IL-6-receptor system induces human chorionic gonadotropin production by activating a tyrosine kinase-dependent signal transduction pathway different from pathways triggered by protein kinase activators including gonadotropin releasing hormone. J Clin Endocrinol Metab 1993; 17:704–709
133. Watson IH, Berck JS, Martinez-Maza O. Growth inhibition of ovarian cancer cells induced by antisense IL-6 oligonucleotides. Gynecol Oncol 1993; 49:8–15
134. Schroder W, Ruppert C, Bender HG. Concomitant measurements of interleukin 6 (IL-6) in serum and peritoneal fluid of patients with benign and malignant ovarian tumors. Eur J Obstet Gynecol Reprod Biol 1994; 56:43–6
135. Marandi MM, Carson LF, Weinberg B, Haney AF, Twiggs LB, Ramakrishnan S. Serum and ascitic fluid levels of interleukin 1, interleukin 6 and tumor necrosis factor alpha in patients with ovarian epithelial cancer. Cancer 1993; 72:2433–40
136. Howard M, O'Garra A, Ishida H, De Waal Malefyt R, de Vries J. Biological properties of interleukin 10. J Clin Immunol 1992; 12:239–47
137. Cadet P, Rody PL, Tyring SK, Yandell RB, Hughes TK. Interleukin-10 messenger ribonucleic acid in human placenta: implications of a role for interleukin-10 in fetal allograft protection. Am J Obstet Gynecol 1995; 173:25–9
138. Yui J, Hemmings D, Garcia-Lloret M, Guilbert LJ. Expression of the human p55 and p75 receptors in primary villous trophoblasts and their role in cytotoxic signal transduction. Biol Reprod 1996; 55:400–409
139. Wang Y, Walsh SW. TNFα concentrations and mRNA expression are increased in pre-eclamptic placentas. J Reprod Immunol 1996; 32:157–69
140. Wegman TG, Lin H, Guilbert L, Massman TR. Bidirectional cytokine interactions in the maternal–fetal relationship: is successful pregnancy a Th2 phenomenon? Immunol Today 1993; 14:353–6
141. Clark DA, Arck PC, Chaouat G. Why did your mother reject you? Immunogenetic determinants of the response to environmental selective pressure expressed at the uterine wall. Am J Reprod Immunol 1999; 41:1–11

17 Protective Role of Human Chorionic Gonadotrophin and Luteinizing Hormone Against Breast Cancer

Z. M. Lei and Ch. V. Rao

Introduction

Human chorionic gonadotropin (hCG) belongs to both the glycoprotein hormone and cystine-knot growth factor families.[1,2] The glycoprotein hormone family includes luteinizing (LH), follicle stimulating and thyroid stimulating hormones.[1] All are heterodimers of non-covalently bound common α-subunit and hormone specific ß-subunit. The ß-subunits of hCG and LH are similar except for thirty additional amino acids at the C-terminus of ß subunit of hCG.[1] The cystine-knot growth factor family consists of platelet derived growth factor ß, nerve growth factor and transforming growth factor ß.[2] Simply through association, hCG can be expected to have growth factor-like actions, which it does.[3,4]

LH binds to the same receptor and has the same biological actions as hCG.[5] The receptor is a single chain transmembrane glycoprotein which is a member of the G protein-coupled receptor family.[5] The receptor consists of an extracellular hormone binding domain, seven transmembrane spanning regions and a short cytoplasmic tail. Cyclic AMP/protein kinase A, and also in some cases, protein kinase C signaling is involved in the LH and hCG actions.[6]

hCG is produced primarily by the placenta and LH by the anterior pituitary gland. The α subunit is encoded by a single gene, whereas the ß subunit of hCG is encoded by a cluster of six genes of which 3, 5 and 8 are transcriptionally more active than the others.[7] The ß subunit of LH is encoded by a single gene.[8] The ß-subunit is rate limiting in the synthesis of dimer hormones. A number of agents, including hCG, can control the synthesis of hCG.[3,9] The synthesis of LH is also regulated by a number of agents, including LH itself, through its actions on GnRH neurons in the hypothalamus and gonadotropes in the anterior pituitary gland.[8,10,11]

Human chorionic gonadotropin also belongs to a family of embryonically related markers that include carcinoembryonic antigen and α-fetoprotein.[12] Thus, a wide variety of cancers and cancer cells contain dimer hCG and/or one of its subunits. In fact, to date, more than 70 different cancer cell lines have been shown to contain them.[13-16] The presence of hCG and/or one of its subunits in cancer cells is probably due to synthesis rather than sequestration. This ectopic expression is considered a recapitulation of the embryonic state as is cancer. The expression of hCG and/or one of its subunits increases in advanced cancers, suggesting that they might be involved in the disease.[17] As a result, a contraceptive hCG vaccine has been tested, especially for cancers of the colon and pancreas.[18-20] It is possible that some of the cancers may also ectopically express LH. Despite these advances, very little is known about how hCG works in the cancers. Like other hormones, hCG acts via binding to its receptors. Until about 13 years ago, LH/hCG receptors had not been demonstrated in nongonadal tissues.[4] The recent demonstration of their presence, including some cancers arising from nongonadal tissues, forced a change in the widely-held belief that LH and hCG are only gonadal regulating hormones.[3,4]

Recent studies suggest that hCG and LH have dual roles in cancers. In some, it promotes (endometrial,[21-25] choriocarcinomas[26] and lung[27]), while in others it inhibits the cancers (for example prostate[28-31] and breast cancers[32-34]). Some contradictions in the literature as to whether hCG prevents or promotes cancers could be due to whether they produce dimer hCG or just its ß subunit, which may have a stimulatory effect probably due to the formation of homodimers.[35-37] Advances with respect to the protective role of dimer hCG and LH in breast cancer have been concisely outlined in this article.

Early Full-Term Pregnancy Protects Against Breast Cancer

Epidemiologic data suggest that young women are highly susceptible to developing breast cancer.[38,39] If they complete a full-term pregnancy before 20 years of age, their risk of developing breast cancer later in life will be reduced by about half .[40.41] This benefit is seen among all ethnic groups worldwide and increases in multiple, as compared to single, pregnancies and then decreases after about 30 years of age. An interruption of pregnancy reduces the protective effect.[40-43] The phenomenon of pregnancy protecting against breast cancer is also seen in rats and mice.[44-47] For example, chemical carcinogen 7,12-dimethylbenz[α]anthracene (DMBA) was much less effective in inducing mammary tumors in non-castrated parous rats as compared with nulliparous animals.[32,48] The nulliparous animals got the same protection as pregnant rats if they were treated with hCG for about 21 days, which is equivalent to full-term pregnancy.[32,48] It is not clear whether rats have chorionic gonadotropin. Nevertheless, it is possible that LH works in the same way as hCG during pregnancy in women.

Although the epidemiological findings suggest that early full-term pregnancy is the most effective natural means of protecting against breast cancer, it does not mean that every woman who completes an early pregnancy is completely immune from developing breast cancer. This is because breast cancer has multiple (genetic, viral, environmental, dietary) etiologies and pregnancy may not be able to override some of their effects.[49]

Evidence That Direct hCG Action May Confer Protection Against Breast Cancer

Pregnancy is a state of chorionic elevation of steroid and protein hormones. Thus, the protective effect of pregnancy can be due to any of these hormones. In order to learn which one, Russo and Russo and their colleagues initiated a number of studies using a rat breast cancer model.[32,48-53] In this model, the administration of DMBA resulted in a consistent induction of mammary tumors. This induction was greatly reduced when rats were pre- or simultaneously treated with hCG. The disease progression also slowed when hCG was administered after the carcinogenesis was first induced by DMBA treatment. These data indicate that hCG worked, but how it worked remained speculative. In the absence of knowledge that rat mammary glands were targets of LH and hCG action, it was speculated that estradiol and progesterone, produced as a result of stimulation of ovaries by hCG, inhibited the carcinogenesis. This logic was counterintuitive because estradiol is mitogenic and thus serves as a risk factor for breast cancer. A recent study simulating pregnancy levels of estradiol alone or estradiol with progesterone demonstrated an inhibitory effect on mammary carcinogenesis induced by N-methyl-N-nitrosourea in nulliparous rats.[54] Whether this benefit could have been due to elevation of LH levels has not been examined. Since LH is a homolog that binds to the same receptors and has the same actions, it could offer the same benefit as hCG. This possibility may explain how early menopause and ovariectomy can also protect women against breast cancer.[42] Thus, protection may come from chronic elevation of LH levels in addition to deprivation of estrogens. The higher incidence of breast cancer in postmenopausal women with elevated LH levels could be the result of not completing a full-term pregnancy at an early age. Moreover, due to other causes, their disease may have begun years or sometimes decades before the clinical manifestation and, by the time they reach menopause, it would have been too late for LH to have any protective effect.

Several laboratories have now demonstrated that rat and sow breast tissues, normal and malignant human breast tissues and human breast cancer cell lines contain LH/hCG receptor transcripts and receptor protein which can bind ^{125}I-hCG.[33,34,55-57] However, the receptor levels are lower in breast tissues and cells than in traditional targets such as ovaries. The receptors are primarily present in epithelial cells which are the origin of a majority of breast cancers.[55,56] Sow breast receptor levels increase from the proliferative to the secretory phase, suggesting that progesterone may upregulate and/or estrogen may downregulate the receptors.[56]

MCF-7 cells contained higher receptor levels than the other human breast cancer cell lines tested.[33,34,56] This was due to an increased transcription of LH/hCG receptor gene which, in turn, appears to be due to higher levels of Ap2 and Egr transcription factors.[57]

It has been shown that hCG can inhibit the growth and invasion and increase the cyclic AMP and decrease ER levels in MCF-7 cells.[33,34,58] LH, but not the other members of the glycoprotein hormone family, can mimic hCG's actions.[33,34] Among the hCG effects, the inhibition of invasion was more dramatic.[34] The effect of hCG on the inhibition of MCF-7 cell growth is probably not due to a decrease in ER levels since hCG can decrease the growth of ER negative MDA-MB-231 cells.[33] It is quite likely that cyclic AMP/protein kinase A signaling may mediate the hCG effects. Using an antisense phosphorothioate oligodeoxynucleotide synthesized from a human LH/hCG receptor sequence to inhibit its synthesis, it was found that hCG cannot work in the absence of normal levels of its receptors in MCF-7 cells.[34]

Mechanism of hCG Action in Breast Cancer

The breasts of nonparous animals and women predominantly contain type 1 and type 2 lobules which mostly contain undifferentiated epithelial cells that are capable of rapid proliferation upon stimulation.[59] The uncontrolled cell proliferation can lead to ductal carcinoma in situ which progresses to invasive carcinoma. The breasts of parous animals or women, on the other hand, mainly contain types 3 and 4 lobules, which contain differentiated, secretory and nonproliferative epithelial cells.[59] When nulliparous rats are treated with hCG, the type 1 lobules can permanently differentiate into type 3 and 4 lobules.[59] Although this differentiation is a physiological phenomenon in preparation of breast for lactation, it also happens to reduce the pool of cells that are most vulnerable to carcinogenic transformation. The differentiation effect alone may not explain the protective role of hCG. For example, placental lactogen, which also can induce the differentiation, does not protect against breast cancer.[45,60] However, whether the differentiation induced by placental lactogen is nonreversible, as is the case with hCG, is not known.

There must be other mechanisms that hCG may also use. One such mechanism could be that hCG directly inhibits cell growth,[33,34,58] invasion[34] and increases apoptosis.[61,62] The inhibition of cell growth could be mediated by increasing inhibin[58,63,64] and/or decreasing insulin-like growth factor (IGF), its receptors and increasing some of the IGF binding proteins (IGFBPs).[65] Like hCG, inhibin decreases cell growth and increases apoptosis. IGF, on the other hand, has opposite effects. Decreasing IGF-1, its receptors and increasing IGFBPs will reduce the availability of IGF and its action. Other possibilities include hCG enhancing the cellular DNA repair mechanisms[66] and increasing the expression of other genes that might prevent and/or decrease the expression of others that might promote the carcinogenic transformation of breast epithelial cells.[67,68]

Clearly, from all the evidence, there is very little room for doubt that breast is another nongonadal target of hCG and LH action and that their action may be relevant to physiological changes in breast in preparation for lactation and at the same time confer protection against cancer.

Summary and Perspective

Recent studies from several laboratories demonstrated that human and animal breast tissues and human breast cell lines contain low levels of functional LH/hCG receptors. The hCG and LH effects are consistent with these hormones protecting breast from carcinogenic transformation. These effects may explain the decreased incidence of breast cancer in women who complete a full-term pregnancy early in life or if they had early menopause or an ovariectomy. This pregnancy-induced protection is also seen in rats and mice which could be due to LH and/or placental gonadotropins that these animals may produce which are similar to CG. These findings suggest that LH and hCG could be used to protect against breast cancer. However, hCG is preferable because of its longer half-life in circulation. Logic from the findings discussed in this article suggests:

1 a better prognosis when breast cancer tissue contains dimer hCG

2 early treatment of women who delay their first pregnancy with hCG may reduce the risk of breast cancer

3 the direct administration of hCG into breast cancer tissue may slow the disease progression.

These predictions can easily be tested in clinical trials. The lower incidence of breast cancer among women who take hCG for weight loss suggests that hCG might work.[69]

References

1. Pierce JG, Parsons TF. Glycoprotein hormones: structure and function. Ann Rev Biochem, 1981; 50:465–495
2. Lapthorn AJ, Harris DC, Littlejohn A, Lustbader JW, Canfield RE, Machin KJ, Morgan FJ, Isaacs NW. Crystal structure of human chorionic gonadotropin. Nature 1994; 369:455–61
3. Rodway MR, Rao ChV. A novel perspective on the role of human chorionic gonadotropin during pregnancy and in gestational trophoblastic disease. Early Pregnancy 1995; 1:176–87
4. Rao ChV. The beginning of a new era in reproductive biology and medicine: expression of low levels of functional luteinizing hormone/human chorionic gonadotropin receptors in nongonadal tissues. J Physiol Pharmacol 1996; 47(Suppl. 2):41–53
5. Segaloff D, Ascoli M. The lutropin/chorio-gonadotropin receptor. 4 years later. Endocrine Rev 1993; 14:324–47
6. Ryu KS, Gilchrist RL, Koo YB, Ji I, Ji TH. Gene, interaction, signal generation, signal divergence and signal transduction of the LH/hCG receptor. Int J Gynecol Obstet 1998; 60:S9–20
7. Policastro PF, Daniels-McQueen S, Carle G, Boime I. A map of the hCG-ß LH-ß gene cluster. J Biol Chem 1986; 261:5907–16
8. Albanese C, Colin IM, Crowley WF, Ito M, Pestell RG, Weiss J, Jameson JL. The gonadotropin genes: evolution of distinct mechanisms for hormonal control. Recent Prog Horm Res 1996; 51:23–58
9. Jameson LJ, Hollenberg AN. Regulation of chorionic gonadotropin gene expression. Endocr Rev 1993; 14:203–21
10. Huang ZH, Lei ZM, Rao CV. Novel independent and synergistic regulation of gonadotropin-α subunit gene by luteinizing hormone/human choriogonadotropin and gonadotropin releasing hormone in the α-T3-1 gonadotrope cells. Mol Cell Endocrinol 1997; 130:23–31
11. Lei ZM, Rao ChV. *Cis*-acting elements and trans-acting proteins in the transcriptional inhibition of gonadotropin-releasing hormone gene by human chorionic gonadotropin in immortalized hypothalamic GT1-7 neurons. J Biol Chem 1997; 272:14365–71
12. Jacobs EL, Haskell CM. Clinical use of tumor markers in oncology. Curr Probl Cancer 1991; 15:299–360
13. Acevedo HF, Krichevsky A, Campbell-Acevedo EA, Galyon EA, Buffo MJ, Hartsock RJ. Flow cytometry method for the analysis of membrane-associated human chorionic gonadotropin, its subunits and fragments on human cancer cells. Cancer 1992; 69:1818–28
14. Acevedo HF, Krichevsky A, Campbell-Acevedo EA, Galyon JC, Buffo MJ, Hartsock RJ. Expression of membrane-associated human chorionic gonadotropin, its subunits, and fragments by cultured human cancer cells. Cancer 1992; 69:1829–42
15. Acevedo HF, Tong JY, Hartsock RJ. Human chorionic gonadotropin-beta subunit gene expression in cultured human fetal and cancer cells of different types and origins. Cancer 1995; 76:1467–75
16. Lazar V, Diez SG, Laurent A, Giovangrandi Y, Radvanyi F, Chopin D, Bidart JM, Bellet D, Vidaud M. Expression of human chorionic gonadotropin ß subunit genes in superficial and invasive bladder carcinomas. Cancer Res 1995; 55:3735–8
17. Acevedo HF, Hartsock RJ. Metastatic phenotype correlates with high expression of membrane-associated complete ß-human chorionic gonadotropin in vivo. Cancer 1996; 78:2388–99
18. Triozzi P, Gochnour D, Martin EW, Aldrich W, Powell J, Kim JA, Young DC, Lombardi J. Clinical and immunologic effects of a synthetic ß-human chorionic gonadotropin vaccine. Int J Oncol 1994; 5:1447–53
19. Trozzi PL, Stevens VC, Aldrich W, Powell J, Todd CW, Newman MJ. Effects of a ß-human chorionic gonadotropin subunit immunogen administered in aqueous solution with a novel nonionic block copolymer adjuvant in patients with advanced cancer. Clin Cancer Res 1997; 3:2355–62
20. Triozzi PL, Stevens VC. Human chorionic gonadotropin as a target for cancer vaccines. Oncol Rep 1999; 6:7–17
21. Lin J, Lei ZM, Lojun S, Rao ChV, Satyaswaroop PG, Day Jr TG. Increased expression of luteinizing hormone/human chorionic gonadotropin receptor gene in human endometrial carcinomas. J Clin Endocrinol Metab 1994; 79:1483–91
22. Bax CMR, Chatzaki E, Davies S, Gallagher CJ. Elucidating the role of gonadotropins in endometrial cancer cell growth. Biochem Soc Trans 1996; 24:S443

23. Konishi I, Koshiyama M, Mandai M, Kuroda H, Yamamoto S, Nanbu K, Komatsu T, Matsushita K, Rao ChV, Mori T. Increased expression of LH/hCG receptors in endometrial hyperplasia and carcinoma in anovulatory women. Gynecol Oncol 1997; 65:273–80
24. Nagamani M, Cao HA. Specific binding and proliferative effects of luteinizing hormone in human endometrial cancer cell lines. J Soc Gynecol Invest 1997; 4:A132
25. Han SW, Zhou XL, Lei ZM, Rao ChV. Role of luteinizing hormone in human endometrial carcinoma. In: Program of the Endocrine Society Annual Meeting, Abstract, 1999: 1–593
26. Lei ZM, Taylor DD, Gercel-Taylor C, Rao ChV. Human chorionic gonadotropin promotes tumorigenesis of choriocarcinoma JAR cells. Trophoblast Res 1999; 13:147–59
27. Sanjeer K, Talwar GP, Biswas DK. Necrosis and inhibition of growth of human lung tumor by anti-α human chorionic gonadotropin antibody. J Natl Cancer Inst 1992; 1:42–7
28. Tao Y-X, Bao S, Ackermann DM, Lei ZM, Rao ChV. Expression of luteinizing hormone/human chorionic gonadotropin receptor gene in benign prostatic hyperplasia and in prostate carcinoma in humans. Biol Reprod 1997; 56:67–72
29. Bao S, Lei ZM, Rao CV.1997; The presence of functional luteinizing hormone/chorionic gonadotropin receptors in human prostate cell lines. In: Program of the Endocrine Society Annual Meeting, Abstract, 1999: 3–403
30. Dirnhofer S, Berger C, Hermann M, Steiner G, Madersbacher S, Berger P. Coexpression of gonadotropic hormones and their corresponding FSH- and LH/CG-receptors in the human prostate. Prostate 1998; 35:212–20
31. Lei ZM, Rao ChV. Direct luteinizing hormone regulation of male reproductive tract. In: Coutinho EM, Spinola P (eds), Reproductive Medicine. A Millenium Review. The Proceedings of the Tenth World Congress on Human Reproduction. Parthenon Publishing, London, England, 2000 (in press)
32. Russo IH, Russo J.Chorionic gonadotropin: a tumoristatic and preventive agent in breast cancer. In: Teicher BA. (ed.), Drug Resistance in Oncology. Marcel Dekker, New York, 1993; 537–60
33. Lojun S, Bao S, Lei ZM, Rao ChV. The presence of functional luteinizing hormone/chorionic gonadotropin receptors in human breast cell lines: Implications supporting the premise that hCG protects women against breast cancer. Biol Reprod 1997; 57:1202–10
34. Li X, Lei ZM, Rao ChV. The actions of human chorionic gonadotropin in MCF-7 cells support the premise that it may protect woman against breast cancer. In: Program of the Endocrine Society Annual Meeting, Abstract, 1999: 3–195
35. Gillott DJ, Iles RK, Chard T. The effects of ßhCG on the in vitro growth of bladder cancer cells. Brit J Can 1996; 73:323–6
36. Bièche I, Lazar V, Noguès C, Poynard T, Giovangrandi Y, Bellet D, Lidereau R, Vidaud M. Prognostic value of chorionic gonadotropin ß gene transcripts in human breast carcinoma. Clin Cancer Res 1998; 4:671–6
37. Butler SA, Laidler P, Porter JR, Kicman AT, Chard T, Cowan DA, Iles RK. The ß-subunit of human chorionic gonadotrophin exists as a homodimer. J Mol Endocrinol 1999; 22:185–92
38. Hildreth N, Shore R, Dvuretski P. The risk of breast cancer after irradiation of the thymus in infancy. N Engl J Med 1989; 321:1281–4
39. Tokunaga M, Land CE, Tokuoka S. Follow-up studies of breast cancer incidence among atomic bomb survivors. J Radiat Res (Tokyo) 1991; 32: Suppl. 201–11
40. MacMahon B, Cole P, Liu M, Lowe CR, Mirra AP, Ravinhar H, Salber EJ, Valaoras VG, Yuasa S. Age at [first] birth and breast cancer risk. Bull WHO 1970; 34:209–21
41. Trapido EJ. Age at first birth, parity, and breast cancer risk. Cancer 1983; 51:946–8
42. Kelsey JL, Gammon MD, John EM. Reproductive factors and breast cancer. Epidemiol Rev 1993; 15:36–47
43. Lambe M, Hsieh C, Tsaih S, Ekbom A, Adami HO, Trichopoulos D. Maternal risk of breast cancer following multiple birth: a nationwide study in Sweden. Cancer Causes Control 1996; 7:533–8
44. Welsch CW. Host factors affecting the growth of carcinogen-induced rat mammary carcinomas: a review and tribute to Charles Brenton Huggins. Cancer Res 1985; 45:3415–43
45. Russo J, Russo IH. Toward a physiological approach to breast cancer prevention. Cancer Epidemiol Biomaker Prev 1994; 3:353–64
46. Russo I, Russo J. Mammary gland neoplasia in long-term rodent studies. Environ Health Perspect 1996; 104:938–67
47. Sinha DK, Pazik JE, Dao TL. Prevention of mammary carcinogenesis in rats by pregnancy: effect of full-term and interrupted pregnancy. Br J Cancer 1988; 57:390– 4
48. Tay LK, Russo J. Effect of human chorionic gonadotropin on 7,12-dimethylbenz[a]anthracene-induced DNA binding and repair synthesis by rat mammary epithelial cells. Chem Biol Interact 1985; 55:13–21

49. Russo J, Yang X, Hu YF, Bove BA, Huang Y, Silva ID, Tahin Q, Wu Y, Higgy N, Zekri A, Russo IH. Biological and molecular basis of human breast cancer. Front Biosci 1998; 3:D944–60
50. Russo IH, Koszalka M, Gimotty PA, Russo J. Protective effect of chorionic gonadotropin on DMBA-induced mammary carcinogenesis. Br J Cancer 1990; 62:243–7
51. Russo IH, Koszalka M, Russo J. Human chorionic gonadotropin and rat mammary cancer prevention. J Natl Cancer Inst 1990; 82:1286–9
52. Russo IH, Koszalka M, Russo J. Effect of human chorionic gonadotropin on mammary gland differentiation and carcinogenesis. Carcinogenesis 1990; 11:1849–55
53. Russo IH, Koszalka M, Russo J. Comparative study of the influence of pregnancy and hormonal treatment on mammary carcinogenesis. Br J Cancer 1991; 64:481–4
54. Guzman RC, Yang J, Rajkumar L, Thordarson G, Chen X, Nandi S. Hormonal prevention of breast cancer: Mimicking the protective effect of pregnancy. Proc Natl Acad Sci 1999; 96:2520–25
55. Tao YX, Lei ZM, Rao ChV. Luteinizing hormone/human chorionic gonadotropin receptors in lactating rat mammary glands. Life Sci 1997; 60:1297–303
56. Meduri G, Charnaux N, Loosfelt H, Jolivet A, Spyratos F, Brailly S, Milgrom E. Luteinizing hormone/human chorionic gonadotropin receptors in breast cancer. Cancer Res 1997; 57:857–64
57. Hu YL, Lei ZM, Rao ChV. *Cis*-acting elements and *trans*-acting proteins in the transcription of luteinizing hormone/human chorionic gonadotropin receptors gene in human breast cells. Breast J 1999; 5:186–93
58. Alvarado MV, Alvarado NE, Russo J, Russo IH. Human chorionic gonadotropin inhibits proliferation and induces expression of inhibin in human breast epithelial cells in vitro. In vitro Cell Dev Biol 1994; 30:A4–8
59. Russo J, Russo IH. Hormonally induced differentiation: a novel approach to breast cancer prevention. J Cell Biochem Suppl 1995; 22:58–64
60. Russo J, Russo I. Biological and molecular bases of mammary carcinogenesis. Lab Invest 1987; 57:112–37
61. Srivastava P, Russo J, Russo IH. Chorionic gonadotropin inhibits rat mammary carcinogenesis through activation of programmed cell death. Carcinogenesis 1997; 18:1799–1808
62. Srivastava P, Russo J, Mgbonyebi OP, Russo IH. Growth inhibition and activation of apoptotic gene expression by human chorionic gonadotropin in human breast epithelial cells. Anticancer Res 1998; 18:4003–10
63. Alvarado MV, Russo J, Russo IH. Immunolocalization of inhibin in the mammary gland of rats treated with hCG. J Histochem Cytochem 1993; 41:29–34
64. Alvarado MV, Ho TY, Russo J, Russo IH. Human chorionic gonadotropin regulates the synthesis of inhibin in the ovary and mammary gland of rat. Endocrine 1994;2:1107–14
65. Huynh H. In vivo regulation of the insulin-like growth factor system of mitogens by human chorionic gonadotropin. Intl J Oncol 1998; 13:571–5
66. Huang Y, Bove B, Wu Y, Russo IH, Yang X, Zekri A, Russo J. Microsatellite instability during the immortalization and transformation of human breast epithelial cells in vitro. Mol Carcinogensis 1999; 24:118–27
67. Ho TY, Russo J, Russo IH. Polypeptide pattern of human breast epithelial cells following human chorionic gonadotropin (hCG) treatment. Electrophoresis 1994; 15:746–50
68. Srivastava P, Silva ID, Russo J, Mgbonyebi OP, Russo IH. Identification of new genes differentially expressed in breast carcinoma cells treated with human chorionic gonadotropin. Int J Oncol 1998; 13:465–9
69. Bernstein L, Hanisch R, Sullivan-Halley J, Ross RK. Treatment with human chorionic gonadotropin and risk of breast cancer. Cancer Epidemiol Biomarkers Prev 1995; 4:437–40

18 Proliferation, Differentiation and Apoptosis in Pregnancy and Cancer

Richard G. Lea

Introduction

The placenta is often compared to a tumour in terms of its rapid growth over a short period of time and its ability to evade maternal immune rejection. In the placenta the processes that regulate cellular proliferation, cell cycle arrest and apoptosis are tightly regulated so that growth and differentiation occur at the right gestational times to the benefit of the pregnancy. In tumour growth, apoptosis is described as being disregulated so that a high proliferative rate is maintained. Since the placenta is a controlled tumour, the basic mechanisms which regulate the growth of both are believed to be similar. It follows therefore that studies of placental growth may enhance our understanding of tumour development and vice versa. The objective of this review is to investigate the extent of this commonality of mechanisms in terms of the regulation of cellular proliferation, differentiation and apoptosis.

Proliferation and Apoptosis: a Delicate Balance

Proliferation, differentiation and apoptosis are normal features of many developmental and homeostatic processes. The balance between cell death and survival is regulated by complex interactions between intrinsic and extrinsic factors which determine cell numbers and indeed the final differentiated cell state.

When DNA damage occurs, cells may respond by either undergoing cell death by apoptosis or imposing a delay in the cell cycle during which the damage is repaired. Normal progression through the cell cycle is regulated by cyclins and cyclin-dependent kinases (CDKs).[1] Cell cycle inhibitory proteins such as p53 (tumour suppresser gene) and p21 counteract the growth promoting activity of cyclins and CDKs and induce cell cycle arrest.[2] The proliferation of cells is therefore counteracted by both cellular apoptosis and cell cycle arrest. The transcription of p21 can be activated by p53 dependent and independent mechanisms.

Cell death by apoptosis (programmed cell death) is a process by which single or small numbers of unwanted cells are removed from a tissue without affecting tissue or organ morphology or function. Apoptotic cell clearance is characterised by distinct morphological changes manifest by condensation of nuclear heterochromatin into a crescent shape, cell shrinkage and condensation and finally the formation of membrane bound apoptotic bodies which are phagocytosed by macrophages or neighbouring cells. This process occurs without the release of noxious substances, thus preventing the stimulation of an inflammatory response. In contrast, necrosis involves the unplanned death of large numbers of cells in a tissue in response to cell injury and this is manifest by cell leakage and lysis leading to the stimulation of an inflammatory response.[3,4]

A key feature of programmed cell death by apoptosis is the activation of endogenous endonucleases which cleave nuclear DNA into oligonucleosomal fragments.[5] This is preceded by the activation of a family of protease molecules known as caspases. These proteases exist in all animal cells and are activated by proteolytic cleavage of their proforms at conserved Asp residues.[6] Since caspases activate each other, they generate a proteolytic cascade with upstream caspases considered as the initiators and downstream caspases considered as the effectors. The effector caspases cleave protein substrates in the cell irreversibly stimulating the morphological changes described.[7]

Caspase activation can occur through various mechanisms. The best documented mechanism is through the tumour necrosis factor (TNF) family of cytokine death receptors. These include Fas (CD95), TNFR1 (CD120a), DR3 (Tramp), DR4 (Trail-R1), DR5 (Trail-R2) and CAR-1.[8] All of these receptors have death domains which recruit and bind adapter proteins such as Fadd/Mort-1. The adapter protein then binds, cleaves and activates one of the upstream caspases (Caspase 8 or 10) and hence the cascade of protease interactions is initiated.[7,8] Another cell signalling system which mediates the effects of apoptotic stimuli such as TNFα and Fas ligand is the sphingomyelin pathway. This system is reported to play a role in cell growth arrest, differentiation and apoptosis and the key second messenger involved is ceramide.[9] The sphingomyelin cycle is initiated upon activation of sphingomyelinases which cleave sphingomyelin into ceramide and phorylcholine. Several sphingomyelinase isoenzymes are present in mammalian tissues and these differ in terms of catalytic properties, subcellular localisation and mode of regulation.[10] Apoptosis is associated with the activation of acid sphingomyelinase and increased intra-cellular ceramide, whereas other cellular responses are associated with the activation of the neutral isoenzyme. Since acid sphingomyelinase is compartmentalised in the cytoplasm, its putative role as a second messenger in apoptosis has raised some controversy.[10] However, sphingolipid metabolites regulate ceramide associated apoptosis, e.g. sphingosine-1-phosphate (S1P) suppresses apoptosis in response to TNFα and Fas ligand. Although TNFα and Fas ligand stimulate the caspase cascade, it is uncertain how the two pathways interact.

Apoptosis is regulated by a large family of protein products many of which are members of the *bcl-2* gene family. At least 17 members of the *bcl-2* family have been detected in humans, some of which inhibit apoptosis (*bcl-2*, *bcl-x-long*, *bcl-w*, *bok*, *mcl-1*) and some of which are pro-apoptotic (*bax*, *bcl-x-short*, *bad*, *bik*, *bim*, *hrk*).[11] Pro- and anti-apoptotic proteins form homo- and heterodimers in which one member enhances or antagonises the activity of the other. The most documented of these interactions is the binding of the pro-apoptotic proteins bax, bak and bok to the anti-apoptotic proteins bcl-2 and bcl-x-long. Consequently, the inhibitory effect of bcl-2 and bcl-x-long is counteracted.[12,13] In studies of apoptosis, the ratio of bcl-2 to bax is considered an important determinant of cell death or survival.[4] The bcl-2 family proteins induce changes in mitochondria resulting in cytochrome c release in the case of bax and reduced release in the case of bcl-2.[7,14,15]

Proliferation and Apoptosis in the Normal and Abnormal Placenta

Apoptosis is a feature of trophoblast cells at all stages of gestation. However, the balance between placental apoptosis, proliferation and differentiation changes according to gestational age. Proliferating cell nuclear antigen (PCNA) expression, indicative of proliferation, is most abundant in early placenta cytotrophoblasts and decreases to low levels at term when cytotrophoblasts are sparse.[16,17] In the first trimester placenta, apoptotic nuclei are predominantly found in the cytotrophoblast although some fragmented nuclei have been observed in the syncytiotrophoblast usually in association with fibrinoid deposits in syncytial knots or sprouts, at terminal villous tips or in the syncytiotrophoblast of large stem villi.[16,18,19] The incidence of placental apoptosis is reported to increase with gestation and detailed histological studies have shown that more than 50% of placental apoptotic nuclei are trophoblast with less than 5% endothelial and the remainder stromal.[20] However, other studies report a decrease in placental apoptosis as gestation progresses. This probably reflects the criteria used to detect apoptosis and/or simply the sparcity of cytotrophoblasts in late gestation.[16,17]

Placenta collected from failing first trimester pregnancies exhibits a higher than normal incidence of apoptosis in the syncytiotrophoblast, particularly at terminal villous tips usually associated with rapid growth.[4,19,21] Although these changes were not associated with human chorionic gonadotrophin or gestational age the apoptosis to proliferation balance is clearly biased towards apoptotic cell death.[21] Intrauterine growth restriction is also associated with increased syncytiotrophoblast apoptosis and this is also a feature of placentas collected from ectopic pregnancies.[20,22]

These findings indicate that throughout gestation placental apoptosis is finely tuned and changes as gestation progresses. These changes are manifest by:

1. a change in the trophoblast lineage predominantly exhibiting apoptosis
2. an apparent increased incidence of apoptosis.

When pregnancy is threatened or failing the localisation and/or the number of apoptotic nuclei increases. Since these changes are evident in placental tissue distant from the normal implant site (ectopic), it would appear that placental apoptosis is influenced or regulated (or both) by local factors produced at the implantation site such as cytokines and growth factors. It follows, therefore, that gestational dependent changes in placental apoptosis are regulated by gestational dependent changes in local regulatory factors.

Proto-oncogenes, bcl-2:bax Ratio and Placental Growth

The protein product of the proto-oncogene *bcl-2* is present in both first and third trimester placental syncytiotrophoblast. In contrast first trimester cytotrophoblasts are bcl-2 negative and bax positive, and this is thought to account for the predominance of apoptotic nuclei in this lineage.[4] Similarly, the increased apoptosis in the syncytiotrophoblast from failing first trimester pregnancies is associated with lower levels of syncytiotrophoblast bcl-2 protein with no apparent change in bax.[4] Interestingly, syncytiotrophoblast bcl-2 protein appears to increase with normal advancing gestation.[17] These data suggest that the ratio of bcl-2 to bax is critical in regulating placental apoptosis. It follows therefore that should this regulation break down then the controlled gestation dependent development of the placenta is likely to be seriously compromised. Indeed the overproliferation of placenta in the situation of complete mole and choriocarcinoma is associated with an increased expression of bcl-2, few apoptotic cells and marked expression of PCNA.[17,23]

The syncytiotrophoblast is dependent on the fusion of the underlying cytotrophoblast cells for growth and regeneration. This process involves the exposure of cytotrophoblast membrane phosphytidylserine (the phosphytidylserine flip) and this is believed to be a signal for cell fusion and syncytium formation. As the phosphitidylserine flip also occurs in the early stages of apoptosis, apoptotic cell death is thought to be involved in syncytium formation. Studies of the apoptotic cascade in this process have shown that a few cytotrophoblasts do exhibit the phosphatidylserine flip; however, further progression along the apoptotic cascade is in most cases thought to be blocked by Bcl-2 or Mcl-1 proteins.[18] Interestingly, the syncytiotrophoblast exhibited variable progression along the cascade. Cells undergoing apoptosis were predominantly detected in syncytial knots and these regions

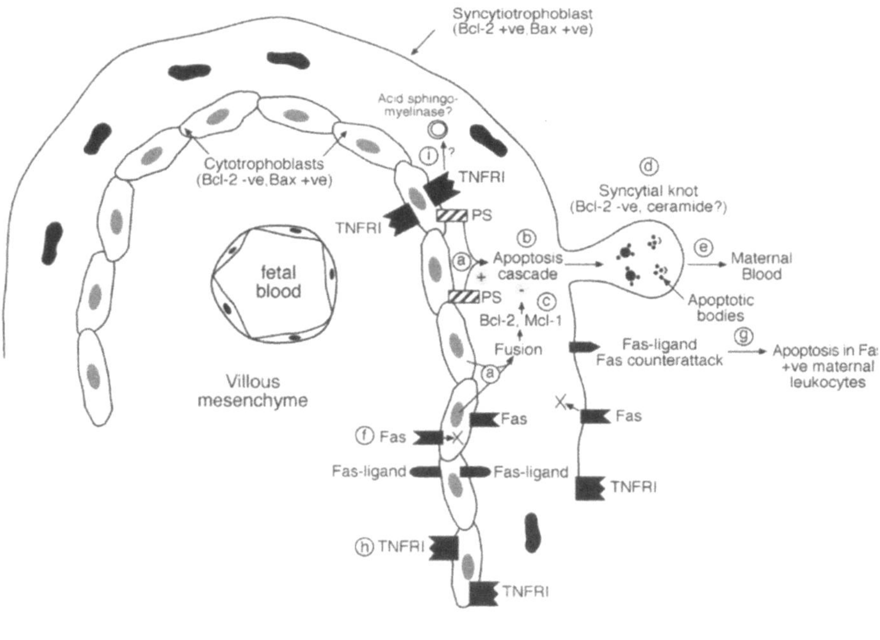

Fig. 18.1. The apoptosis cascade in placental chorionic villi. (a) The fusion of cytotrophoblasts exposes phosphytidylserine [PS] (the phoshytidylserine flip) which initiates the apoptosis cascade (b). (c) Bcl-2 and Mcl-1 donated by the cytotrophoblasts to the syncytium block the cascade from progressing further. (d) The specialised syncytial knots are bcl-2-negative and the apoptosis cascade continues resulting in nuclear fragmentation and the generation of apoptotic bodies. It is unknown if ceramide plays a role in this process. (e) The syncytial knot containing groups of apoptotic nuclei is extruded into the maternal circulation where it is thought to be phagocytosed in the maternal lung. (f) The Fas receptor located in the cytotrophoblasts and syncytiotrophoblast is unable to initiate apoptosis on stimulation [X = Fas signalling block]. (g) Placental Fas ligand is thought to induce apoptosis in Fas-positive maternal leukocytes but can not initiate apoptosis through placental Fas receptor [Fas counterattack]. (h) The TNFR1 is able to initiate the apoptotic cascade if levels of pro-inflammatory cytokines are increased. (i) The activation of the TNFR1 receptor may also induce apoptosis through the sphingomyelin pathway; compartmentalised acid sphingomyelinase is thought to be present in the syncytiotrophoblast. However, apoptosis occurs predominantly in the syncytial knots.

were also characterised by the phosphotidylserine flip but no nuclear proteins (Fig. 18.1). In other areas Bcl-2 and Mcl-1 were predominant and nuclear proteins were detectable.[18] The authors conclude that the apoptotic cascade starts in the cytotrophoblast cells thus promoting fusion into the syncytium. Bcl-2 and Mcl-1 in the syncytium prevent further progression along the cascade in this lineage with the exception of the syncytial knots. In these Bcl-2-negative, Mcl-1-negative specialised regions, the cascade is completed and clusters of apoptotic nuclei are extruded into the maternal circulation after which they lodge in the maternal lungs and are phagocytosed.[18] It follows therefore that failure of cytotrophoblast cell fusion increases syncytiotrophoblast apoptosis and breakdown.

The tumour suppressor gene p53 is present at low levels in normal villous and extravillous trophoblast and at high levels in some cytotrophoblasts.[24,25] There is little evidence for the expression of the mutant form of p53 in placenta. Surprisingly, the analysis of complete and partial hydatidiform moles and choriocarcinomas revealed only one p53 mutation.[23] In contrast, choriocarcinoma cell lines (JAR, JEG-3 and BeWo) do express the mutant form of p53.[24] Levels of p53 as well as p21 and mdm2 were however higher in complete moles and choriocarcinomas as compared to normal placentas. In the normal placenta, therefore, wild type p53 may limit trophoblast invasive activity. However, as higher levels of wild type p53 appear to be present in at least some placental tumours, the normal tumour suppressing activity of p53 appears not to be functional and may therefore be inactivated at a different level.

Death Receptors and Placental Apoptosis

The death receptors Fas, TNFR1 and more recently the TRAIL receptor DR4 have been identified in the human placenta.[26,27,28] The TNFR1 has been detected on cytotrophoblasts and also the syncytiotrophoblast.[26,29] Studies of term cultured villous cytotrophoblasts show that TNFα is able to induce apoptosis of these cells and that interferonγ (IFNγ) enhanced this effect.[30] Fas is expressed by first and third trimester syncytiotrophoblast as well as term cytotrophoblasts.[18,26] However, in contrast to TNF, neither Fas antibody nor Fas ligand was able to induce placental apoptosis. It appears therefore that Fas mediated killing is inactivated in trophoblast.[26] Also in the placenta is the anti-apoptotic molecule Flip which is able to compete with pro-caspase 8 for binding to the adaptor protein Fadd (see earlier) and thus block Fas signalling.[31] However, since TNFR1 activation activates the same signalling pathway as Fas, this does not appear to be the mechanism. The mechanism by which Fas signalling is blocked remains to be elucidated.

Of note is that the placenta also expresses Fas ligand predominantly in the cytotrophoblasts and invasive interstitial trophoblast (first trimester) within maternal tissue, with low levels in the syncytiotrophoblast.[32,33,34] The blocked Fas R signalling mechanism may therefore prevent autocrine/juxtacrine Fas mediated placental damage. The role of Fas ligand in the placenta is uncertain. One possibility is that it may protect invasive trophoblast from maternal immune attack by inducing apoptosis in FasR positive decidual or circulating maternal leukocytes.[34] However, as fetal development is maintained in Fas/Fas ligand knock out mice even after immune stimulation, the Fas/Fas ligand system does not seem to be mandatory for pregnancy success.[35] Indeed, in experimental situations, Fas ligand can induce a pro-inflammatory response, e.g. Fas ligation can induce secretion of the chemokine IL-8.[36] This may account for the relatively low level of Fas ligand expression in the syncytiotrophoblast. The mechanism involved is unknown, however it is clear that Fas ligand is expressed at sites of immune privilege, e.g. the eye and testis. It is likely therefore that Fas ligand functions in an environment where immune privilege is mediated by a number of other factors. The related TRAIL DR4 receptor mRNA has been detected in the human placenta but not in trophoblast cell lines, whereas the TRAIL protein has been immunolocalised to the syncytiotrophoblast. It is not known if DR4 protein is present on placenta.[28]

The ceramide system has also been implicated as playing a role in trophoblast apoptosis. Payne and colleagues have shown that apoptosis in primary cultures can be induced with ceramide or acid sphingomyelinase.[37] Further, EGF was shown to inhibit ceramide and acid sphingomyelinase induced apoptosis and this was associated with reduced levels of ceramide. Furthermore, recent studies have shown that acidic sphingomyelinase, and therefore increased ceramide, is required for TNFR1 (p55) mediated trophoblast apoptosis (L. Guilbert, personal communication). The mechanism by which compartmentalised acid sphingomyelinase is activated in trophoblast cells is not clear; however, it is thought to involve membrane bound caveolae which concentrate plasma membrane lipids and trap external molecules for delivery to the acidic cellular compartment.[37,38]

Proto-oncogenes, bcl-2:bax Ratio and Tumour Development

Although many of the regulatory factors which are important in placental development play a similar role in the development of tumours, cancer is characterized by uncontrolled proliferation and a defect in apoptosis. Indeed, the balance of apoptosis and proliferation in a developing tumour is highly indicative of the severity and overall prognosis. In human cancers, there are many examples of changes in the bcl-2 to bax ratio or of alterations in other apoptosis-suppressing or promoting bcl-2 family members.[7,13] Furthermore, a shift in the bcl-2 to bax ratio in favour of bcl-2 is frequently associated with decreased apoptosis, increased histological abnormality and poorer prognosis, e.g. in oral, esophageal, squamous cell carcinoma of the tongue, ameloblastomas, breast cancer and adenocarcinoma of the uterine cervix.[39-46] Alpha-fetoprotein (AFP), producing gastric cancers, associated with a much poorer prognosis than AFP negative tumours, have higher proliferative activity, weaker apoptosis and better neovascularization.[47] An inverse relationship has also been reported between bcl-2 and lung cancer metastasis.[48]

Chemotherapeutic strategies effective against breast cancer are reported to derive their efficacy through changes in the expression of apoptotic regulatory genes, e.g. increased bax and decreased bcl-2 are reported in breast cancer cells.[49,50] In addition, bcl-2 antisense treatment of non-small cell lung cancer cells decreased bcl-2, reduced proliferation, decreased cell viability and increased apoptosis.[51] Changes in the bcl-2 to bax ratio or ratios of other pro- to anti-apoptotic proteins is known to induce tumour resistance to many cell death stimuli.[7] These include chemotherapeutic strategies and even tumour suppressor genes such as *p53* which promote apoptosis and oncogenes which promote proliferation.[7,11]

In tumours, apoptosis inducing stimuli can induce the tumour suppressor protein p53 which in turn can induce bax and cell death. However, while *p53* and its protein product are associated with reduced tumour growth, the *p53* gene becomes inactivated by gene mutations and other mechanisms in more than half of human cancers, thus favouring continued proliferation e.g. in oral and lung cancer.[39,52] Placental site trophoblastic tumours have a higher proliferative index and a wider distribution of cyclins and cdks than intermediate trophoblast. In this study p53 was localised only to the tumour cells.[53]

Death Receptors and Tumour Apoptosis

Non-lymphoid tumours usually express both Fas and Fas ligand and this system has been proposed as one mechanism by which tumours may evade the immune system. There is now substantial evidence that tumour Fas ligand can induce apoptosis in Fas-receptor positive leukocytes including tumour infiltrating lymphocytes.[54] However, unlike normal cells, tumours are relatively resistant to Fas-mediated apoptosis. Consequently, the tumour is protected from its own Fas ligand and from the Fas ligand positive lymphocytes. The tumour thus has a defensive strategy (Fas resistance) and an offensive strategy against immune cells termed the Fas counterattack.[55]

One mechanism by which Fas receptor signalling is blocked is through the antiapoptotic proteins that block caspase activation (see above). Indeed, in contrast to the placenta (see above) Fas resistance in some types of tumour has been attributed to elevated levels of Flip.[31] Alternative mechanisms of Fas resistance reported in specific tumours are:

1 downregulation of Fas expression

2 mutations in the genes that encode the receptors and the downstream effectors, e.g. caspase 8

3 the expression of an antagonistic soluble Fas lacking a transmembrane domain.[7,55]

Members of the bcl-2 family regulate Fas mediated apoptosis in some cell types; indeed Fas resistance has been associated with increased bcl-2 and decreased bax and bak. However, in other cells Fas mediated apoptosis is not blocked by bcl-2. Impaired Fas receptor signalling has also been associated with the mutant form of p53.[56] Further, the proto-oncogene *c-myc*, associated with driving proliferation in tumour cells, can induce Fas mediated apoptosis in cells deprived of survival factors.[57] It follows therefore that tumour Fas resistance will facilitate the proliferative role of c-myc while limiting apoptosis should the local cytokine environment change.

The association of elevated ceramide and tumour apoptosis has been studied largely through the use of tumour cell lines. Indeed, studies of the MCF7 human breast carcinoma cells have shown that blocking ceramide glycosylation increases the sensitivity of the cells to apoptosis inducing drugs.[58] Recent studies have shown that the induction of apoptosis in a neuroblastoma cell line in response to a phosphatase inhibitor is associated with elevated ceramide levels.[59] The authors suggest that in conjunction with phosphatase inhibition, ceramide facilitates caspase activation. Although there are many other examples in the literature of an association between increased cellular ceramide and apoptosis, the mechanism by which apoptosis is triggered in this way and the interactions with the caspase pathway require further clarification.[10,60]

The Role of Cytokines in Placental Growth

The balance between apoptosis, proliferation and differentiation is influenced by cytokines. Indeed, the profile of cytokines at the healthy maternal–fetal interface are compatible with those produced by Th2 cells whereas elevated levels of inflammatory cytokines (Th1 type) are detrimental to pregnancy.[4,61] Pregnancy itself is often described as a Th2 phenomenon where maternal immunity is biased against cell mediated Th1 type immunity and Th2 type immunity (antibody mediated) predominates.[62,63] It follows therefore that changes in levels of placental cytokines will affect the regulation of placental apoptosis and/or proliferation. However, the effects of such changes are dependent on the extent of the changes and the stage of gestation at which it occurs.

Studies of the effects of epidermal growth factor (EGF) on placental growth in vitro have shown that at 4 to 5 weeks both EGF and its receptor are present in the cytotrophoblast, and that EGF stimulated cytotrophoblast proliferation but did not affect syncytiotrophoblast human chorionic gonadotrophin (hCG) and human placental lactogen (hPL) secretion. However, at 6 to 12 weeks EGF and its receptor were present in syncytiotrophoblast and EGF stimulated hCG and hPL secretion without affecting proliferation.[17] Further, thyroid hormone (T3) enhanced secretion of EGF in cultured placental explants. These findings indicate that EGF is important in the regulation of placental growth and function in synergy with thyroid hormone.

Increased levels of the pro-inflammatory cytokine TNFα in reproductive tissues is detrimental to pregnancy and elevated TNFα levels characterise IUGR, a condition also associated with increased placental apoptosis.[64,65] Both TNFα and its receptors are expressed in villous trophoblast and thus lower levels of this cytokine appear to be beneficial.[27,29,64] Studies by Guilbert and colleagues have shown that TNFα induces apoptosis in primary cultures of cytotrophoblasts and syncytiotrophoblasts and this effect is enhanced by IFNγ.[30,66] Furthermore, TNFα acts through the p55 receptor in the induction of apoptosis and TNFα/IFNγ induced trophoblast apoptosis can be inhibited by EGF.[30,66] The mechanisms by which TNFα, IFNγ and EGF regulate trophoblast apoptosis are unknown. However, TNFα/IFNγ do not induce the production of reactive oxygen and nitrogen intermediates[67] and the cytokines (TNFα, IFNγ, EGF) do not modulate cellular expression levels of bcl-2 in cultures of cytotrophoblasts.[68] However, cells which express high bcl-2 levels are more resistant to TNFα induced apoptosis than cells with low bcl-2 levels.[68] Interestingly, placentas from first trimester failing pregnancies from a subset of women with a history of recurrent miscarriage have lower levels of placental TNFα than placentas from sporadically failing pregnancies. In contrast, placental bcl-2 levels were reduced in all failing first trimester pregnancies regardless of the clinical history.[64,69] These data support the conclusion of Guilbert and colleagues that placental bcl-2 and TNFα are independently regulated.[4,64,68,69] It is possible however that cytokines may induce post-translational modification of bcl-2.

The Role of Cytokines in Tumour Growth

The immune privileged environment in which tumours grow exhibits a number of similarities to the Th2-like environment of the placenta. The immunosuppressive Th2 cytokine IL-10 is produced by the placenta and by human gliomas.[70,71]. Its anti-inflammatory role is important for the development of both, indeed in the latter it also stimulates cell proliferation and motility.[71,72] Transforming growth factor beta (TGFß) is also important for successful pregnancy and induces a switch from Th1 to Th2 in tumour bearing mice partially through an IL-10 dependent mechanism.[73,74] In breast cancer, TGFß is important for immune surveillance and appears to protect against DNA damage.[75,76] Tumour infiltrating lymphocytes isolated from human gliomas express high levels of IL-4 and GM-CSF but no IFNγ, IL-2 or TNFß.[77] In addition, an imbalance in circulating Th1 and Th2 subsets in favour of Th2 has been reported in patients with colorectal cancer.[78,79]

A bias towards Th2 is therefore beneficial for both tumour and placental development. Since the pro-inflammatory cytokines can induce apoptosis of tumour cells, it is clearly advantageous to the tumour not to elicit such an inflammatory response. Such is the effectiveness of pro-inflammatory cytokines in combating cancers, TNFα and IFNγ are used in combination with chemotherapy to treat cancers and this has been shown to be particularly effective if administered through isolated limb perfusion.[80] TNFα and IFNγ have been shown to upregulate Fas antigen in a colorectal cell line (COLO 201) and to induce apoptosis in a dose dependent manner.[81] Similar results have been reported for myeloid leukemia cell lines and TNFα in combination with IFNγ are reported to induce apoptosis in murine colon carcinoma cells through the TNFR1 receptor.[82,83] In total, the bias towards a Th2-like environment characterising the 'immune privileged' environment of tumours will enhance tumour survival by limiting apoptosis induced by pro-inflammatory cytokines.

Conclusion

The developing placenta and tumour are able to grow and develop effectively while evading maternal or host immune rejection reactions. The mechanisms by which the placenta and tumour survive are closely related to those which facilitate growth and development. Consequently, some of the strategies are common to both (Table 18.1). These include a block on Fas or Fas ligand mediated apoptosis, enabling Fas ligand to induce apoptosis in potentially threatening immune cells (Fas counterattack). Different tumours, however, appear to exhibit different mechanisms in blocking this apoptotic trigger. Ceramide associated apoptosis is also a feature of both placental and tumour apoptosis. Pro-inflammatory cytokines are generally detrimental to the developing placenta and tumour, indeed apoptosis can be induced in both via the TNFαR1 receptor. Consequently both develop in an immune privileged environment where the profile of local cytokines is largely compatible with those produced by Th2 immune cells. The proliferative activity of more than half of cancers is facilitated by the mutation of the p53 tumour suppressor gene. In contrast only the wild type gene appears to be present in the normal placenta indicative of a role in limiting trophoblast invasion and/or proliferation. Finally the bcl-2:bax ratio plays a critical role in controlling the development of both the placenta and tumour. In the situation of pregnancy, however, it is likely that all the above mechanisms operate to a greater or lesser extent throughout gestation. Gestation dependent changes in endocrine and immune status will clearly have direct and indirect effects on these processes. In contrast, the local environment of cancerous tumours is not subject to the same degree of controlled environmental change. A greater understanding of the mechanisms controlling placental and tumour growth may enable further clinical intervention so that growth is altered in a way that benefits the mother and/or cancer patient.

Table 18.1 Apoptosis in the placenta and tumour: similarities and differences

Features	Placenta	Tumour
Fas R signalling	Blocked, mechanism unknown (possible Fas counterattack)	Blocked, several mechanisms (Fas counterattack)
TNFαR1 (p55) signalling	TNFα induces apoptosis in villous cytotrophoblasts (IFNγ enhances effect)	TNFα induces apoptosis in some tumours. (IFNγ enhances effects in some cases)
Ceramide mediated apoptosis	Increased ceramide associated with apoptosis in term placenta TNFα increases and EGF decreases ceramide levels*	Increased ceramide associated with apoptosis in tumour cell lines
Bax:bcl-2 ratio	Cytotrophoblast: bcl-2-ve, bax+ve Syncytiotrophoblast: bcl-2+ve, bax+ve Gestational increase in syncytium bcl-2 Apoptosis associated with syncytium formation	Ratio in favour of bcl2 (apoptosis↓, proliferation↑)
p53	Wild type expressed in cytotrophoblasts Limits proliferative activity	Mutant form in >50% of tumours Allows proliferative activity
Proliferation	Cytotrophoblasts: 1st trim ↑, 3rd trim ↓	Usually high
Local cytokine environment	Bias towards Th2 type cytokines	Immune privilege conferred by Th2 type cytokines

* L. Guilbert, personal communication.

References

1. Pestell RG, Albanese C, Reutens AT, Segall JE, Lee RJ, Arnold A. The cyclins and cyclin-dependent kinase inhibitors in hormonal regulation of proliferation and differentiation. Endocr Rev 1999; 20:501–34
2. Gartel AL, Serfas MS, Tyner AL. P21 – negative regulator of the cell cycle. Proc Soc Exp Biol Med 1996; 213:138–49
3. Savill J. Apoptosis in disease. Eur J Clin Invest 1994; 24:715–23
4. Lea RG, Riley SC, Antipatis C et al. Cytokines and the regulation of apoptosis in reproductive tissues: a review. Am J Reprod Immunol 1999; 42:100–109
5. Arrends MJ, Morris RG, Wyllie A. Apoptosis: the role of the endonuclease. Am J Pathol 1990; 136: 593–608
6. Alnemri ES. Mammalian cell death proteases: a family of highly conserved aspartate specific cysteine proteases. J Cell Biochem 1997; 64:33–42
7. Reed JC. Dysregulation of apoptosis in cancer. J Clin Oncol 1999; 17:2941–53
8. Wallach D, Boldin M, Varfolomeev E, Beyaert R, Vandenabeele P, Fiers W. Cell death induction by receptors of the TNF family: towards a molecular understanding. FEBS Lett 1997; 410:96–106
9. Perry DK, Hannun YA. The role of ceramide in cell signaling. Biochim Biophys Acta 1998; 1436:233–43

10. Hofmann K, Dixit VM. Ceramide in apoptosis – does it really matter? Trends Biochem Sci 1998; 23:374–7
11. Reed JC. Bcl-2 and the regulation of programmed cell death. J Cell Biol 1994; 124:1–6
12. Oltavi ZN, Korsmeyer SJ. Checkpoints of dueling dimers foil death wishes Cell 1994;79:189–92
13. Reed JC. Double identity for proteins of the bcl-2 family. Nature 1997; 387: 773–6
14. Yang J, Liu X, Bhalla K et al. Prevention of apoptosis by bcl-2: release of cytochrome c from mitochondria blocked. Science 1997; 275:1129–32
15. Reed JC. Cytochrome c: can't live with it – can't live without it. Cell 1997; 91:559–62
16. Chan CC, Lao TT, Cheung AN. Apoptotic and proliferative activities in first trimester placentae. Placenta 1999; 20:223–7
17. Mochizuki M, Maruo T, Matsuo H, Samoto T, Ishihara N. Biology of human trophoblast. Int J Gynaecol Obstet 1998; 60:Suppl. 1:S21–8
18. Huppertz B, Frank HG, Kingdom JC, Reister F, Kaufmann P. Villous cytotrophoblast regulation of the syncytial apoptotic cascade in the human placenta. Histochem Cell Biol 1998; 110:495–508
19. Lea RG, Riley SC, Tulppala M, Critchley HOD. Placental apoptosis and pregnancy failure. J Reprod Fert, Abstract Series 1997; 20:Abstr. 3:4
20. Smith SC, Baker PN, Symonds EM. Placental apoptosis in normal human pregnancy. Am J Obstet Gynaecol 1997; 177:57–65
21. Kokawa K, Shikone T, Nakano R. Apoptosis in human chorionic villi and decidua during normal embryonic development and spontaneous abortion in the first trimester. Placenta 1998; 19:21–6
22. Kokawa K, Shikone T, Nakano R. Apoptosis in human chorionic villi and decidua in normal and ectopic pregnancy. Mol Human Reprod 1998; 4:87–91
23. Fulop V, Mok SC, Genest DR, Szigetvari I, Cseh I, Berkowitz RS. C-myc, c-erbB-2, c-fms and bcl-2 oncoproteins. Expression in normal placenta, partial and complete mole, and choriocarcinoma. J Reprod Med 1998; 43:101–10
24. Aboagye-Mathiesen G, Zdravkovic M, Toth FD, Graham CH, Lala PK, Ebbesen P. Altered expression of the tumor suppressor/oncoprotein p53 in SV40 Tag-transformed human placental trophoblast and malignant trophoblast cell lines. Early Pregnancy 1996; 2:102–12
25. Haidacher S, Blaschitz A, Desoye G, Dohr G. Immunohistochemical evidence of p53 protein in human placenta and choriocarcinoma cell lines. Hum Reprod 1995; 10:983–8
26. Payne SG, Smith SC, Davidge ST, Baker PN, Guilbert LJ. Death receptor Fas/Apo-1/CD95 expressed by human placental cytotrophoblasts does not mediate apoptosis. Biol Reprod 1999; 60:1144–50
27. Yui J, Hemmings D, Garcia-Lloret M, Guilbert LJ. Expression of the human p55 and p75 tumor necrosis factor receptors in primary villous trophoblasts and their role in cytotoxic signal transduction. Biol Reprod 1996; 55:400–409
28. Phillips TA, Ni J, Pan G et al. TRAIL (Apo-26; and TRAIL receptors in human placentas: implications for immune privilege. J Immunol 1999; 162:6053–9
29. Yelavarthi KK, Hunt JS. Analysis of p60 and p80 tumor necrosis factor-alpha receptor messenger RNA and protein in human placentas. Am J Pathol 1993; 143:1131–41
30. Yui J, Garcia-Lloret M, Wegmann T, Guilbert L. Cytotoxicity of tumour necrosis factor-alpha and gamma-interferon against primary human placental trophoblasts. Placenta 1994; 15:819–35
31. Irmler M, Thome M, Hahne M et al. Inhibition of death receptor signals by cellular Flip. Nature 1997; 388:190–95
32. Kauma SW, Huff TF, Hayes N, Nilkaeo A. Placental Fas ligand expression is a mechanism for maternal immune tolerance to the fetus. J Clin Endocrinol Metab 1999; 84(6):2188–94
33. Hammer A, Dohr G. Apoptotic nuclei within the uterine decidua of first trimester pregnancy arise from CD45 positive leukocytes. Am J Reprod Immunol 1999; 42:88–94
34. Runic R, Lockwood CJ, Ma Y, Dipasquale B, Guller S. Expression of Fas ligand by human cytotrophoblasts: implications in placentation and fetal survival. J Clin Endocrinol Metab 1996; 81:3119–22
35. Chaouat G, Cayol V, Mairovitz V, Dubanchet S. Localization of the Th2 cytokines IL-3, IL-4, IL-10 at the fetomaternal interface during human and murine pregnancy and lack of requirement for Fas/Fas ligand interaction for a successful allogeneic pregnancy. Am J Reprod Immunol 1999; 42:1–13
36. Abreu-Martin MT, Vidrich A, Lynch DH, Targan SR. Divergent induction of apoptosis and IL-8 secretion in HT-29 cells in response to TNF-alpha and ligation of Fas antigen. J Immunol 1995; 155:4147–54
37. Payne SG, Brindley DN, Guilbert LJ. Epidermal growth factor inhibits ceramide-induced apoptosis and lowers ceramide levels in primary placental trophoblasts. J Cell Physiol 1999; 180:263–70
38. Lee RJ, Wang S, Low PS. Measurement of endosome pH following folate receptor-mediated endocytosis. Biochim Biophys Acta 1996; 1312:237–42

39. Ito T, Fujieda S, Tsuzuki H et al. Decreased expression of bax is correlated with poor prognosis in oral and oropharyngeal carcinoma. Cancer Lett 1999; 140:81-91
40. Ravi D, Ramadas K, Mathew BS, Nalinakumari KR, Nair MK, Pillai MR. De novo programmed cell death in oral cancer. Histopathology 1999; 34:241-9
41. Loro LL, Vintermyr OK, Liavaag PG, Jonsson R, Johannessen AC. Oral squamous cell carcinoma is associated with decreased bcl-2/bax expression ratio and increased apoptosis. Hum Pathol 1999; 30:1097-1105
42. Soslow RA, Remotti H, Baergen RN, Altorki NK. Suppression of apoptosis does not foster neoplastic growth in Barrett's esophagus. Mod Pathol 1999; 12:239-50
43. Xie X, Clausen OP, De Angelis P, Boysen M. The prognostic value of spontaneous apoptosis, bax, bcl-2, and p53 in oral squamous cell carcinoma of the tongue. Cancer 1999; 86:913-20
44. Kumamoto H, Ooya K. Immunohistochemical analysis of bcl-2 family proteins in benign and malignant ameloblastomas. J Oral Pathol Med 1999; 28:343-9
45. Schorr K, Li M, Krajewski S, Reed JC, Furth PA. Bcl-2 gene family and related proteins in mammary gland involution and breast cancer. J Mammary Gland Biol Neoplasia; 1999; 4:153-64
46. Kokawa K, Shikone T, Otani T, Nakano R. Apoptosis and the expression of bax and bcl-2 in squamous cell carcinoma and adenocarcinoma of the uterine cervix. Cancer 1999; 85:1799-809
47. Koide N, Nishio A, Igarashi J, Kajikawa S, Adachi W, Amano J. Alpha-fetoprotein-producing gastric cancer: histochemical analysis of cell proliferation, apoptosis, and angiogenesis. Am J Gastroenterol 1999; 94:1658-63
48. Volm M, Koomagi R. The implications of proliferation and apoptosis for lung cancer metastasis. Oncol Rep 1999; 6:373-6
49. Gibson LF, Fortney J, Magro G, Ericson SG, Lynch JP, Landreth KS. Regulation of bax and bcl-2 expression in breast cancer cells by chemotherapy. Breast Cancer Res Treat 1999; 55:107-17
50. Suzuki K, Kazui T, Yoshida M et al. Drug-induced apoptosis and p53, bcl-2 and bax expression in breast cancer tissues in vivo and in fibroblast cells in vitro. Jpn J Clin Oncol 1999; 29:323-31
51. Chen Y, Sato M, Fujimura S et al.Expression of bcl-2, bax, and p53 proteins in carcinogenesis of squamous cell lung cancer. Anticancer Res 1999; 19:1351-6
52. Koty PP, Zhang H, Levitt ML. Antisense bcl-2 treatment increases programmed cell death in non-small cell lung cancer cell lines. Lung Cancer 1999; 23:115-27
53. Ichikawa N, Zhai YL, Shiozawa T et al. Immunohistochemical analysis of cell cycle regulatory gene products in normal trophoblast and placental site trophoblastic tumor. Int J Gynecol Pathol 1998; 17:235-40
54. Bennett MW, O'Connell J, O'Sullivan GC et al.1998; The Fas counterattack in vivo: apoptotic depletion of tumor-infiltrating lymphocytes associated with Fas ligand expression by human esophageal carcinoma. J Immunol 160:5669-75
55. O'Connell J, Bennett MW, O'Sullivan GC, Collins JK, Shanahan F. The Fas counterattack: cancer as a site of immune privilege. Immunol Today 1999; 20:46-52
56. O'Connell J, Bennett MW, O'Sullivan GC, Collins JK, Shanahan F. The Fas counterattack: a molecular mechanism of tumor immune privilege. Mol Med 3: 1997; 294-300
57. Shi Y, Guilbert JM, Cotter TG, Bissonnette RP, Green DR. Role for c-myc in activation-induced apoptotic cell death in T cell hybridomas. Science 1992; 257:212-15
58. Lucci A, Han TY, Liu YY, Giuliano AE, Cabot MC. Modification of ceramide metabolism increases cancer cell sensitivity to cytotoxics. Int J Oncol 1999; 15:541-6
59. Spinedi A, Di Bartolomeo S, Di Sano F, Rodolfo C, Ambrosino A, Piacentini M. Ceramide accumulation precedes caspase-dependent apoptosis in CHP-100 neuroepithelioma cells exposed to the protein phosphatase inhibitor okadaic acid. Cell Death Differ 1999; 6:618-23
60. Hannun YA, Linardic CM. Sphingolipid breakdown products: anti-proliferative and tumor-suppressor lipids. Biochim Biophys Acta 1993; 1154:223-36
61. Lea RG, Calder A. The immunology of pregnancy. Curr Op Infect Dis 1997; 10:171-6
62. Wegmann TG, Lin H, Guilbert L, Mossman TR. Biderectional cytokine interactions in the maternal-fetal relationship: is successful pregnancy a Th2 phenomenon? Immunol Today 1993; 14:353-6
63. Piccinni MP, Beloni L, Livi C, Maggi E, Scarselli G, Romagnani S. Defective production of both leukemia inhibitory factor and type 2 T-helper cytokines by decidual T cells in unexplained recurrent abortions. Nat Med 1998; 4:1020-24
64. Lea RG, Tulppala M, Critchley HOD. Deficient syncytiotrophoblast TNF-α characterises failing first trimester pregnancies in a subgroup of recurrent miscarriage patients. Human Reprod 1997; 12:1313-20
65. Smith SC, Baker PN, Symonds EM. Increased placental apoptosis in intrauterine growth retardation. Am J Obstet Gynaecol 1997; 177:1395-401

66. Garcia-Lloret MI, Yui J, Winkler-Lowen B, Guilbert LJ. Epidermal growth factor inhibits cytokine-induced apoptosis of primary human trophoblasts. J Cell Physiol 1996; 167:324–32
67. Smith SC, Guilbert LJ, Yui J, Baker PN, Davidge ST. The role of reactive nitrogen/oxygen intermediates in cytokine-induced trophoblast apoptosis. Placenta 1999; 20:309–15
68. Ho S, Winkler-Lowen B, Morrish DW, Dakour J, Li H, Guilbert L. The role of bcl-2 expression in EGF inhibition of TNF-a/IFN-g-induced villous trophoblast apoptosis. Placenta 1999; 20:423–30
69. Lea RG, Al-Sharekh N, Tulppala M, Critchley HOD. The immunolocalisation of bcl-2 at the maternal–fetal interface in healthy and failing pregnancies. Human Reprod 1997; 12:153–8
70. Bennett WA, Lagoo-Deenadayalan S, Whitworth NS et al. First-trimester human chorionic villi express both immunoregulatory and inflammatory cytokines: a role for interleukin-10 in regulating the cytokine network of pregnancy. Am J Reprod Immunol 1999; 41:70–78
71. Huettner C, Czub S, Kerkau S, Roggendorf W, Tonn JC. Interleukin 10 is expressed in human gliomas in vivo and increases glioma cell proliferation and motility in vitro. Anticancer Res 1997; 17:3217–24
72. Chaouat G, Assal Meliani A, Martal J et al. IL-10 prevents naturally occurring fetal loss in the CBA x DBA/2 mating combination, and local defect in IL-10 production in this abortion-prone combination is corrected by in vivo injection of IFN-tau. Immunol 1995; 154:4261–68
73. Lea RG, Underwood J, Flanders KC et al. A subset of patients with recurrent spontaneous abortion is deficient in transforming growth factor beta-2-producing "suppressor cells" in uterine tissue near the placental attachment site. Am J Reprod Immunol 1995; 34:52–64
74. Maeda H, Shiraishi A. TGF-beta contributes to the shift toward Th2-type responses through direct and IL-10-mediated pathways in tumor-bearing mice. Immunol 1996; 156:73–8
75. Arteaga CL, Hurd SD, Winnier AR, Johnson MD, Fendly BM, Forbes JT. Anti-transforming growth factor (TGF)-beta antibodies inhibit breast cancer cell tumorigenicity and increase mouse spleen natural killer cell activity. Implications for a possible role of tumor cell/host TGF-beta interactions in human breast cancer progression. J Clin Invest 1993; 92:2569–76
76. Ohmori T, Yang JL, Price JO, Arteaga CL. Blockade of tumor cell transforming growth factor-betas enhances cell cycle progression and sensitizes human breast carcinoma cells to cytotoxic chemotherapy. Exp Cell Res 1998; 245:350–59
77. Roussel E, Gingras MC, Grimm EA, Bruner JM, Moser RP. Predominance of a type 2 intratumoural immune response in fresh tumour-infiltrating lymphocytes from human gliomas. Clin Exp Immunol 1996; 105:344–52
78. Pellegrini P, Berghella AM, Del Beato T, Cicia S, Adorno D, Casciani CU. Disregulation in TH1 and TH2 subsets of CD4-positive T cells in peripheral blood of colorectal cancer patients and involvement in cancer establishment and progression. Cancer Immunol Immunother 1996; 42:1–8
79. Mullen CA. Review: analogies between trophoblastic and malignant cells. Am J Reprod Immunol 1998; 39:41–9
80. Lejeune FJ, Ruegg C, Lienard D. Clinical applications of TNF-alpha in cancer. Curr Opin Immunol 1998; 10:573–80
81. Koshiji M, Adachi Y, Sogo S et al. Apoptosis of colorectal adenocarcinoma (COLO 201) by tumour necrosis factor-alpha (TNF-alpha) and/or interferon-gamma (IFN-gamma), resulting from downmodulation of Bcl-2 expression. Clin Exp Immunol 1998; 111:211–8
82. Munker R, Andreeff M. Induction of death (CD95/FAS), activation and adhesion (CD54) molecules on blast cells of acute myelogenous leukemias by TNF-alpha and IFN-gamma. Cytokines Mol Ther 1996; 2:147–59
83. Sveinbjornsson B, Rushfeldt C, Olsen R, Smedsrod B, Seljelid R. Cytotoxic effect of cytokines on murine colon carcinoma cells involves TNF-mediated apoptosis. Biochem Biophys Res Commun 1997; 233:270–75

19 Controlled vs Uncontrolled Angiogenesis: Color Doppler Studies

Asim Kurjak, Sanja Kupesic and Tina Zodan

At first sight, cancer and pregnancy cannot be more opposite. The result of pregnancy is a new life and the result of cancer is very often death. However, when observed closely, mechanisms that act in the beginning of life are just the same as those that lead to cancer. Hyperplasia, increased metabolic turnover and, above all, angiogenesis, are the features of both conditions. Pregnancy and cancer are both highly angiogenic conditions. It is incredible how the same molecules, angiogenic substances and growth factors can produce so different result on the vasculature.

All organs of the human body have a physiological duty to form certain compounds and molecules while disintegrating others, with the aim of maintaining the frail molecular equilibrium. In order to perform their task, all the organs and body parts must be connected by a single vascular network. As with any other live tissue, vascular endothelium has the ability to regenerate and to spread through other tissues in order to perfuse them.

The formation of new blood vessels is called angiogenesis and it results in neovascularization. It has been discovered that new blood vessels arise from post-capillary venules in response to angiogenic stimulus. After proteolysis of the basement membrane and interstitial matrix degradation, endothelial cells migrate towards the angiogenic stimulus. These cells form capillary buds, which are later canalized to form a tubule. As the endothelial cells of the tubule proliferate, they join the adjacent capillary bud and form a loop. At this point, blood begins to flow and a new vessel is formed.

Where pregnancy and events leading to pregnancy are concerned, angiogenesis happens in folliculogenesis, corpus luteum formation, during the endometrial cycle and early placentation. On the other hand, chronic inflammation, certain immune reactions and many malignant diseases are also characterized by angiogenesis. However, solid tumor angiogenesis differs from physiological angiogenesis. In physiological processes, such as corpus luteum development or ovulation, angiogenesis subsides, or terminates, once the process is completed. Contrariwise, tumor angiogenesis is never self-limited. Once tumor-induced angiogenesis is initiated, it continues indefinitely until tumor growth is restrained and neovascularization interrupted[1-4] (see Table 19.1). Whilst in healthy adult tissues endothelial cells have a

Table 19.1. Normal and abnormal angiogenesis.

Angiogenic factors	
Angiogenesis in physiological and pathophysiological condition	
Ovulation	Cancer and metastasis
Corpus luteum formation	
Implantation	
Placentation	
Embryogenesis	
Ectopic pregnancy	
Wound healing	
Arthritis	
Chronic inflammation	

low mitotic rate and form a quiescent population, tumor induced endothelium undergoes rapid mitosis and proliferation.

Being formed in this rapid and hectic way, tumor vessels must necessarily differ from those formed in self-limiting events. It is now known that tumor vessels have their special characteristics:

1 a single branch varies in caliber, being formed of narrow and dilated segments
2 elongation and coiling
3 non-hierarchical vascular network, vascular rings and sinusoids
4 no normal precapillary architecture with dichotomous branching, and no decrease in size or diameter of the higher-order branches
5 incomplete vascular wall: various gaps in the endothelium, discontinuity of basal membrane, and scarce muscular layer except in pre-existing vessels encased by the tumor. The amount of structural abnormalities depends on how rapidly a tumor grows.

Well-differentiated, slow-growing tumors are expected to have less disturbed vessel architecture because angiogenesis can keep pace with the slow tumor growth. Anaplastic, poorly differentiated tumors grow so rapidly that the angiogenic process only manages to create chaotic, vessel-like spaces lacking mature elements.

After the nature of tumoral vessels was established, the question spontaneously arose: "Is there a diagnostic tool that could give us the insight into vessel quality?" The answer came with the improvement of ultrasound machines and the invention of Doppler machines, later developed into color Doppler apparatus. This technique makes it possible to locate the vessels and to study their characteristics. The working principles of this tool are based on shift of frequency discovered by Doppler. The emitted sound wave reflects from the erythrocyte membrane and returns to the transducer with changed frequency. Color indicates the direction of blood flow: towards or away from the transducer. The software in the Doppler equipment can calculate velocity, resistance index, pulsatility index and other parameters. As mentioned above, if angiogenesis is physiological or even tumoral, but is progressing slowly, the newly formed vessels will have smooth muscle layer within their walls. This means that these vessels are able to contract, either under the influence of vegetative regulatory mechanisms, or when stimulated by vasoactive molecules. When the vessel wall contracts, the diameter of the vessel decreases and the resistance to blood flow increases. In rapidly growing tumors, newly formed vessels have disturbed architecture and hardly any muscular cells. The vessel wall cannot contract, the lumen remains wide open and the resistance to blood flow is low. In a vessel with a regular wall, blood flow rises in systole when blood is forced through by heart contraction. The blood pushes aside the vessel walls, but as the pressure drops in time of diastole, the smooth muscle cells contract and reduce the lumen to its previous diameter. In contrast, vessels formed in the process of rapid tumor neovascularization remain wide open throughout the heart cycle. The Resistance Index (RI) and Pulsatility Index (PI) describe the vessel dynamics. In general, malignant, fast growing tumors display low RI and PI, while benign, slow growing masses display moderate to high RI and PI.

However, pregnancy-related conditions with their high metabolic turnover, growth-rate and angiogenesis share some Doppler characteristics of malignant growths and we review them here in succession.

Folliculogenesis

The fundamental unit of the ovary is the follicle, which consists of the female germ cell (oocyte) surrounded by a series of specialized cell layers, the granulosa and theca cells. Every month during the woman's reproductive life, one oocyte is released from the single mature follicle that has completed development. A number of biochemical, morphological and vascular changes occur within the cell layers during this process.

The pattern of angiogenesis around the developing follicle and corpus luteum can be visualized using an injection–corrosion technique that produces three-dimensional vascular casts of the ovary, which are then observed with scanning electron microscopy. The characteristic vascular pattern starts as a simple capillary network around the primary follicles (Fig. 19.1). With follicular development, a multilayered and complicated vascular system develops surrounding the follicles, the largest vascular network being that around the Graafian follicle (Fig. 19.2). Just before rupture, marked dilatation of the vessels occurs and the new blood vessels become "leaky" (Fig. 19.3). Angiogenesis in the follicle is limited to the theca, but following follicular rupture the thecal vessels invade the granulosa layer to give rise to the luteal vascular network.[5-8]

Although we know that angiogenesis occurs in the early follicular phase of the cycle, it is possible that at this time the density of blood vessels is too low to allow detection of blood flow in these areas. The dramatic rise in peak systolic velocity observed is consistent with the marked dilatation of new blood vessels just before follicular rupture noted in studies of corrosion casts of ovarian follicles.[5,6]

The ovary receives its arterial vascularization from two sources: the ovarian artery and the utero-ovarian branch of the uterine artery.[9] These arteries anastomose, forming an arch parallel to the ovarian hilus, and constitute the vascular genital arcade. The ovarian artery emerges from the abdominal aorta beneath the renal arteries. From there, it descends obliquely and, crossing the ureter and iliac vessels, enters into the infundibulopelvic ligament.

The ovary has an arterial supply known for its special pattern and obvious functional changes. From the ovarian hilus, arterial branches penetrate the stroma[10] and

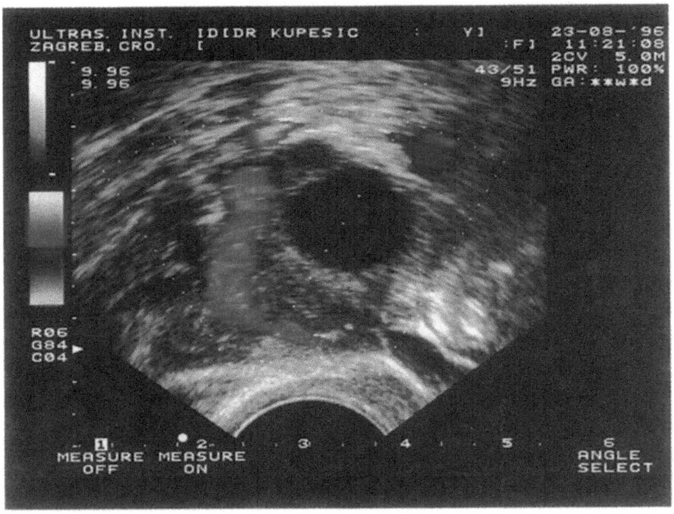

Figure 19.1. Transvaginal color Doppler scan of the follicle. Note perifollicular capillaries and ovarian and iliac vessels in close proximity to the ovary.

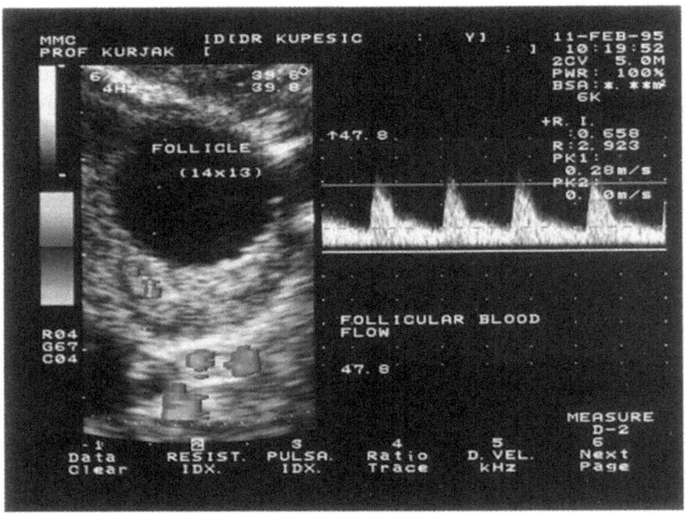

Figure 19.2. Transvaginal color Doppler scan of the growing follicle. Blood flow signals obtained from the periphery of the follicle demonstrate moderate-to-high resistance index (RI=0.66).

acquire a tortuous and helicoid pathway (they roll up around their own axis). For such a special pattern, they are named spiral or helical arteries. Getting further into the ovarian stroma, spiral arteries divide more and more and become progressively smaller in diameter. In the cortical zone the diameter becomes 40–60 micrometers and dividing at a right or sharp angle from the principal branch they successively form arterioles of the first capillary system.[11]

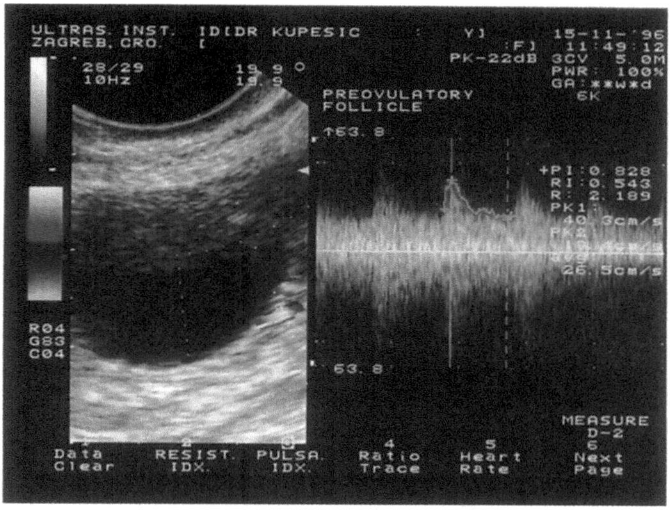

Figure 19.3. Transvaginal color Doppler scan of the preovulatory follicle. As a result of vasodilatation of perifollicular capillaries resistance index drops to the value of 0.54.

Table 19.2. Ovarian perfusion in physiological and pathophysiological conditions.

Ovarian blood flow in various conditions	
Ovarian blood flow	Resistance Index (RI±SD)
follicular phase	0.54±0.04
early luteal phase	0.43±0.04
late luteal phase	0.49±0.02
polycystic ovaries (PCOS)	0.54±0.08
luteal phase defect	0.55±0.10
endometriosis	0.45±0.12
pelvic inflammatory disease:	
acute inflammation	0.55±0.09
chronic inflammation	0.55±0.10
benign ovarian tumors	>0.40
malignant ovarian tumors	±0.40

The cyclic vascular changes can be studied by color Doppler (Table 19.2). With this modality, areas of vascularity on the follicular rim can be detected when the dominant follicle reaches 10 mm in diameter. In the early follicular phase the intraovarian blood flow shows resistance index of 0.54±0.04 (Figs 19.2 and 19.3).

A decline in RI begins 2 days before ovulation and reaches its nadir at ovulation (0.44±0.04).[12] The increase in the peak systolic blood velocity within the follicle in the presence of a relatively constant RI is a particularly interesting finding that might herald impending ovulation. Increased vascularity on the innermost rim of the follicle[13] may represent the dilatation of new vessels that have developed between the relatively vascular theca cell layer and the normally hypoxic granulosa cell layer of the follicle. Disruption of these vascular changes has profound effects on the oxygen concentration across the follicular epithelium.

Transvaginal sonography coupled with color flow and Doppler waveform analysis appears to be very reliable in confirming ovulation once it has occurred. A marked drop in blood flow impedance in the early luteal phase, added to changing ovarian morphology, accurately confirms the ovulation and allows the diagnosis of some ovulatory problems.[14,15]

Corpus Luteum Formation

The formation of a corpus luteum is an important event in the reproductive cycle and one of the crucial factors in early pregnancy support. Its clinical importance is strongly supported by many lines of investigation.[16] After ovulation, blood vessels of the theca layer invade the cavity of the ruptured follicle, starting the formation of the corpus luteum. Once formed, the corpus luteum consists of several cell types: K cells, large luteal cells and small luteal cells. Large luteal cells originate from granulosa cells, whereas small luteal cells originate from theca cells. Large luteal cells produce more progesterone than small luteal cells, but the latter seem to be more responsive to stimulation by LH or human chorionic gonadotropin. In addition, small luteal cells are thought to produce the so-called corpus luteum angiogenic factor, responsible for the neovascularization of the luteal tissue. Possibly, this function of small luteal cells is totally independent from their steroidogenic function. It has been shown that human luteal cells in culture produce prostaglandin I2, prostaglandin E2 and prostaglandin F2alfa. Prostaglandins, the production of which is under the control of lypoxygenase products of arachidonic acid such as 5-hydroxyeicosatetraenoic acid (5-HETE) and not under the control of hCG, have a direct impact on progesterone production.

The luteal phase of the cycle begins with ovulation and formation of the corpus luteum, and ends with the beginning of menstruation. The first event is a significant FSH and LH surge. After that the formation of the corpus luteum takes place. Small luteal cells produce more and more LH receptors and thus amplify the production of progesterone. This chain reaction continues until the mid-luteal phase, which is characterized by peak values of blood LH and progesterone, and the lowest resistance index (RI) in the corpus luteum blood vessels, as proven by transvaginal color and pulsed Doppler ultrasonography by Kupesic and colleagues.[16] Consequently, progesterone suppresses the secretion of gonadotropins, LH and progesterone levels decrease, and the RI in the vessels of the corpus luteum increases.

The qualitative postovulatory changes in intraovarian flow velocity waveforms are exciting: increased turbulent flow accompanying morphological changes in the intraovarian vascular network[17] (Fig. 19.4) and the appearance of numerous arteriovenous shunts during the luteal phase.[18] After ovulation, the RI shows a significant difference from the preovulatory values. Each woman with documented ovulation showed a RI of 0.43 ± 0.04 shortly after ovulation.[19] It remains at the low level for 4 to 5 days and then gradually climbs to a value of 0.50, still lower than that seen in the early follicular phase (Fig. 19.5). Luteal conversion can be detected in all normal ovulatory cycles[12] independently of corpus luteum identification. Converted blood flow signals are maintained throughout the luteal phase and are not observed on the non-dominant side, or in patients with anovulatory cycles or luteinized unruptured follicles.[20]

Changes in the intraovarian flow velocity therefore occur before ovulation, implying a complexity of these changes that may involve both angiogenesis and hormonal factors, while postovulatory vascular accommodation is potentially important in the luteal phase. Using transvaginal color Doppler, corpus luteum blood flow,

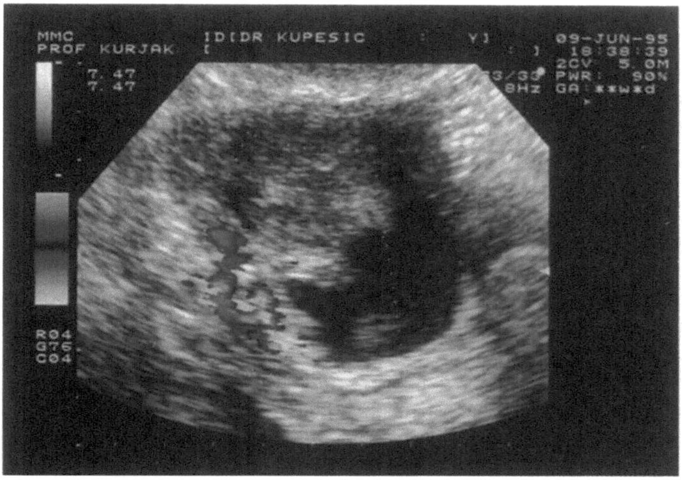

Figure 19.4. Transvaginal color Doppler scan of the corpus luteum. Note irregular contours of the ruptured follicle and peripheral distribution of the vessels.

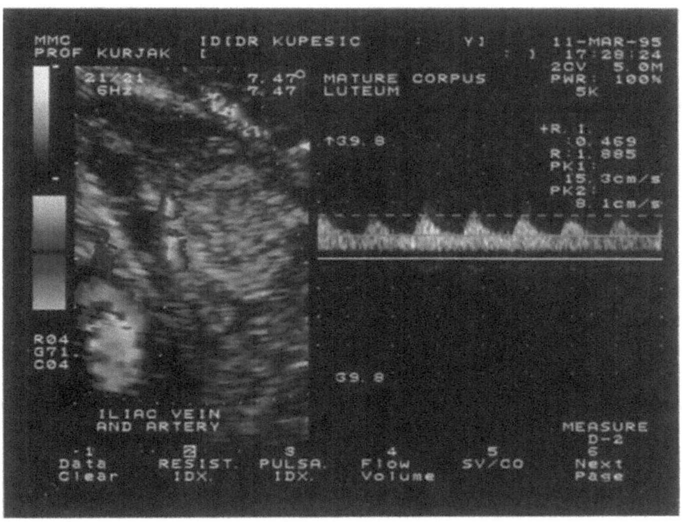

Figure 19.5. Transvaginal color Doppler scan obtained from mature corpus luteum. Low-to-moderate vascular resistance (RI=0.47) indicates normal corpus luteum function.

characterized by low impedance and high flow requirements, can easily be detected in normal early pregnancy, ectopic pregnancy and non-pregnant women.[21]

The importance of vasculature in the ovarian cycle is best noticed in the condition called luteal phase defect. The main features of this condition are lack of progesterone, a luteal phase of the cycle shorter than 11 days, and, when related to the endometrium, an endometrium out of phase by more than 2 days. Ultrasound and hormonal parameters have been used to evaluate this condition but without greater success.[22]

A new era in the study of luteal phase defect began with the advent of color Doppler. Kupesic and Kurjak[23] tried to evaluate the intraovarian resistance index in patients with normal corpus luteum function and those with luteal phase defect. A significant decline of the RI ($p<0.001$) occurred on the day of the LH peak (RI 0.44 ± 0.04). The lowest RI values were obtained during the mid-luteal phase (RI 0.42 ± 0.06), with a return to higher vascular resistance (0.50 ± 0.04) during the late luteal phase. In 15 patients, endometrial biopsy was performed, and normal endometrial dating was detected. In the LPD group, no difference ($p>0.05$) was obtained in terms of intraovarian RI during the follicular phase. However, the mean RI throughout the luteal phase (0.56 ± 0.04) was significantly higher ($p<0.001$) compared to that in the normal women. Mean progesterone levels were significantly lower in the LPD group.

Glock and Brumsted[24] correlated ovarian blood flow with values of progesterone throughout the cycle. Mean progesterone levels were significantly lower for LPD patients than for normal women throughout the luteal phase ($p<0.001$). The whole study showed a correlation between the resistance index of corpus luteum blood flow and plasma progesterone in the natural cycle. Contrary to previously presented data, Merce and colleagues[25] did not detect any significant correlation between the resistance index values and serum progesterone levels. Similarly, Tinkanen[26] found no difference between the blood flow in the corpus luteum in controls with a normal luteal phase, and infertility patients with an abnormal luteal phase.

In the light of controversial data it is not clear whether inadequate vascularization plays a role in luteal phase deficiency and whether luteal flow can be used as an accurate predictor for the evaluation of normal and pathological pregnancy.

Endometrial Changes

The menstruating portion of the endometrium in normal fertile women is characterized by disintegration and exfoliation of the two functional layers of the endometrium (the compacta and spongiosa).[27] Only the basal layer, wherefrom regeneration and resurfacing of the endometrium occur, remains intact. Hormonal deprivation as well as the alterations of the spiral arteriolar system are essential parts of the mechanism. The increased coiling of the spiral arterioles creates circulatory stasis, leading to further tissue ischemia. Vasoconstriction of the spiral arterioles and necrosis of their walls result in bleeding.[28]

The distal portion of the arteriolar system, as well as the capillary and venous beds are then shed in the functionalis. The local arteries, which are relatively insensitive to decreasing estrogen and progesterone levels, are unaffected and serve to maintain the integrity of the stratum basalis throughout the menstrual cycle. As the endometrium thickens 4–5-fold during the next menstrual cycle the remnants of the spiral arteries in the basalis must undergo substantial growth and give rise to a completely new capillary bed in order to maintain the integrity of the rapidly growing stroma. This process is initiated by the growth of new capillaries from the existing vasculature in the basalis.

Endometrial thickness less than 5 mm is usually associated with early follicular phase. The endometrial glands, lined by moderately low columnar cells, are narrow and tubular. Mitotic figures become numerous and blood vessels begin to run upward from the basal layer toward the surface area of the endometrium, where a capillary network develops. As ovulation approaches the glands become more numerous and expected endometrial thickness is about 10 mm. Triple-line endometrium is typical for follicular phase. During the secretory phase there is a significant increase of glycogen, acid phosphatase and lipids in the endometrium. It becomes hyperechoic, homogenous with a loss of the triple-line morphology and surrounding anechoic halo.

By using transvaginal color and pulsed Doppler sonography (TVCD) it becomes possible to study the alterations of endometrial perfusion in physiological and patophysiological conditions. Increased endometrial vascularity during the menstrual cycle depends on the changes of the uterine, arcuate and radial artery blood flow (Fig. 19.6). Transvaginal color Doppler enables evaluation of the blood flow changes in spiral arteries during the normal ovulatory cycle[29] (Fig. 19.7). The day before ovulation, spiral artery blood flow velocity starts increasing with a resistance index of 0.54 ± 0.03. It reaches its nadir of 0.49 ± 0.05 between days 16 and 18 (Fig. 19.8).

It seems that endometrial perfusion presents more accurate non-invasive assay of uterine receptivity than uterine artery perfusion alone. Therefore, blood flow velocity waveform changes of spiral arteries may be used to predict implantation success rate, to reveal unexplained infertility problems and to select patients for correction of endometrial perfusion abnormalities by an appropriate treatment.[30]

In postmenopausal women the endometrium should appear relatively hypovascular. With hyperplasia or cancer, the endometrium becomes vascular.

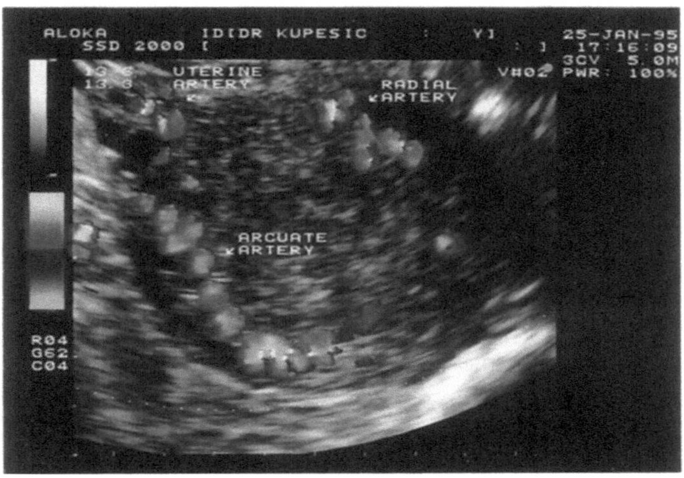

Figure 19.6. Transvaginal color Doppler scan of the uterus demonstrating entire uterine vasculature. Uterine arteries are visualized laterally from the cervix at the level of cervico-corporeal junction, arcuate arteries encircle the uterus and radial arteries run within the myometrial portion.

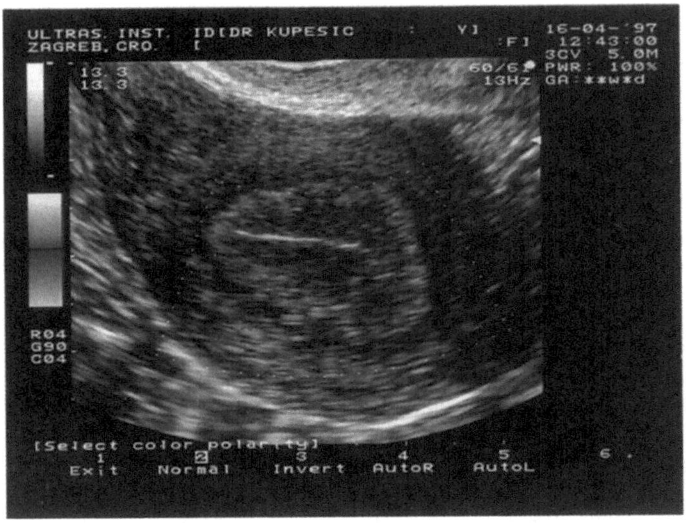

Figure 19.7. Transvaginal color Doppler scan of the periovulatory transformed endometrium. Note endometrial and subendometrial vascularity representing radial and spiral arteries.

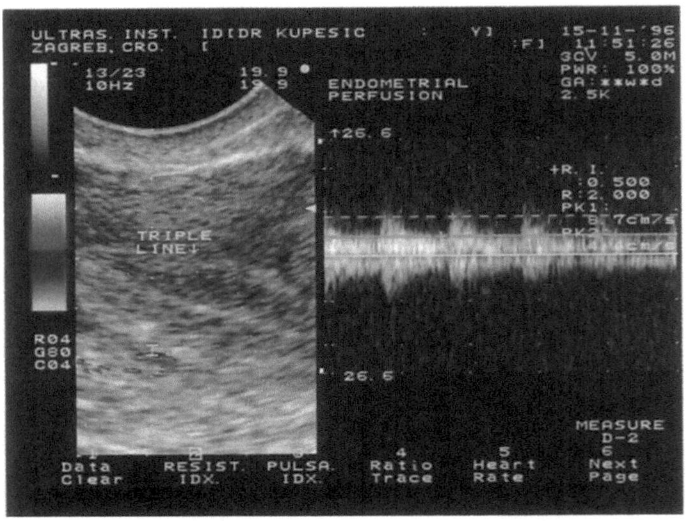

Figure 19.8. Blood flow signals obtained from the triple-line endometrium demonstrate moderate vascular resistance typical for periovulatory phase.

Instead of spontaneously regressing, the endometrial microvascularity in hyperplasia becomes more intense.

There have been ultrastructural observations that the endometrial microvascularity in hyperplasia consists of extensive proliferation of immature capillaries that are disorganized when compared to those of usual endometrium.[31]

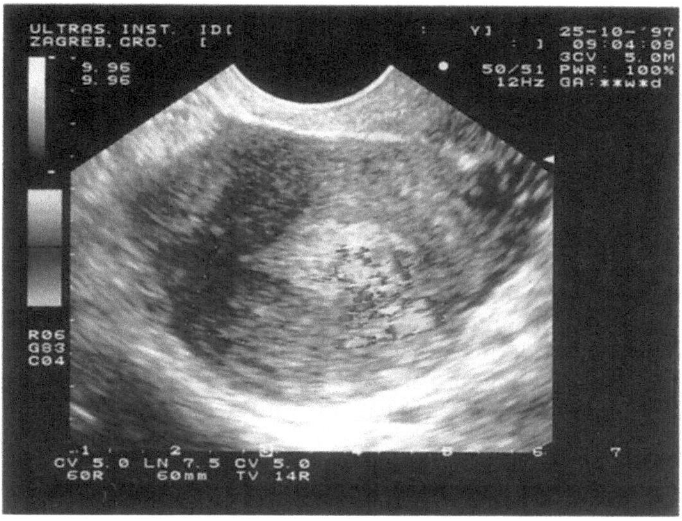

Figure 19.9. Transvaginal color Doppler scan of the uterus in a postmenopausal patient. Note thickened, richly vascularized endometrium.

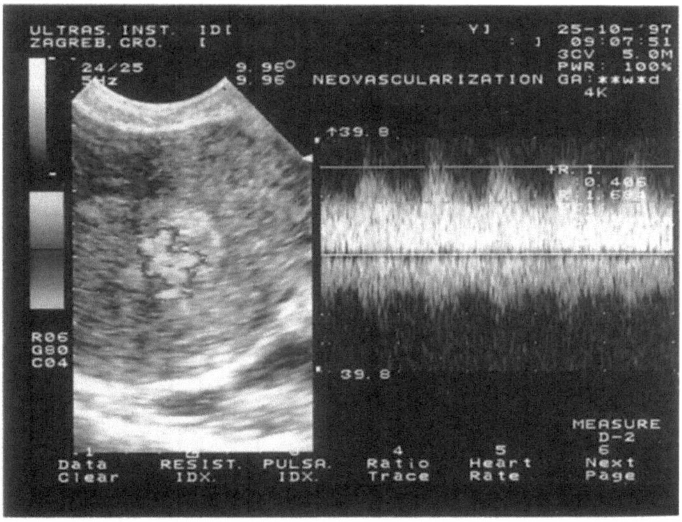

Figure 19.10. The same patient as in Fig. 19.9. Low vascular resistance signals obtained from the central parts of the endometrial lesion (RI=0.41) indicate endometrial malignancy which was proved by histopathology.

Although incompletely understood, the angiogenesis that occurs with endometrial hyperplasia and carcinoma is probably initiated by elaboration of growth factors and/or reduced production of an inhibitory regulator. Microscopically, the tumor vessels have incomplete basement membranes and are leaky. These features may become increasingly apparent on color Doppler ultrasound.[32]

Endometrial thickness greater than 14 mm in premenopausal and greater than 5 mm in postmenopausal women, should be an indicator for further investigation.[33] Morphology itself can not be used to discriminate benign from malignant conditions since the problem of differentiating endometrial hyperplasia is still unsolved by B-mode transvaginal sonography alone.

Endometrial hyperplasia and endometrial carcinoma are angiogenic, and should therefore be detected by sensitive Doppler units (Fig. 19.9). The peripheral distribution of the regularly separated vessels is typical of endometrial hyperplasia. Color flow and pulsed Doppler signals are usually obtained from the border of the hyperplastic endometrium. A significant difference has been found in terms of the RI value between endometrial malignancy (mean RI=0.42) (Fig. 19.10) and endometrial hyperplasia (mean RI=0.50).[34] Some clinicians have begun to utilize sonographic and Doppler evaluation to decide which patients should undergo biopsy and which patients can simply be followed. This can be particularly useful in elderly patients in poor medical condition, as well as in patients with stenotic cervical os.

Placentation

One of the most intriguing angiogenic events is placentation. An increase in color mapping of this endometrial circulation has been reported as an early sign of pregnancy.[30] The first clearly objective sign of the beginning of uteroplacental circulation is the visualization of the gestational sac which, according to our statistics, happens on average day 32 of amenorrhea or at 4.5 weeks with a mean diameter of 3.8 mm

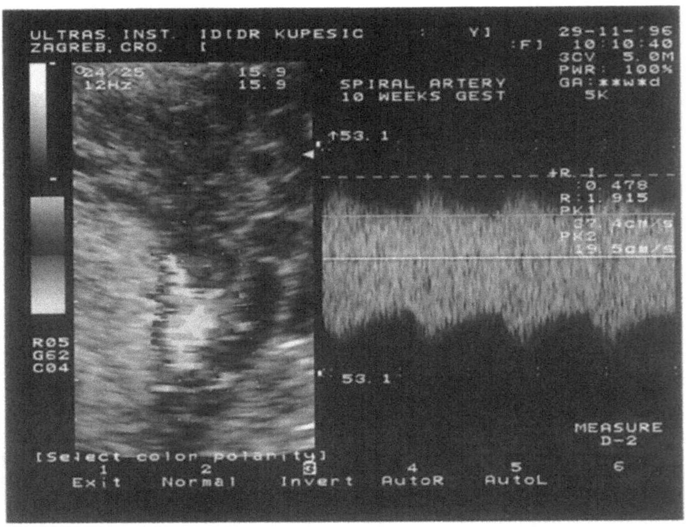

Figure 19.11. Transvaginal color Doppler scan of the spiral arteries at 10 weeks' gestation. Note low-to-moderate vascular resistance (RI=0.48) typical for dilated spiral arteries due to trophoblastic invasion and hormonal influence.

(ranges from 2.7 to 5.2 mm).[35] Color Doppler shows a signal from the periphery of the sac that penetrates the endometrium and the adjacent myometrium like a comet, so it could be called the "color comet" sign. Pulsed Doppler in this area demonstrates a low resistance velocity waveform. Both features show the transformation of the spiral arteries (Fig. 19.11) and, to a lesser degree, the radial arteries into arteries of low impedance due to the trophoblast invasion. These changes occur and can be seen at a specific place in the gestational sac, from which the chorion frondosum will develop. In this way color Doppler discovers the site of placental development before it is visualized in a real time image.[35]

Placental vascularization develops gradually, and although the placental villi are completely vascularized at the end of the third week of embryonic development (week 5 of amenorrhea), the feto-placental circulation starts when embryonic and placental vessels join through the umbilical vessels and the heart begins to beat. In the intervillous space fetomaternal exchanges take place. This is because the uteroplacental arteries flow into it and the placental villi are suspended like an upside-down tree. According to embryological studies uteroplacental circulation is established around day 12 of the embryo development, when maternal blood flows into the syncytiotrophoblast lacunae.[36] Histological studies of the intervillous space can only examine the existence of maternal blood in the intervillous space or the permeability of the spiral arteries. They cannot, however, recognize the existence of a true intervillous flow as it can be demonstrated by in vivo studies. Kurjak et al.[37] and Merce et al.[38] were first to report the possibility of recording the intervillous flow using transvaginal color Doppler during the first trimester of normal pregnancy. The venous blood flow

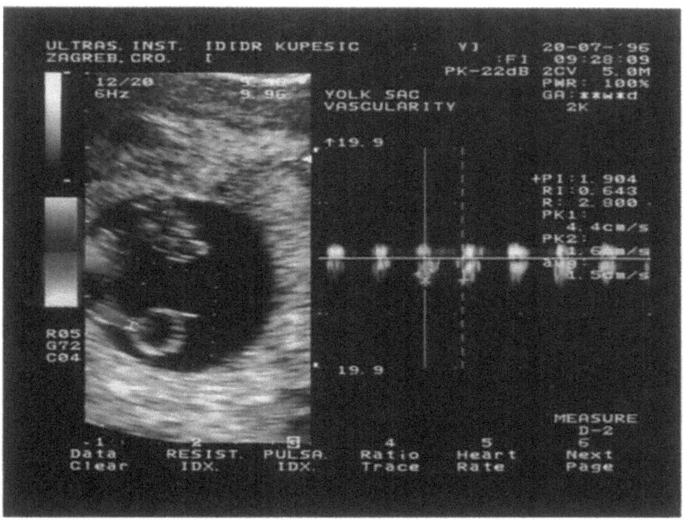

Figure 19.12. Transvaginal color Doppler scan at 6–7 weeks' gestation. Blood flow signals are clearly displayed from the wall of the yolk sac. Absence of the diastolic flow and low velocity are typical features of yolk sac vascularity.

signal can be recognized at 6 weeks of pregnancy in the chorionic ring segment where the uteroplacental or retrochorionic arteries flow, coinciding with the first recording of the fetoplacental and umbilical circulation.[30,38]

The yolk sac is the first structure that is visualized within the gestational sac upon ultrasound examination, and it should be recognized in all gestational sacs exceeding 10 mm. Kurjak and Kupesic[39] were first to report the importance of this circulation in evaluation of the early pregnancy. A characteristic waveform profile of the yolk sac vessels included low velocity (5.8±1.7 cm/s) and inconsistent diastolic flow (PI=3.24±0.94) (Fig. 19.12). Vitelline stalk vessels showed similar peak systolic velocity (5.4±1.8 cm/s) and PI values (3.14±0.91). As yolk sac vascularity decreases with the advancement of pregnancy the placental vascularity rises. This is another detail that explains how one vascular system (placenta) takes over the nutrition from another (yolk sac).

There are numerous data provided by histological and color Doppler studies proving that the intervillous circulation begins early in normal pregnancy, which is in accordance with classical embryological theories. This is possible because the trophoblastic invasion is a progressive process and although some of the spiral arteries are totally occluded, the majority of them are opened or only partially occluded. In this way the inflow of blood in the intervillous space is controlled and increases progressively during the first trimester.[40]

Apart from spiral arteries, changes of diameter happen also in other uterine vessels. RI and PI gradually drop from the first day of implantation to the twelfth week of gestation and then remain on these low levels (Fig. 19.13). Trophoblastic infiltration of the placental bed is probably not the only factor that regulates the transformation of the uterine vessels. The final action of vasodilatation is performed through the influence of hormones and prostaglandins.[41]

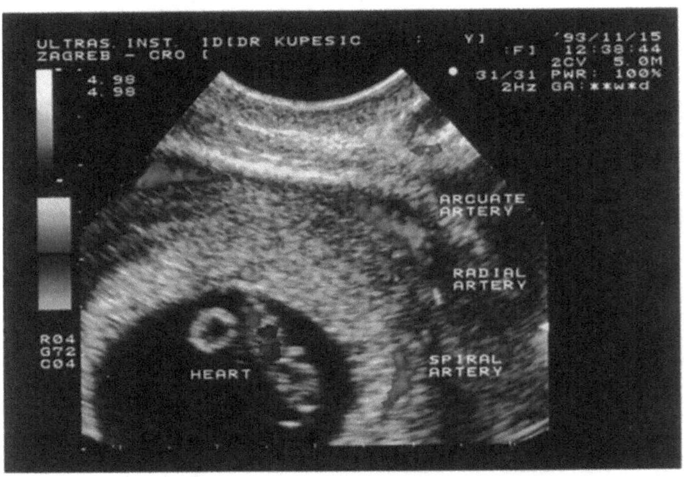

Figure 19.13. Transvaginal color Doppler scan of an early pregnancy. Both maternal and embryonic side of circulation are displayed using this technique. Color Doppler facilitates visualization of embryonic heart activity.

Malignant Angiogenesis

Angiogenesis is a common phenomenon in malignant neoplasms, but the intensity of neovascularization may depend on the characteristics of the individual tumor.[42] An incremental decrease of the impedance indices in the tumoral vessels may reflect the increase in angiogenesis and be an indicator of the tumor's malignant potential.[43]

Macroscopically, the tumor vasculature can be categorized as peripheral or central vascularization[44] (Fig. 19.14). Although this classification is not appropriate and anatomically correct, it may help in the assessment of an ultrasonically detectable vascular position within tumor tissue. It is believed that peripherally located vessels within the tumor originate from pre-existing host vasculature, while centrally located vessels develop in response to angiogenic tumor cell activity and/or because of necrotic processes.

Very few studies have tried to evaluate or quantify the amount of vascularity within the tumor.[45-47] In one of the early series, we described vessel arrangement in adnexal lesions as diffuse or having a regularly separated vascular pattern.[48] A diffuse vessel arrangement was categorized as more than one colored spot displayed over the tumor tissue. We found that compared to isolated vessels, diffuse vessels located within the central solid parts of the tumor were almost three times higher in malignant tumors than in benign lesions, suggesting that the area demonstrating a diffuse vascular pattern has high angiogenic activity (Fig. 19.15).

Structural abnormalities of tumoral capillaries cause various functional impairments. The transcapillary permeability is increased (up to eight times normal). Mural defects may even be large enough to allow extravasation of red blood cells. Generally, increased permeability causes haemoconcentration and increased viscous flow resistance. Vascular endothelial growth factor (VEGF) has been shown to be increased in cases with high vascular permeability.[49]

In highly vascularized tumors the total vascular cross-sectional area is increased, which lowers the peripheral flow resistance. However, lumen irregularities may regionally increase flow resistance. The interstitial space is usually three to five times larger than normal. High interstitial pressure leads to compression of vessels inside

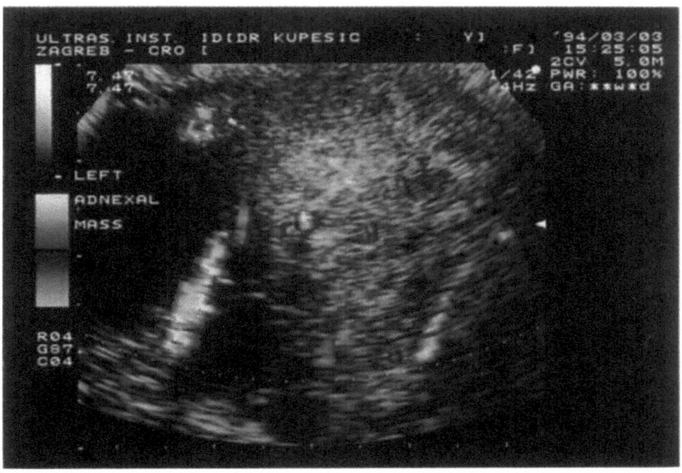

Figure 19.14. Transvaginal color Doppler scan of a huge adnexal mass. Color Doppler facilitates detection of the randomly dispersed vessels, feature typical of ovarian malignancy.

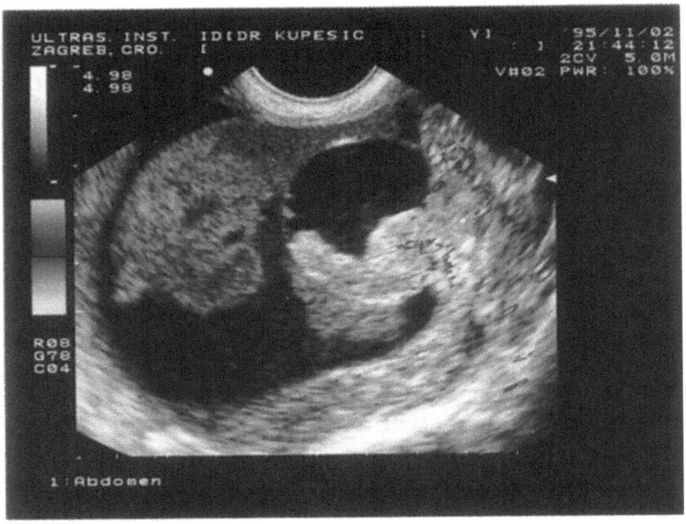

Figure 19.15. Transvaginal color Doppler scan of a complex adnexal mass. Color Doppler displays irregular course of the vessels within the central solid portion of the tumor.

the tumor. Where arteriovenous shunts develop, a fraction of blood will bypass the capillary bed. Consequently, despite a low global flow resistance and a high global blood flow, a variable proportion of the tumor may be deprived of its blood supply. Generally, four regions can be recognized in a tumor: an avascular (necrotic) region; a seminecrotic (ischemic) region; a stabilized microcirculation; and an advancing front as a region of tumor hyperemia.

Pulsed Doppler and vascular resistance to blood flow has been and still is one of the major features in the assessment of tumor vascular characteristics. It is a fact that difference in vascularity exists and blood vessels in malignant adnexal lesions show lower resistance to blood flow that in benign adnexal masses. Although different authors suggest different cut-off values, we have found that levels of 0.40 for RI and 1.0 for PI are the best discriminatory values between benign and malignant adnexal tumors[50-52] (Fig. 19.17).

Angiogenesis is also required for endometrial neoplasms. Abulafia and coworkers[53] evaluated angiogenesis in endometrial hyperplasia and Stage I endometrial carcinoma, as well as the relationship between angiogenesis and tumor grade and depth of invasion. Areas close to deepest myometrial invasion or those with the highest grade of endometrial hyperplasia and the highest angiogenic intensity were selected. Their study demonstrated increased angiogenicity of complex endometrial hyperplasia compared with controls or simple hyperplasia; similar angiogenic capability of complex hyperplasia compared with Stage Ia endometrial carcinoma; increased angiogenesis in invasive (Stages Ib and Ic endometrial carcinoma compared with complex hyperplasia or Stage Ia) endometrial carcinoma; and increasing angiogenesis with higher tumor grade. This suggests that angiogenic capacity may be one of the biological characteristics associated with endometrial tumor grade.

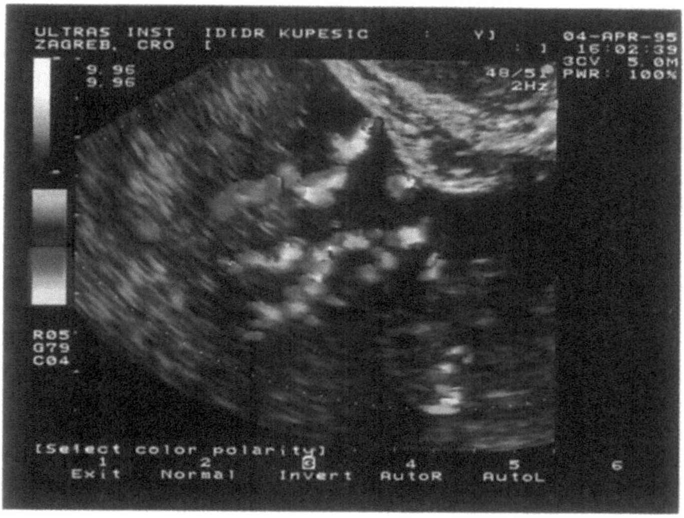

Figure 19.16. Neovascularization in an ovarian tumor as seen by transvaginal color Doppler. Note irregular course of the intratumoral vessels.

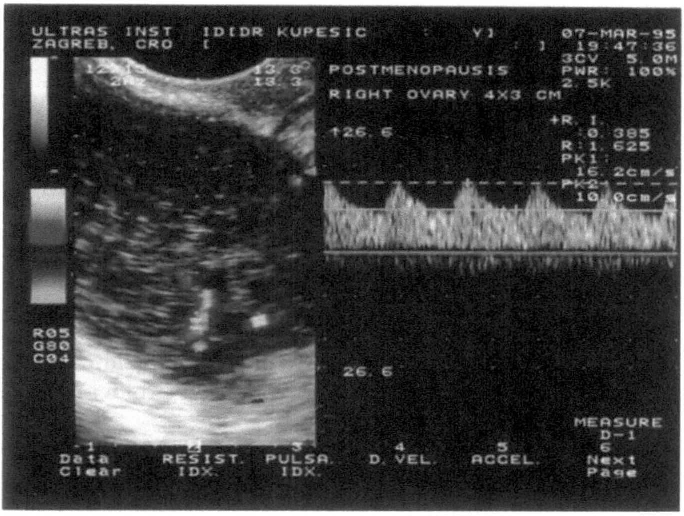

Figure 19.17. Transvaginal color Doppler scan of a slightly enlarged ovary (4×3×3 cm) in a postmenopausal patient. Low vascular resistance (RI=0.39) was the only parameter suspective of ovarian malignancy. Histopathology proved ovarian cystadenocarcinoma.

Kupesic et al.[34] analyzed 267 patients with uterine lesions before hysterectomy. Angiogenesis was detected in 167 (67%) benign masses, while in all malignant lesions (n=26) areas of neovascularization were detected. Arterial blood flow signals were derived from areas of neovascularization showing significantly lower ($p<0.05$) resistance index (RI=0.37±0.07) in the cases of endometrial carcinoma than in patients with benign uterine cavity lesions (RI=0.54±0.09). Central vessels within endometrial carcinoma tended to have lower velocity and impedance compared to peripheral ones. Significant difference was detected in the vascular resistance of the uterine artery between patients with endometrial malignancy and those with benign lesions (RI=0.64±0.08) vs RI=0.74±0.09). This study corroborated our previous results.[54]

In recent years, cancer scientists have used molecular and biochemical knowledge, as well as insights into tumor physiology, to bridge the gap between preclinical and clinical work. The main field of interest was angiogenic factors. The first indication of the importance of angiogenesis for tumor growth came from observations in the early 1980s that tumors secreted soluble factors that could stimulate endothelial growth.[55] The basic and acidic fibroblast growth factors were among the first to be identified and were soon followed by many others such as vascular endothelial growth factor/vascular permeability factor and transforming growth factors (TGF-alpha).

It is believable that a major role in vasodilatation and angiogenesis during ovulation may be attributed to the action of prostaglandins; PGE2 and PGI2 are assumed to be potent vasodilators[56] but also angiogenic stimulants, especially PGE1 and PGE2.[57] Based on the assumption that angiogenesis is a uniform process, a newly formed vascular network should yield no difference in blood flow parameters if detected in the early stage of its development in folliculogenesis, corpus luteum or benign and malignant lesions. Regarding the blood flow characteristics of early angiogenesis taken together with the vasodilatation and opening of arterio-venous shunts by the action of prostaglandins at the local level, it is reasonable to believe that certain benign tumors, and some normal conditions, have high angiogenic potential and/or intense local production of prostaglandins. The micromolecular events that lead to the rupture of Graafian follicle are also based on vasoactive events.

When Doppler parameters are compared it is obvious that RI values in benign and malignant conditions are much alike. That is why angiogenesis of corpus luteum can look like a malignant ovarian lesion. In this case, the Doppler machine is set to detect angiogenic, well perfused tissue, and it performs its task extremely well. Angiogenesis of corpus luteum can sometimes look like the "ring of fire" seen in cases of ectopic pregnancy. For all these reasons corpus luteum is also called "the great imitator".

Endometrial changes in perfusion may consequently lead to proliferation, secretion or shedding. Endometrial hyperplasia is a condition between normal endometrium and endometrial cancer. Again, the more disturbed the endometrial cells are, the bigger the amount of angiogenesis and the perfusion rate. Therefore, in cases of endometrial malignancy one can detect intensive proliferation of the immature capillaries and low RI values.

In order to metastasize, tumor cells must degrade the extracellular matrix, then penetrate the vessel wall and force itself into the circulation. Consequently, upon reaching the target organ they must do the same actions again. A very similar process happens during trophoblast invasion. Trophoblast destroys spiral arteries and transforms them into non-contractile channels.

Future Prospects

A new tool for study of angiogenesis is 3D power Doppler. This three-dimensional imaging modality allows the clinician to visualize the many overlapping vessels easily and quickly, and to assess their relationship to other vessels or surrounding tissues. The implementation of the three-dimensional display permits the physician to view

Table 19.3. Parameters for the assessment of tumors and various imaging tools.

Conventional B-mode and 3D Ultrasound	Transvaginal color Doppler	3D power Doppler
morphology	blood flow	angiogenic properties
relation to other organs	vessels quality (RI,PI,Vel)	branching pattern
		overall vascularity and perfusion

structures in three dimensions interactively, rather than having to assemble the sectional images mentally.[58] The three-dimensional power Doppler system may thus improve the information available on tumor vascularity and speed up the entire patient management process (Table 19.3).

Our initial results show that 3D power Doppler accurately detects characteristic structural abnormalities of the malignant tumor vessels such as microaneurysms, arteriovenous shunts, tumoral lakes, disproportional calibration, elongation, coiling and dichotomous branching.[59,60] The vessel pattern is distinctly chaotic. All these vascular features are shown in their true spatial relations (Fig. 19.18). While color Doppler was useful in detecting vascularized structures, 3D power is excellent in the study of vascular morphology.

Morphological analysis of the blood vessel system represents another approach to tumor diagnosis which, so far, has not been extensively evaluated. However, there is a distinct impression that the distribution and branching pattern of blood vessels that supply a fast-growing tumor differ from those of the normal blood supply to normal organs. This means that blood vessel distribution seems to carry additional

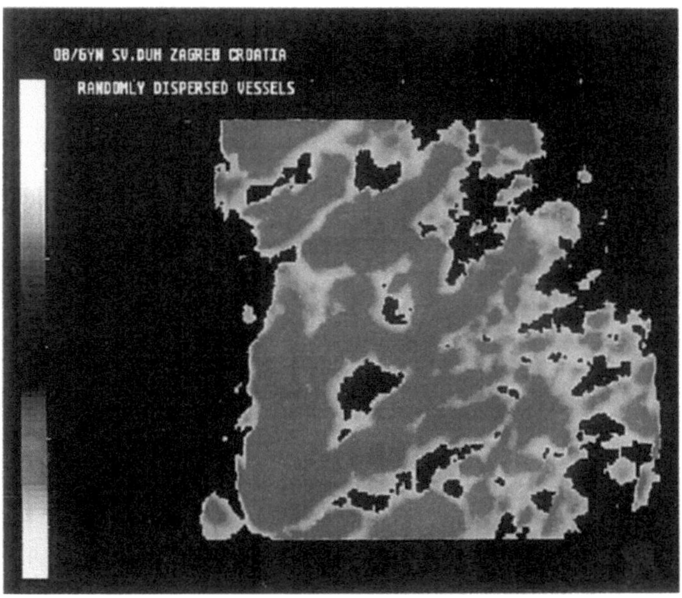

Figure 19.18. Three-dimensional power Doppler scan of the malignant ovarian tumor vasculature. Instillation of the echo enhancing contrast enables depiction of irregular tumoral vessels with chaotic arrangement and disproportional calibration and branching.

Table 19.4. Difference between benign and malignant angiogenesis as seen by 3D power Doppler

Benign conditions	Malignant lesions
linear arrangement	chaotic vessel arrangement
regular branching	irregular branching

information that is missed in the present diagnostic approaches. However, describing branching structures like the blood vessel tree is a mathematically complicated task that calls for the most recent mathematical apparatus.

The branching pattern is the result of some principle (mathematical law) that acts repeatedly upon the blood vessels, so that they branch out in similar ways at different scale factors. Such objects that are self-similar at different scales are called fractals. The process is, presumably, similar to processes that govern the branching in an actual tree. If the underlying rule changes, the branching pattern must change too.

Our hypothesis is that the general view of the pattern of branching in blood vessels within 1 cm^3 generally resembles that of the branching in 50 cm^3 of the same tissue. We postulate that blood vessel trees are an example of fractal[61,62] geometry. The normal blood vessel trees (arteries and veins) form branched structures with ever-smaller branches and diameters. They provide blood to the whole body while taking up less than 6% of the available space. The underlying proposition of our hypothesis is that there is a change in fractal dimension when the branching becomes unregulated by normal processes, i.e. when the ordered growth is replaced by disordered growth[58] (Table 19.4). This study is still in progress.

Finally, there is no good or bad angiogenesis. There is only angiogenesis, that so miraculously produces such opposite results. It is only our ability to recognize physiologic and pathologic vessel formation based on Doppler and clinical data, and patients' history and age, that allows us to distinguish between them.

References

1. Folkman, J., Long, D. and Becker, F. Growth and metastasis of tumor in organ culture. Tumor Res. 1963; 16:453–67
2. Folkman, J., Cole, P. and Zimmerman, S. Tumor behavior in isolated perfused organs: in vitro growth and metastasis of biopsy material in rabbit thyroid and canine intestinal segment. Ann. Surg. 1966; 164:491–502
3. Folkman, J. and Gimbrone, M. Perfusion of the thyroid. Acta Endocrinol. 1971; 4:237–48
4. Folkman, J. The Intestine As An Organ Culture. In: Burdette, J. and Thomas, C.C. (eds), Carcinoma of the Colon and Antecedent Epithelium. Illinois: Springfield, 1970: 113–27
5. Kanzaki, H., Okamura, H., Okuda, Y. Scanning electron microscopic study of rabbit ovarian follicle microvasculature using resin injection-corrosion casts. J. Anat. 1982; 134:697–704
6. Murakami, T., Ikebuchi, Y., Ohtsuka, A. The blood vascular wreath of rat ovarian follicle, with special reference to its changes in ovulation and luteinization: a scanning electron microscopic study of corrosion casts. Arch. Histol. Cytol. 1988; 51:299–313
7. Bassett, D.L. The changes in the vascular pattern of the ovary of the albino rat during the estrous cycle. Am. J. Anat. 1943; 73:252–92
8. Brambell F.W.R. Ovarian Changes. In: Parkes A.S. (ed.), Marshall's Physiology of Reproduction, Vol 1 (1). London: Longmans and Green, 1956: 397–542
9. Ginther, O.J., Diersche, D.K.J., Walsh, S.W. and Del Campi, C.H. Anatomy of arteries and veins of uterus and ovaries in rhesus monkeys. Biol. Reprod. 1974; 11:204–19
10. Reynolds, S.R.M. Blood and Lymph Vascular Systems of the Ovary. In: Greep, S.R. (ed.) Female Reproductive System, Part I. Washington: American Physiological Society 1973: 261–316

11. Gillet, J.Y., Koritke, J.G., Muller, P. and Juliens, C. On the microvascularization of the rabbit ovary. Compt. Rend. Soc. Biol. 1968; 162:762–6
12. Kurjak, A. and Kupesic-Urek, S. Infertility. In: Kurjak, A. (ed.), Transvaginal Color Doppler, Carnforth, UK: Parthenon Publishing, 1991: 33–8
13. Bourne, T.H., Jurkovic, D., Waterstone, J., Campbell, S. and Collins, W.P. Intra-follicular blood flow during human ovulation. Ultrasound Obstet. Gynecol 1991; 1:53–9
14. Collins, W., Jurkovic, D., Bourne, T.H., Kurjak, A. and Campbell, S. Ovarian morphology, endocrine function and intra-follicular blood flow during preovulatory period. Hum. Reprod. 1991; 6:319–24
15. Sladkevicius, P., Valentin, L. and Marsal, K. Blood flow velocity in the uterine and ovarian arteries during the normal menstrual cycle. Ultrasound Obstet Gynecol. 1993; 3:199–201
16. Kupesic, S., Kurjak, A., Vujisic, S. and Petrovic, Z. Luteal phase defect: comparison between Doppler velocimetry, histological and hormonal markers. Ultrasound Obstet. Gynecol. 1997; 9:1–8
17. Reynolds, R.M. Morphological determinations of the flow characteristics between an artery and its branch with special reference to the ovarian spiral artery in the rabbit. Acta. Anat. 1948; 5:1–6
18. Niswender, G.D., Reiners, T.J., Dickmann, M.A. and Nett, Y.T.M. Blood flow: a mediator of ovarian function. Biol. Reprod. 1976; 14:64–81
19. Kurjak, A., Kupesic-Urek, S., Schulman, H. and Zalud, I. Transvaginal color Doppler in the assessment of ovarian and uterine blood flow in infertile women. Fertil. Steril. 1992; 56:870–3
20. Merce, L.T., Andrino, R., Barco, M.J. and De la Fuente, P. Cyclic changes of the functional ovarian compartments: echographic assessment. Acta. Obstet. Gynecol. Scand 1990; 69:327–32
21. Zalud, I. and Kurjak, A. The assessment of luteal blood flow in pregnant and non-pregnant women by transvaginal color Doppler. J. Perinat. Med. 1990; 18:215–18
22. Glock, J.L., Blackman, J.A., Badger, G. J. and Brumsted, J.R. Prognostic significance of morphologic changes of the corpus luteum by transvaginal ultrasound in early pregnancy monitoring. Obstet. Gynecol. 1995; 85:37–41
23. Kupesic, S. and Kurjak, A. The assessment of normal and abnormal luteal function by transvaginal color Doppler sonography. Eur. J. Obstet. Gynecol. Reprod. Biol. 1997; 72:83–7
24. Glock, J.L. and Brumsted, J.R. Color flow pulsed Doppler ultrasound in diagnosing luteal phase defect. Fertil. Steril. 1995; 64:500–4
25. Merce, L.T., Garces, D. and De la Fuente, F. Conversion lutea de la onda de velocigrafico de ovulacion y function lutea. Acta. Obstet. Gynecol. Scand. 1989; 2:113–4
26. Tinkanen, H. The role of vascularization of the corpus luteum in the short luteal phase studied by Doppler ultrasound. Acta. Obstet. Gynecol. Scand. 1994; 73:321–3
27. Lawn, A.M. The ultrastructure of the endometrium. J. Reprod. Fertil. 1974; 37:239–42
28. Keye, W.R., Yuen, B.H. and Jaffe, R.B. New concepts in the physiology of the menstrual cycle. Clin. Endocrinol. Metab. 1973; 2:251–8
29. Kupesic, S. and Kurjak, A. Uterine and ovarian perfusion during the periovulatory period assessed by transvaginal color Doppler. Fertil. Steril. 1993; 60:439–43
30. Kupesic, S. The first three weeks assessed by transvaginal color Doppler. J. Perinat. Med. 1996; 24:301–17
31. Horbelt, D., Roberts, D., Parmley, T., Walker, N. Ultrastructure of the microvasculature in human endometrial hyperplasia. Am J. Obstet. Gynecol. 1996; 174:174–83
32. Fleischer, A.C. Tumor Angiogenesis In Ovarian and Endometrial Cancer: Sonographic Depiction and Clinical Implications. In: Kurjak, S., Fleischer A.C. (eds). Doppler Ultrasound in Gynecology. London: Parthenon Publishers, 1998: 101–12
33. Kurjak, A., Kupesic, S., Zalud, I. and Predanic, M. Transvaginal color Doppler. In: Dodson, M.G. (ed.), Transvaginal Ultrasound, New York: Churchill Livingstone, 1995: 325–39
34. Kupesic-Urek, S., Shalan, H. and Kurjak, A. Early detection of endometrial cancer by transvaginal color Doppler. EUROBS 1993; 49:46–9
35. Merce, L.T., Barci, M.J., de la Fuente, F. Doppler velocimetry measured in retrochorionic space and uterine arteries during early human pregnancy. Acta. Obstet. Gynecol. Scan. 1989; 8:603–7
36. Kurjak, A., Kupesic, S., Kostovic, Lj. Vascularization of yolk sac and vitelline duct in normal pregnancies studied by transvaginal color and pulsed Doppler. J. Perinat. Med. 1994; 22:433–40
37. Kurjak, A., Laurini, R., Kupesic, S., Kos, M., Latin, V., Bulic, K. A combined Doppler and morphopathological study of intervillous circulation. Fifth World Congress of Ultrasound in Obstetrics and Gynecology, Book of Abstracts. Ultrasound Obstet. Gynecol. 1995; 6 (Suppl. 2):116
38. Merce, L.T., Barco, M.J., Bau S. Color Doppler sonographic assessment of placental circulation in the first trimester of normal pregnancy. J. Ultrasound Med. 1996; 15:135–42
39. Kupesic, S., Kurjak, A., Ivancic-Kosuta, M. Volume and vascularity of the yolk sac studied by three-dimensional ultrasound and color Doppler. J. Perinat. Med. 1999; 27: 91–6

40. Kurjak, A., Kupesic, S., Hafner, T., Kos, M., Kostovic-Knezevic, L.J., Grbesa, D. Conflicting data on intervillous circulation in early pregnancy. J Perinat. Med. 1997; 25:373–80
41. Kurjak, A., Kupesic, S., Zudenigo, D. Transvaginal color Doppler assessment of the early pregnancy. Arch. Perinatal Med. 1998; 68:29–34
42. Borune, T.H. Should clinical decisions be made about ovarian masses using transvaginal color Doppler? Ultrasound Obstet. Gynecol. 1994; 4:257–60
43. Wu, J.C.C., Lee, C.N., Chen, T.M., Shyu, M.K., Hsieh, C.Y., Chen, H.Y., Hsieh, F.J. Incremental angiogenesis assessed by color Doppler ultrasound in the tumorigenesis of ovarian neoplasms. Cancer 1994; 73:1251–6
44. Fleischer, A.C., Rodgers, W.H., Rao, B.J., Keppler, D.M., Worell, J.A., Wiliams, J., Jones III, H.W. Assessment of ovarian tumor vascularity with transvaginal color Doppler sonography. J. Ultrasound Med. 1991; 10:563–8
45. Rubin, J.M., Adler, R.S., Fowlkes, J.B., Spratt, S., Pallister, J.E., Chen, J.F., Carson, P.L. Fractional moving blood volume: estimation with power Doppler. US Radiol. 1995; 197:183–90
46. Cameron, J.R., Waren, S.E., Laurence, A.M., Dale, R.C., Yongimin, K. Three-dimensional ultrasonic angiography using power-mode Doppler. Ultrasound Med. Biol. 1996; 3:277–86
47. Pairleitner, H., Steiner, G., Hasenoehrl, G. Staudach, A. Three-dimensional power Doppler sonography: imaging and quantifying blood flow and vascularization. Ultrasound Obstet. Gynecol. 1999; 14:139–43
48. Kurjak, A. Predanic, M. New scoring system for prediction of ovarian malignancy based on transvaginal color Doppler. J. Ultrasound Med. 1992; 11:631–8
49. Dvorak, H.F., Brown, L.F., Detmar, M., Dvorak, A.M. Vascular permeability factor/vascular endothelial growth factor, microvascular hyperpermeability, and angiogenesis. Am. J. Pathol. 1995; 146:1029–39
50. Kurjak, A., Zalud, I., Alfireviæ, Z. Evaluation of adnexal masses with transvaginal color Doppler ultrasound. J. Ultrasound. Med. 1991; 10:295–7
51. Kurjak, A., Schulman, H., Sosic, A., Zalud, I. Shalan, H. Transvaginal ultrasound, color flow and Doppler waveform of the postmenopausal adnexal mass. Obstet. Gynecol. 1992; 80:917–21
52. Kurjak, A., Shalan, H., Matijevic, R, Predaniæ, M., Kupesic, S. Stage I ovarian cancer by transvaginal color Doppler sonography – a report of 18 cases. Ultrasound Obstet. Gynecol. 1993; 3:1958
53. Abulafia, O., Triest, W.E., Sherer, D.M., Hansen, C.C. and Ghezzi, F. Angiogenesis in endometrial hyperplasia and Stage I endometrial carcinoma. Obstet. Gynecol. 1995; 86:479–85
54. Kurjak, A., Shalan, H., Sosic, A., Benic, S., Zudenigo, D., Kupesic, S. Predanic, M. Endometrial carcinoma in postmenopausal women: evaluation by transvaginal color Doppler ultrasonography. Am. J. Obstet. Gynecol. 1993; 169:1597–653
55. Folkman, J., Klagsburn, M. Angiogenic factors. Science 1987; 235:442–7
56. Raud, J. Vasodilatation and inhibition of mediator release represent two distinct mechanisms for prostaglandin modulation of acute mast cell dependent inflammation. Br. J. Pharm. 1990; 99:449–54
57. Jaffe, B.M. Prostaglandins and cancer. An update. Prostaglandins 1974; 6:453–61
58. Kurjak, A., Kupesic, S., Breyer, B., Sparac, V. Jukic S. The assessment of ovarian tumor angiogenesis: what does three-dimensional power Doppler add? Ultrasound Obstet. Gynecol. 1998; 12:136–46
59. Kurjak, A., Kupesic, S. Three-dimensional ultrasound and power Doppler in assessment of uterine and ovarian angiogenesis: a prospective study. Croatian Med. J. 1999; 40(3):413–20
60. Kurjak, A., Kupesic, S., Anic, T., Kosuta, D. Three-dimensional ultrasound and power Doppler improve the diagnosis of ovarian lesions. Gynecol. Oncol. 2000; 76; 28-32
61. Breyer, B., Kurjak, A. Tumor vascularization Doppler measurements and chaos: what to do? Ultrasound Obstet Gynecol 1995; 5:209–10
62. Schoenfeld, A, Levavi, H., Tepper, R., Breslavski, D., Amir, R., Ovadia, J. Assessment of tumor induced angiogenesis by three-dimensional display: confusing Doppler signals in ovarian cancer screening? Ultrasound Obstet Gynecol 1994; 4:516–8

20 Angiogenesis and Vasculogenesis in Pregnancy and in Tumor Development

Marek Zygmunt

Investigation of the mechanisms regulating development of new vessels is crucial to our understanding of both tumor biology and early pregnancy development. There are striking similarities between, on the one hand, tumor invasion and tumor vascularization and, on the other, blastocyst implantation and placental development. These two different sets of events share two important features:

1 migration and invasion through extracellular matrix (ECM)
2 the ability to access the host vasculature and recruit a blood supply.

Despite these common features, at least two major differences occur:

1 invasion and new vessel formation during pregnancy is self-limited, compared to uncontrolled tumor growth and vessel formation during oncogenesis
2 the implanting embryo not only accesses the maternal vasculature, but also forms its own vascular system, whereas a tumor does not generate vessels of its own.

This chapter will provide a general overview of the recent work on vascular development during early pregnancy and a short comparision of the molecular mechanisms governing physiologic vascularisation in the female reproductive tract and aberrant vascular development in cancer.

Processes of Angiogenesis and Vasculogenesis

The vascular system develops through two distinct processes: vasculogenesis and angiogenesis (Polle and Coffin 1989). During vasculogenesis, endothelial progenitor cells (angioblasts) form a primitive vascular network. This process occurs mainly during fetal development, although recruitment of angioblasts from bone marrow and peripheral blood in response to ischemic insult have been described in adults (Risau and Flamme 1995, Takahashi et al. 1999). Vasculogenesis consists of three major steps: induction of hemangioblasts and angioblasts (mediated mainly through fibroblast growth factor, FGF), assembly of primordial vessels (mediated mainly by vascular endothelial growth factor/ vascular endothelial growth factor receptor system, VEGF/VEGF R) and transition from vasculogenesis to angiogenesis (Flamme, Frolich and Risau 1997).

Angiogenesis represents the development of new vessels from pre-existing vessels. Two forms of angiogenesis have been described: sprouting and nonsprouting angiogenesis (intussusception) (Folkman and Shing, 1992). Physiologic angiogenesis plays an important role in wound and fracture healing, formation of corpus luteum, endometrial growth, embryo implantation and placentation. In contrast, pathologic angiogenesis underlies pathophysiology of the following conditions: tumor growth and metastasis, rheumatoid arthritis, retinopathies, chronic inflammation and psoriasis (Folkman 1995). Therapeutic angiogenesis, defined as the use of biological agents or bioactive materials to stimulate the growth of new blood vessels, was developed for the treatment of ischemic heart disease, cerebrovascular disease and delayed wound healing (Hockel et al. 1993, Thompson, Li and Maragoudakis 2000). Inhibition of angiogenesis appears to be a very important approach to the treatment of neoplasia (Denekamp 1990).

In general, the angiogenic process is initiated by growth factors (such as basic fibroblast growth factor (bFGF), vascular endothelial growth factor (VEGF), placental growth factor (PlGF), tumor necrosis factor alpha (TNFα), etc.) (Folkman and Klagsbrun 1987). These growth factors increase the permeability of the vessels, stimulate proteolytic degradation of the extracellular matrix (basal and reticular lamina) by specific proteases (collagenases and plasminogen activators), and cause proliferation of endothelial cells. The process is compleated by chemotactic migration of the endothelial cells and invasion of the ECM, formation of a lumen (through intra- or extracellular mechanisms either from intracellular vacuoles or extracellular channels), and the functional maturation of the endothelium (recruitment of pericytes and smooth muscle cells) (Reynolds, Killilea and Redmer 1992, Torry and Rongish 1992, Risau 1997). The angiogenic phenotype of proliferating and migrating endothelial cells is characterized by the cell adhesion molecules expressed, particularly alpha V integrins, which mediate cell adherence and spreading on matrix containing vitronectin and fibrinogen and thereby ensure cell survival. In vitro blockage of these integrins by high affinity antagonists resulted in effective inhibition of neovascularization (Brooks, Clark and Cheresh 1994, Hammes et al. 1996).

Regulation of Angiogenesis

A broad spectrum of factors play a crucial role in the initiation and regulation of angiogenesis, and the switch to angiogenesis is regulated by a change in the local equilibrium between angiogenic factors and their inhibitors. The list of inducers of angiogenesis includes:

- cytokines, hormones and growth factors (see Table 20.1.)
- hypoxia and hypoglycemia
- shear stress and stretch
- components of ECM (e.g. laminin, fibronectin) and their receptors (integrins alphaV, alpha 5)
- matrix metalloproteinases (MMPs) and their tissue inhibitors (TIMPs) as regulators of MMPs
- other proteases (e.g. urokinase-type and tissue-type plasminogen activator, uPA, tPA)

Table 20.1. Regulatory factors of angiogenesis.

(a) angiogenic factors	(b) angiostatic factors (natural)
Angiopoietins	Angiostatin
aFGF, bFGF	Thrombospondin
VEGF-A, -B, -C, -D	Endostatin
PlGF	TNFα
PDGF	Prolactin
G-CSF	TXA_2
GM-CSF	
Leptin	**(c) angiostatic factors (therapeutic)**
IL-8	
Proliferin	Thalidomide
IGF-I	CM101 (bacterial polysacharide from GBS)
TGF α, TGF β	Fumagillin (from Aspergillus fumigatus)
hCG	TNP-470 (derivated from fumagillin)
IGF-II	RU-486
Estrogens	Steroids (?)
PGE_1, PGE_2	
TNFα	
Hepatocyte growth factor (HGF)/ scatter factor (SF)	

- fibrin
- inflammatory cells and pericytes

The most important positive regulators of angiogenesis are VEGF, FGF and the angiopoietins.

Vascular Endothelial Growth Factor (VEGF)

VEGF (-A) is a highly specific mitogen for the vascular endothelial cells. Five different isoforms have been described: $VEGF_{121}$, $VEGF_{145}$, $VEGF_{165}$, $VEGF_{189}$ and $VEGF_{206}$ Five further members of the VEGF family are: VEGF-B, VEGF-C, VEGF-D and placental growth factor (PlGF). Two specific VEGF receptors, VEGFR-1 (Flt-1) and VEGFR-2 (KDR/ murine analog Flk-1) are expressed on the endothelial cells and in soluble form in maternal serum during pregnancy (only sVEGFR-1). VEGFR-2 is responsible for the mitogenic, anti-apoptotic and permeability-enhancing actions of VEGF, whereas VEGFR-1 is thought to act as a negative regulator of VEGF actions on the vascular endothelium by sequestering the ligand (Ferrara and Davis-Smyth 1997). Recently, two other VEGF receptors have been discovered: neuropilin-1 and VEGFR-3 (Flt-4) (Galland et al. 1993, Soker et al. 1998). VEGF actions include not only mitogenic activation of endothelial cells but also induction of serine proteases (uPA and tPA) and collagenases, increased endothelial chemotaxis and vasodilation. VEGF gene expression is regulated by oxygen tension, various growth factors and cytokines (EGF, TGF beta, PGE_2, IL-1, IL-6) as well as placental hormones (e.g. hCG) (Zygmunt, Mazzuca and Han 2000).

Fibroblast Growth Factor (FGF)

FGF represents a large family of growth and differentiation factors with at least 18 members.

The two most important are FGF-1 (acidic FGF) and FGF-2 (basic FGF), which share more than 50% structural homology. Both FGFs stimulate proliferation and modulate the functions of endothelial cells, inhibit apoptosis and are chemotactic. There are both high and low affinity receptors for FGF. The high affinity receptor family is represented by FGFR-1 to -4, which are tyrosine kinase receptors and are responsible for signaling functions. Low affinity receptors are involved in the sequestration and stabilization of the ligand and most of them are heparan sulfate proteoglycans (HSPG). They are also present in soluble form in biological fluids and extracellular matrix (ECM) (Baird and Klagsbrun 1991, Klagsbrun 1992).

Angiopoietins

The angiopoietins (Ang-1 and Ang-2) are critically involved in the formation of vasculature during vasculogenesis. Both are ligands for the Tie2 receptor (a tyrosine kinase receptor, expressed on endothelial and hematopoietic cells). A previously described receptor of this class, Tie1, remains an orphan receptor since the search for its ligand has been unsuccessful.

Angiopoietins are mainly involved in the stabilization and remodeling of the primary capillary plexus and are responsible for survival of endothelial cells (Sato et al. 1995, Suri et al. 1998, Hayes et al. 1999). Ang-1 was shown to be expressed in cyto- and syncytiotrophoblast, whereas Ang-2 and Tie2 are predominantly expressed in cytotrophoblast (Dunk et al. 2000).

Inhibitors of Angiogenesis

The two most potent natural inhibitors of angiogenesis are angiostatin and thrombospondin (see Table 20.1.). Angiostatin is a proteolytic fragment of plasminogen which has a strong antiproliferative action on endothelial cells and also suppresses the growth of primary tumors in mice (O'Reilly et al. 1994). Thrombospondin (TSP) is released from thrombin activated platelets and is known to be produced by many cell types including endothelial and smooth muscle cells, macrophages, neutrophils and fibroblasts. Soluble TSP is antiproliferative for endothelial cells, modulates endothelial cell adhesion and has an anti-chemotactic effect both in vitro and in vivo, whereas bound TSP might promote angiogenic responses (DiPietro et al. 1993).

Models for Studying Angiogenesis

Since inadequate vasculogenesis and angiogenesis are associated with a number of physiological and pathological processes, several in vivo and in vitro techniques have been developed to study and reliably quantify the angiogenic response.

The Microsurgical Corneal Pocket Method

This method was developed to study the angiogenic reaction of normally avascular cornea in rabbits, rats or mice (Gimbrone et al. 1974, Muthukkarupan and Auerbach 1979). After embbeding the test substance, cell suspension or tissue sample in a slow-release polymer (Hydron, ELVAX), the test material is microsurgically placed within 2 mm of the corneoscleral junction and vascular sprouting detected and quantified using a computerized image analysis system (Langer and Folkman 1976). The two most important limitations of the corneal pocket assay are high cost and time consumption as well as the fact that surgical manipulation of the cornea can stimulate angiogenesis on its own (Wilting and Christ 1992).

The Chick Chorioallantoic Membrane Assay (CAM)

CAM assay was originally used to study angiogenesis by grafting tumor samples into a chick chorionic membrane (Ausprunk, Knighton and Folkman 1975). In this model CAM is detached from the shell by aspiration of albumin, a window is scissored out and underlying CAM vessels are exposed. On day 8 of the incubation grafts are placed on the CAM and the vasoproliferative response is evaluated. CAM assay is characterized by technical simplicity and low cost, making it a favorite tool for screening purposes.

Subcutaneous Disk Implantation Angiogenesis Assay

Nelson, Conley and Fajardo (1993) described an assay in which a polyvinyl sponge with angiogenic factors in its centre is introduced under the skin of a host animal. The disc system can also be modified to introduce tumor cells into the sponge. Histological and morphological examination of disc area allows evaluation of the disc-bound host-derived blood vessel penetration. Due to the surgical procedure and subsequent inflammatory response, this assay is an appropriate model to study angiogenesis in wound-healing processes.

The Mesenteric Window Angiogenesis Assay (MWAA)

Another model for quantitative studies of mammalian angiogenesis, exploiting the membranous part of the mesentery in rats, was proposed by Norrby, Jakobsson and Sorbo (1986). The angiogenic response to different substances after intraperitoneal injection is quantified at sacrifice using morphometric techniques. One major advantage of MWAA is the physiological environment (including natively vascularized tissue lacking significant physiologic angiogenesis). On the other hand, this model does not allow direct studies of antiangiogenic process.

In vitro Angiogenesis Assay

The introduction of endothelial cell culture techniques resulted in the development of several two- and three-dimensional culture systems for studying the cellular and molecular mechanisms of various steps of the angiogenic response. In these assays plastic beads coated with endothelial cells or whole tissue segments are embedded in fibrin, ECM or collagen gels and cultivated. Test substances or their combinations can be added to the assay at this point. After 1–4 days of incubation, the vascular sprouts migrating into the gel are quantified (Nehls and Drenckhahn, 1995).

Clinical Investigation on Angiogenesis

A number of techniques have been described for the measurement of tissue perfusion and evaluation of vascular development. The most important invasive methods are: radioisotopic clearance techniques, laser Doppler flowmetry and thermal clearance. Non-invasive techniques, such as positron emission tomography (PET), dynamic computered tomography (DCT) and Xenon-enhanced computer tomography, have been used to provide quantitative functional information on blood perfusion in the region of interest. In addition, recent developments in Doppler ultrasonography and Dynamic Magnetic Resonance Imaging allow non-invasive flow detection and evaluation of vascular development in small vessels of human subjects (Feldmann et al. 1993, Madjar et al. 1994, Kurjak et al. 1997, Francis et al. 1998, Dennie et al. 1998, Taylor et al. 1999, Yagel et al. 1999 a, b).

Angiogenesis in the Female Reproductive Tract

The cyclic development of new vasculature plays a crucial role in normal reproductive processes (e.g. follicular and endometrial development) and pathologic reproductive processes (e.g. ovarian hyperstimulation, follicular cyst formation, polycystic ovary, endometriosis, dysfunctional uterine bleeding). During follicular growth and the subsequent development of a corpus luteum, a complex vascular network develops within the thecal cell layer and, after ovulation, additional vessels develop towards ruptured follicle. Three angiogenic factors appear to play major role in ovarian angiogenesis: VEGF and angiopoietin-1 and -2 (Findlay 1986, Reynolds et al. 1992, Cooper et al. 1995, Jaffe 2000). Distinct angiogenic factors (VEGF and angiopoietins) were shown not only to be important for the physiological changes but also to be associated with the pathogenesis of ovarian hyperstimulation syndrome (Levin et al 1998).

The growth of the endometrial vasculature begins during the proliferative phase and continues throughout the secretory phase of the menstrual cycle in preparation for implantation. The changes in the endometrial vasculature comprise an increase in the length, branching and coiling of the spiral arteries as the endometrium regenerates during each menstrual cycle. Sex steroids and other angiogenic factors regulate vascular function during the menstrual cycle. VEGF was shown to increase 3-fold in the secretory phase and rise toward menstruation as compared with the proliferative phase (Torry et al. 1996). Both progesterone and estrogen have been shown to induce VEGF expression in human uterine stromal cells, whereas RU-486 blocked this effect (Hyder and Stancel 1999). FGF was shown to be upregulated by progesterone and prolactin in rat endometrium (Srivastava et al. 1998, Rider and Psychyos, 1994).

The Role of Vasculogenesis and Angiogenesis in Placental Development and Uterine Adaptation

Uterine Adaptation to Pregnancy

An adequate nutrient and substrate supply is essential for the normal intrauterine development of the fetus. Disturbances in uterine blood supply are associated with higher perinatal morbidity and mortality due to preterm delivery, pre-eclampsia and pregnancy disorders such as intrauterine growth restriction (IUGR).

Adaptation of the uterine vasculature to the rising needs of the fetus occurs through both vasodilation and the growth and development of new vessels. Angiogenesis, which is the process of blood vessel formation in direct response to tissue demands, plays an important role in the pregnancy-associated changes in the reproductive tract. The endometrium, decidua and placenta are rich sources of angiogenic growth factors (Folkman and Klagsbrun 1987, Reynolds, Killilea and Redmer 1992, Torry and Rongish 1992, Hyder and Stancel 1999).

Since the uterus and its contents demand an increased supply of blood during pregnancy, its vasculature undergoes three main adaptative changes: vasodilation; increased permeability; and growth and development of new vessels (Reynolds, Killilea and Redmer 1992, Torry and Rongish 1992).

In the early stages of human pregnancy (7–11 days), intact capillaries grow and surround the syncytiotrophoblast layer. These capillaries form a capillary plexus connected to the syncytiotrophoblast lacunae and constitute the first very simple vascular system supplying the embryo (Harris and Ramsay 1966, Burton, Jauniaux and Watson 1999). Concurrent with the growth of the uterus and vascular adaptation at the fetomaternal interface, there are also profound changes in the vascular system of the deeper part of the uterus supplied by basal arteries. The extent of these changes was demonstrated by Horn (1918), who compared the uterine vasculature of nulliparae and non-pregnant multiparae and multiparae in the first month of pregnancy. His data clearly demonstrated permanent angiogenic changes of the uterine vasculature in response to pregnancy (Horn 1918).

The idea that these physiological changes in the uterine circulation are hormonally regulated, by a factor of trophoblast origin, was first advanced by Beker (1948). In our recent studies we focused on human chorionic gonadotropin (hCG), a hormone responsible for numerous pregnancy-related and pregnancy-maintaining changes (Rao 1998). We were able to show that hCG, in addition to its invasion-stimulating action on the trophoblastic cells (Zygmunt et al. 1998), has a direct angiogenic effect and that hCG/LH receptor-expressing uterine endothelial cells respond to hCG treatment with increased capillary formation in vitro. These findings support the hypothesis that hCG may have a key regulatory role in angiogenesis and vascular function in the female reproductive tract (Keller et al. 1999). In subsequent experiments, we demonstrated that phorbol ester (a kinase C activator), but not cAMP or forskolin (a kinase A activator) mimicked hCG actions in our model, indicating that protein kinase C (PKC) is part of the signal transduction pathway utilized during hCG-induced tube formation. Possible subsequent events of signal transduction may involve activation of extracellular signal-regulated kinases (ERK-1 and ERK-2), mitogen-activated protein kinases (MAP) as well as myosin light chain kinase (MLCK) (McKinnon and Zygmunt, unpublished observations). In addition to its direct angiogenic function, we showed that hCG might also act as an indirect angiogenic factor within the female reproductive tract by inducing VEGF in human macrophages (Zygmunt et al. 2000).

We have also shown that insulin-like growth factor-II (IGF-II), which is highly expressed in cytotrophoblast, promotes uterine angiogenesis. We hypothesized that these actions of IGF-II are mediated through IGF-type 2 receptor (IGF-IIR), which is expressed on the endothelium of myometrial and endometrial vasculature (Herr et al. 2000).

Placental Vasculogenesis and Angiogenesis

Placental vascular growth begins as early as 21 days post-conception (Demir et al. 1989, Asan et al. 1999) and continues throughout gestation. At this stage the primary villi are composed of a massive core of cytotrophoblast covered by a thick layer of syncytiotrophoblast. With the development of the secondary villi a core of irregularly dispersed, homogeneous connective tissue cells can be recognized beneath the cytotrophoblast layer. Vasculogenesis can first be observed at the stage of early tertiary villi. At this stage, roundish or cord-like masses of hemangiogenetic cells can be distinguished. At 28 days post-conception a clearly defined lumen is visible. In later stages of development (32 days post-conception and more) erythrocytes can be observed within the vascular lumen, as well as a still incomplete layer of pericytes. There is sprouting of new vessels from the distal ends of existing capillaries at this stage. At six weeks of gestation, a basal lamina can be detected around the villous vessels. The development of villous capillaries from hemangioblastic cells can be observed until 10–12 weeks of gestation. From 12 weeks onwards, the capillaries coil, bulge, form sinusoids and protrude towards the trophoblastic layer, forming a so-called syncytio-capillary membrane. Although reliable signs of formation of new vessels are absent in the second half of pregnancy, some capillary sprouts can be seen. It is possible to differentiate between stem, intermediate and terminal villi at this stage of gestation, the latter being responsible for nutrient and gas exchange between fetus and mother.

Human placenta is a rich source of angiogenic substances and these may play an important role in the regulation of placental vessel formation as well as in maternal vascular adaptation to pregnancy. VEGF expression has been described in villous trophoblast and fetal macrophages within villous stroma, although the villous endothelium lacked immunostaining for VEGF (Jackson et al. 1994, Sharkey et al. 1993, Shiraishi et al. 1996). VEGFR-1 and VEGFR-2 are expressed on both villous endothelial cells and cytotrophoblast, suggesting a possible role of VEGF not only in vessel formation but also in trophoblastic invasion (Charnock-Jones et al. 1994, Cooper et al. 1995, Clark et al. 1996). Recently, a circulating antagonist of VEGF was described in maternal circulation (Clark et al. 1998). Another member of the VEGF family, PlGF, has been also detected in the villous trophoblast and in the tunica media of larger stem vessels (Khaliq et al. 1996). It has been shown that bFGF is expressed in the villous trophoblast and could be detected in the conditioned medium of the villous tissue explants (Hamai et al. 1998). Proliferin (PLF) and proliferin-related protein (PRP) – two prolactin related peptides expressed by trophoblast giant cells – have been identified as potent regulators of angiogenesis in the murine placenta (Jackson et al. 1994), although the role of these placental proteins has yet to be evaluated in humans (for review see Linzer and Fisher 1999). Recent studies by Goldman-Wohl and collegues (2000) revealed the presence of another receptor–ligand pair in the feto-maternal interface. Angiopoietin-1 was shown to be expressed in the syncytiotrophoblast during the first trimester, whereas Tie-2 receptor was observed in fetal and maternal endothelium as well as in endovascular trophoblast, suggesting an involvement in fetal and maternal vasculature development. Also another recently described angiogenic factor, leptin, is expressed in the placenta and serum during pregnancy and may play a role in vascular development during pregnency (Tamura et al. 1998, Bouloumie et al. 1998, Sierra-Honigmann et al. 1998).

Impaired Angiogenesis and Pregnancy Associated Disorders

Early Pregnancy Wastage

Vascularization of the human embryo takes place very early in pregnancy (second week post-conception) and is initiated in the extraembryonic areas. It has been shown that there is a close relationship between embryonic development and the state of vascularization of the chorionic villi and that normal chorionic villous vascularization is essential for the undisturbed development of pregnancy (te Velde et al. 1997). Meegdes and collegues (1988) described a poor vascular development in cases of intrauterine embryonic death and blighted ova compared to normal villous tissue obtained from legal abortions. These villi were characterized by significantly lower vascular density, fibrosis and hydropic degeneration. Since early pregnancy wastage is often associated with chromosomal, metabolic or endocrine disorders, further studies are necessary to establish defective vasculature development as a causal factor in these cases. A recent study by Vuorela and colleagues (2000) described diminished placental trophoblastic VEGF immunoreactivity, reduced placental trophoblastic Tie-1 and Tie-2 expression and weaker VEGFR-1, VEGFR-2, Tie-1 and Tie-2 expression in decidual endothelium of spontaneous abortions. The group also noted differences in the expression of von Willebrand factor (vWF) in the villous vessels of spontaneous and artificial abortions. On the other hand, increased blood vessel density in the parietal decidua was associated with early pregnancy losses, stressing the crucial role of vascular development in early pregnancy (Qiao et al. 1997, Vailhe et al. 1999).

Pre-eclampsia

Pre-eclampsia is a leading cause of perinatal morbidity and mortality. Although its exact etiology remains unknown, regulation of vascular growth in the fetomaternal unit seems to be disturbed, leading to defective placentation (van Beck and Peeters 1998, Dekker and Sibai 1998). Salafia and colleagues (1995) demonstrated a positive correlation between the occurrence of uteroplacental vascular lesions and related villous lesions (avascular villi, chronic villitis, hemorrhagic endovasculitis) and pre-eclampsia. Recent studies have demonstrated a selective deficit of angiogenic factors – VEGF and PlGF – in the blood of pre-eclamptic women (Torry et al. 1998, Reuvenkamp et al. 1999) and of VEGF in umbilical vein blood of pre-eclamptic pregnancies (Lyall et al. 1997). However, Sharkey and colleagues (1996) found increased VEGF levels in women with pre-eclampsia and speculated that VEGF may be involved in the maternal endothelial cell dysfunction that is associated with this condition. Also the expression of the Tie receptor (an angiogenin receptor essential in the process of angiogenesis) is significantly higher in healthy women compared to pre-eclamptic women at term (Vuorela et al. 1998).

Alterations in the expression of angiogenic factors were also demonstrated within the placenta. Cooper and colleagues (1996) showed that mRNA for VEGF and its receptor flt-1 are significantly lower in placental biopsies from pre-eclamptic placentae, suggesting that this abnormality in the expression of growth factors may lead to reduced fetal capillary branching.

Intrauterine Growth Restriction (IUGR)

Disturbances in the development of the villous tree and pathological changes in the villous vascular system characterized by chronic villitis, infarctions and haemorrhagic endovasculitis with subsequent insufficient utero-placental blood flow, have been linked to the pathogenesis of IUGR (Morrow et al. 1989, Nordenvall et al. 1991, Macara et al. 1996, Sato et al. 1995).

Evaluation of the structure of the vascular tree in IUGR revealed a significantly lower number of terminal villi as compared to normal term placentae (Teasdale 1984, Krebs et al. 1996). Furthermore, a reduction in the surface areas and volumes of terminal villi in growth-restricted pregnancies was described by Jackson et al. (1995). Previous studies showed that the degree of vascularization within terminal villi was significantly lower in the IUGR placentae. IUGR cotyledonary arteries were thin and less branched, whereas villous vessels exhibited fewer branches and a majority of their loops were uncoiled (Hitschold et al. 1993, Krebs et al. 1996, Jackson et al. 1995). Recent spectral Doppler-imaging studies have determinated abnormal placental blood flow associated with vascular abnormalities in 60% of cases (Todros et al. 1999, Yagel et al. 1999b), strongly indicating a relationship between placental vascular pathology and IUGR.

Gestational Diabetes and Maternal Diabetes Mellitus

A number of light microscopic, electron microscopic and histochemical studies have been performed on the placentae from women with diabetes mellitus and gestational diabetes. Some of these studies showed a significant increase in the length, diameter and surface area of the placental capillary bed (Jones and Fox 1976, Jacomo et al. 1976, Mayhew et al. 1994), whereas these capillaries appeared unduly immature to other authors (Kami and Mitsui, 1984). In addition, signs of diabetic angiopathy with capillary proliferation, accelerated aging, thickening of the capillary basement membrane and increased fibrosis have been described (Asmussen 1982). Other groups have demonstrated slightly decreased villous vessel cross-sectional area and a reduced degree of vascularization in diabetic placentae (Stoz, Schuhmann and Schmid 1987).

Physiological and Pathological Angiogenesis: A Brief Comparision

Since physiologic neovascularization is tightly regulated, both temporally and spatially, and tumor angiogenesis is characterized by uncontrolled neovascularization, knowledge of the molecular differences in the initiation and termination of the two processes should prove important in developing strategies for the treatment of angiogenesis-related diseases, including anti-tumor therapy. Although the master regulator of neovascularization has yet to be found, the switch to angiogenesis is most likely regulated by a change in the local equilibrium between angiogenic factors and their inhibitors (Holmgren, O'Reilly and Folkman 1995, Hanahan and Folkman 1996). It seems that the induction of angiogenesis is part of the tumor phenotype, rather than being a consequence of uncontrolled tumor growth, and it is initiated very early in the development of the tumor. A number of angiogenic factors are upregulated in tumors. These include VEGF, FGF, TNFα and IL-8. It has been shown that VEGF mRNA and protein are upregulated in response to both oxygen and glucose deprivation, a common situation during tumor development. There is a strong correlation between the degree of vascularization of a tumor and VEGF expression (Berkman et al. 1993). In addition, VEGF R-1 and -2 mRNA are upregulated in tumor-associated endothelial cells (Plate and Risau 1995). Elevated levels of FGF have been reported in a number of different tumors (Arbeit, Olson and Hanahan 1996, Smith et al. 1999). FGF receptors are also overexpressed in a variety of neoplastic tumors (Jacquemier et al. 1994). Other factors like TGFβ, TNFα, IL-1 and IL-8 are also differently regulated in tumors and might contribute to the tumor-associated vascularisation.

A number of oncogenes and tumor suppressor genes are also expressed differently by a variety of tumors and may play an important role in the induction and regulation of angiogenesis. Oncogenes are genes whose products (e.g. growth factors, growth factor receptors, members of different intracellular signaling proteins, transcriptional factors) have the ability to influence functions directly or indirectly related to cellular growth and to transform eukariotic cells to tumorgenic cells. It has been shown that *Ras* oncogene and c-ets-1 oncogenic transcriptional factor are involved in the regulation of endothelial cell motility and the expression of genes involved in matrix degradation. The *Ras*, *fos*, *v-myc* and *c-jun* oncogenes might also stimulate the expression of VEGF or downregulate the expression of inhibitors of angiogenesis (e.g. thrombospondin). Several tumor suppressor genes (e.g. p53) also negatively regulate angiogenesis, and mutation or loss of these genes might be responsible for the angiogenic switch (Rak et al. 1995, Rastinejad and Bouck 1997).

The vessels that result from tumor-induced angiogenesis differ in several important points from normal vessels. In general, tumor vasculature is immature and poorly differentiated, due to rapid growth and development (Blood and Zetter, 1990). The endothelial cells are larger, thicker and irregular in shape and there are less cells in the cross-section of the vessels. The basement membranes of these vessels are frequently discontinuous, pericytes, smooth muscle cells and innervation are missing and there is a increased occurence of dilatation and sinuses (Denekamp, 1990, Blood and Zetter 1990). The composition of ECM is also different in tumor-induced vessels. Tumor-induced ECM is characterized by a high concentration of hyaluronic acid and low concentration of heparan sulphate normally responsible for the sequestration and modulation of the angiogenic heparin-binding growth factors and cytokines (e.g. bFGF, VEGF, TGF beta) (Blood and Zetter 1990).

These morphological changes account for functional differences and lead to an increase in microvascular permeability and decreased flow velocity (Endrich, Hammersen and Messmer 1988), further facilitating tumor growth and metastasis.

Conclusion

There are striking similarities between, on the one hand, tumor invasion and tumor-induced vascularization and, on the other hand, trophoblast invasion and placental development. However, our understanding of the different molecular and functional aspects of these two different processes, in particular the self-limitation of the trophoblastic invasion and vessel formation during gestation, might allow the establishment of new therapeutic strategies for the treatment of both tumor and pregnancy related pathology and tumor.

Acknowledgements

The author thanks Dr. Anthony M. Carter and Dr. Petra M. Zygmunt for useful discussion and comments and reviewing of the manuscript. The work of our laboratory was supported by a grant from the German Research Council (DFG).

References

Arbeit JM, Olson DC, Hanahan D. Upregulation of fibroblast growth factors and their receptors during multi-stage epidermal carcinogenesis in K14-HPV16 transgenic mice. Oncogene 1996; 13(9):1847–57

Asan E, Kaymaz FF, Cakar AN, Dagdeviren A, Beksac MS. Vasculogenesis in early human placental villi: an ultrastructural study. Anat Anz 1999; 181(6):549–54

Asmussen I. Vascular morphology in diabetic placentas. Contrib Gynecol Obstet 1982; 9:76–85

Ausprunk DH, Knighton DR, Folkman J. Vascularization of normal and neoplastic tissues grafted to the chick chorioallantois. Role of host and pre-existing graft blood vessels. Am J Pathol 1975; 79(3):597–628

Baird A, Klagsbrun M. The fibroblast growth factor family. Cancer Cells 1991; 3(6):239–43

Beker JC. Aetiology of eclampsia. Br J Obstet Gynaecol 1948; 756–65

Berkman RA, Merrill MJ, Reinhold WC, Monacci WT, Saxena A, Clark WC, Robertson JT, Ali IU, Oldfield EH. Expression of the vascular permeability factor/vascular endothelial growth factor gene in central nervous system neoplasms. J Clin Invest 1993; 91(1):153–9

Blood CH, Zetter BR. Tumor interactions with the vasculature: angiogenesis and tumor metastasis. Biochim Biophys Acta 1990; 1032(1):89–118

Bouloumie A, Drexler HC, Lafontan M, Busse R. Leptin, the product of Ob gene, promotes angiogenesis. Circ Res 1998; 83(10):1059–66

Brooks PC, Clark RA, Cheresh DA. Requirement of vascular integrin alpha v beta 3 for angiogenesis. Science 1994; 264(5158):569–71

Burton GJ, Jauniaux E, Watson A. Maternal arterial connections to the placental intervillous space during the first trimester of human pregnancy: the Boyd collection revisited. Am J Obstet Gynecol 1999; 181(3):718–24

Charnock-Jones DS, Sharkey AM, Boocock CA, Ahmed A, Plevin R, Ferrara N, Smith SK. Vascular endothelial growth factor receptor localization and activation in human trophoblast and choriocarcinoma cells. Biol Reprod 1994; 51(3):524–30

Clark DE, Smith SK, He Y, Day KA, Licence DR, Corps AN, Lammoglia R, Charnock-Jones DS. A vascular endothelial growth factor antagonist is produced by the human placenta and released into the maternal circulation. Biol Reprod 1998; 59(6):1540–8

Clark DE, Smith SK, Sharkey AM, Charnock-Jones DS. Localization of VEGF and expression of its receptors flt and KDR in human placenta throughout pregnancy. Hum Reprod 1996; 11(5):1090–8

VEGF mRNA levels in placentae from pregnancies complicated by pre-eclampsia. Br J Obstet Gynaecol 1996; 103(12):1191–6.

Cooper JC, Sharkey AM, McLaren J, Charnock-Jones DS, Smith SK. Localization of vascular endothelial growth factor and its receptor, flt, in human placenta and decidua by immunohistochemistry. J Reprod Fertil 1995; 105(2):205–13

Dekker GA, Sibai BM. Etiology and pathogenesis of pre-eclampsia: current concepts. Am J Obstet Gynecol 1998; 179(5):1359–75

Demir R, Kaufmann P, Castellucci M, Erbengi T, Kotowski A. Fetal vasculogenesis and angiogenesis in human placental villi. Acta Anat (Basel) 1989; 136(3):190–203
Denekamp J. Vascular attack as a therapeutic strategy for cancer. Cancer Metastasis Rev 1990; 9(3):267–82
Dennie J, Mandeville JB, Boxerman JL, Packard SD, Rosen BR, Weisskoff RM. NMR imaging of changes in vascular morphology due to tumor angiogenesis. Magn Reson Med 1998; 40(6):793–9
DiPietro LA, Polverini PJ. Angiogenic macrophages produce the angiogenic inhibitor thrombospondin 1. Am J Pathol 1993; 143(3):678–84
Dunk C, Shams M, Nijjar S, Rhaman M, Qiu Y, Bussolati B, Ahmed A. Angiopoietin-1 and angiopoietin-2 activate trophoblast Tie-2 to promote growth and migration during placental development. Am J Pathol 2000; 156(6):2185–99
Endrich B, Hammersen F, Messmer K. Capillary ultrastructure and microcirculatory function of malignant tumors. Adv Exp Med Biol 1988; 242:205–14
Feldmann HJ, Sievers K, Fuller J, Molls M, Lohr E. Evaluation of tumor blood perfusion by dynamic MRI and CT in patients undergoing thermoradiotherapy. Eur J Radiol 1993; 16(3):224–9
Ferrara N, Chen H, Davis-Smyth T, Gerber HP, Nguyen TN, Peers D, Chisholm V, Hillan KJ, Schwall RH. Vascular endothelial growth factor is essential for corpus luteum angiogenesis. Nat Med 1998; 4(3):336–40
Ferrara N, Davis-Smyth T. The biology of vascular endothelial growth factor. Endocr Rev 1997; 18(1):4–25
Findlay JK. Angiogenesis in reproductive tissues. J Endocrinol 1986; 111(3):357–66
Flamme I, Frolich T, Risau W. Molecular mechanisms of vasculogenesis and embryonic angiogenesis. J Cell Physiol 1997; 173(2):206–10
Folkman J. Angiogenesis in cancer, vascular, rheumatoid and other disease. Nat Med 1995; 1(1):27–31
Folkman J, Klagsbrun M. Angiogenic factors. Science 1987; 235(4787):442–7
Folkman J, Shing Y. Angiogenesis. J Biol Chem 1992; 267(16):10931–4
Francis ST, Duncan KR, Moore RJ, Baker PN, Johnson IR, Gowland PA. Non-invasive mapping of placental perfusion. Lancet 1998; 351(9113):1397–9
Galland F, Karamysheva A, Pebusque MJ, Borg JP, Rottapel R, Dubreuil P, Rosnet O, Birnbaum D. The FLT4 gene encodes a transmembrane tyrosine kinase related to the vascular endothelial growth factor receptor. Oncogene 1993; 8(5):1233–40
Gimbrone MA Jr, Cotran RS, Leapman SB, Folkman J. Tumor growth and neovascularization: an experimental model using the rabbit cornea. J Natl Cancer Inst 1974; 52(2):413–27
Goldman-Wohl DS, Ariel I, Greenfield C, Lavy Y, Yagel S. Tie-2 and angiopoietin-2 expression at the fetal-maternal interface: a receptor ligand model for vascular remodelling. Mol Hum Reprod 2000; 6(1):81–7
Hamai Y, Fujii T, Yamashita T, Kozuma S, Okai T, Taketani Y. Evidence for basic fibroblast growth factor as a crucial angiogenic growth factor, released from human trophoblasts during early gestation. Placenta 1998; 19(2-3):149–55
Hammes HP, Brownlee M, Jonczyk A, Sutter A, Preissner KT. Subcutaneous injection of a cyclic peptide antagonist of vitronectin receptor-type integrins inhibits retinal neovascularization. Nat Med 1996; 2(5):529–33
Hanahan D, Folkman J. Patterns and emerging mechanisms of the angiogenic switch during tumorigenesis. Cell 1996; 86(3):353–64
Harris J, Ramsay E. The morphology of human uteroplacentare vasculature. Contrib Embryo 1966; 230:45–57
Hayes AJ, Huang WQ, Mallah J, Yang D, Lippman ME, Li LY. Angiopoietin-1 and its receptor Tie-2 participate in the regulation of capillary-like tubule formation and survival of endothelial cells. Microvasc Res 1999; 58(3):224–37
Herr F, Lang U, Han VKM, Zygmunt M. Insulin-like Growth Factor-II and its receptors in vascular adaptation to pregnancy. Placenta (2000) 21:78A 22
Hitschhold-T, Weiss-E, Beck-T et al. Low target birthweight in growth retardation? Umbilical Doppler velocity waveforms and histomorphic analysis of fetoplacental vascular tree. Am J Obstet and Gynecol 1993; 168:1260–4
Hockel M, Schlenger K, Doctrow S, Kissel T, Vaupel P. Therapeutic angiogenesis. Arch Surg 1993; 128(4):423–9
Holmgren L, O'Reilly MS, Folkman J. Dormancy of micrometastases: balanced proliferation and apoptosis in the presence of angiogenesis suppression. Nat Med 1995; 1(2):149–53
Horn O. Histologische Studien über den menschlichen. Uterus 1918; Karger Berlin
Hyder SM, Stancel GM. Regulation of angiogenic growth factors in the female reproductive tract by estrogens and progestins. Mol Endocrinol 1999; 13(6):806–11
Jackson MR, Carney EW, Lye SJ, Ritchie JW. Localization of two angiogenic growth factors (PDECGF and VEGF) in human placentae throughout gestation. Placenta 1994; 15(4):341–53
Jackson MR, Walsh AJ, Morrow RJ, Mullen JB, Lye SJ, Ritchie JWK. Reduced placental villous tree elaboration in small-for-gestational-age pregnancies: Relationship with umbilical artery Doppler waveforms. Am J Obstet Gynecol 1995; 172 (2):518–25

Jacomo KH, Benedetti WL, Sala MA, Alvarez H. Pathology of the trophoblast and fetal vessels of the placenta in maternal diabetes mellitus. Acta Diabetol Lat 1976; 13(5-6):216–35
Jacquemier J, Adelaide J, Parc P, Penault-Llorca F, Planche J, de Lapeyriere O, Birnbaum D. Expression of the FGFR1 gene in human breast-carcinoma cells. Int J Cancer 1994; 59(3):373–8
Jaffe RB. Importance of angiogenesis in reproductive physiology. Semin Perinatol 2000; 24(1):79–81
Jones CJ, Fox H. Placental changes in gestational diabetes. An ultrastructural study. Obstet Gynecol 1976; 48(3):274–80
Kami K, Mitsui T. Ultrastructural observations of chorionic villi at term in diabetic women. Tokai J Exp Clin Med 1984; 9(1):53–67
Keller S, Wienhard J, Lang U, Zygmunt M. Human chorionic gonadotropin (hCG) is an angiogenetic factor for uterine endothelial cells in vitro. Placenta 1999; (20):A37
Khaliq A, Li XF, Shams M, Sisi P, Acevedo CA, Whittle MJ, Weich H, Ahmed A. Localisation of placenta growth factor (PIGF) in human term placenta. Growth Factors 1996; 13(3-4):243–50
Klagsbrun M. Mediators of angiogenesis: the biological significance of basic fibroblast growth factor (bFGF)-heparin and heparan sulfate interactions. Semin Cancer Biol 1992; Apr.3(2):81–7
Krebs C, Macara LM, Leiser R, Bowman AW, Greer IA, Kingdom JCP. Intrauterine growth restriction with absent end-diastolic flow velocity in the umbilical artery is associated with maldevelopment of the placental tree. Am J Obstet and Gynecol 1996; 175:1534–42
Kurjak A, Dudenhausen JW, Hafner T, Kupesic S, Latin V, Kos M. Intervillous circulation in all three trimesters of normal pregnancy assessed by color Doppler. J Perinat Med 1997; 25(4):373–80
Langer R, Folkman J. Polymers for the sustained release of proteins and other macromolecules. Nature 1976; 263(5580):797–800
Levin ER, Rosen GF, Cassidenti DL, Yee B, Meldrum D, Wisot A, Pedram A. Role of vascular endothelial cell growth factor in Ovarian Hyperstimulation Syndrome. J Clin Invest 1998; 102(11):1978–85
Linzer DI, Fisher SJ. The placenta and the prolactin family of hormones: regulation of the physiology of pregnancy. Mol Endocrinol 1999; 13(6):837–40
Lyall F, Young A, Boswell F, Kingdom JC, Greer IA. Placental expression of vascular endothelial growth factor in placentae from pregnancies complicated by pre-eclampsia and intrauterine growth restriction does not support placental hypoxia at delivery. Placenta 1997; 18(4):269–76
Macara L, Kingdom JCP, Kaufmann P et al. Structural analysis of placental terminal villi from growth-restricted pregnancies with abnormal umbilical artery Doppler waveforms. Placenta 1996; 17:37–48
Madjar H, Prompeler HJ, Sauerbrei W, Wolfarth R, Pfleiderer A. Color Doppler flow criteria of breast lesions. Ultrasound Med Biol 1994; 20(9):849–58
Mayhew TM, Sorensen FB, Klebe JG, Jackson MR. Growth and maturation of villi in placentae from well-controlled diabetic women. Placenta 1994; Jan.15(1):57–65
Meegdes BH, Ingenhoes R, Peeters LL, Exalto N. Early pregnancy wastage: relationship between chorionic vascularization and embryonic development. Fertil Steril 1988; 49(2):216–20
Morrow RJ, Adamson SL, Bull SB et al. Effect of placental embolization on the umbilical artery waveforms in fetal sheep. Am J Obst and Gynecol 1989; 161:1055–60
Muthukkaruppan V, Auerbach R. Angiogenesis in the mouse cornea. Science 1979; 205(4413):1416–8
Nehls V, Drenckhahn D. A novel, microcarrier-based in vitro assay for rapid and reliable quantification of three-dimensional cell migration and angiogenesis. Microvasc Res 1995; 50(3):311–22
Nelson MJ, Conley FK, Fajardo LF. Application of the disc angiogenesis system to tumor-induced neovascularization. Exp Mol Pathol 1993; 58(2):105–13
Nordenvall M, Ullberg U, Laurin G et al. Placental morphology in relation to umbilical artery blood velocity waveforms. Eur J Obstet and Gynecol and Reprod Biol 1991; 40:179–90
Norrby K, Jakobsson A, Sorbo J. Mast cell-mediated angiogenesis: a novel experimental model using the rat mesentery. Virchows Arch B Cell Pathol Incl Mol Pathol 1986; 52(3):195–206
O'Reilly MS, Holmgren L, Shing Y, Chen C, Rosenthal RA, Moses M, Lane WS, Cao Y, Sage EH, Folkman J. Angiostatin: a novel angiogenesis inhibitor that mediates the suppression of metastases by a Lewis lung carcinoma. Cell 1994; 79(2):315–28
Plate KH, Risau W. Angiogenesis in malignant gliomas. Glia 1995; 15(3):339–47
Poole TJ, Coffin JD. Vasculogenesis and angiogenesis: two distinct morphogenetic mechanisms establish embryonic vascular pattern. J Exp Zool 1989; 251(2):224–31
Qiao S, Nagasaka T, Nakashima N. Numerous vessels detected by CD34 in the villous stroma of complete hydatidiform moles. Int J Gynecol Pathol 1997 16(3):233–8
Rak J, Filmus J, Finkenzeller G, Grugel S, Marme D, Kerbel RS. Oncogenes as inducers of tumor angiogenesis. Cancer Metastasis Rev 1995; 14(4):263–77
Rao CV. Novel Concepts iIn Neuroendocrine Regulation of Reproductive Tract Functions. In: The Endocrinology of Pregnancy, Totowa NJ: Humana Press, 1998: 125–44

Rastinejad F, Bouck N. Oncogenes and tumor suppressor genes in the regulation of angiogenesis. In: Bicknell R, Lewis C, Ferrara N (eds), Tumor Angiogenesis. Oxford University Press, 1997: 101–10
Reuvekamp A, Velsing-Aarts FV, Poulina IE, Capello JJ, Duits AJ. Selective deficit of angiogenic growth factors characterises pregnancies complicated by pre-eclampsia. Br J Obstet Gynaecol 1999; 106(10):1019–22
Reynolds LP, Killilea SD, Redmer DA. Angiogenesis in the female reproductive system. FASEB J 1992; 6(3):886–92
Rider V, Psychoyos A .Inhibition of progesterone receptor function results in loss of basic fibroblast growth factor expression and stromal cell proliferation during uterine remodelling in the pregnant rat. J Endocrinol 1994; 140(2):239–49
Risau W. Mechanisms of angiogenesis. Nature 1997; 386(6626):671–4
Risau W, Flamme I. Vasculogenesis. Annu Rev Cell Dev Biol 1995; 11:73–91
Salafia CM, Pezzullo JC, Lopez-Zeno JA, Simmens S, Minior VK, Vintzileos AM. Placental pathologic features of preterm pre-eclampsia. Am J Obstet Gynecol 1995; 173(4):1097–105
Salafia CM, Pezzullo JC, Minior VK, Divon MY. Placental pathology of absent and reversed end-diastolic flow in growth-restricted fetuses. Obstet Gynecol 1997; 90(5):830–6
Sato TN, Tozawa Y, Deutsch U, Wolburg-Buchholz K, Fujiwara Y, Gendron-Maguire M, Gridley T, Wolburg H, Risau W, Qin Y. Distinct roles of the receptor tyrosine kinases Tie-1 and Tie-2 in blood vessel formation. Nature 1995; 376(6535):70–4
Sharkey AM, Charnock-Jones DS, Boocock CA, Brown KD, Smith SK. Expression of mRNA for vascular endothelial growth factor in human placenta. J Reprod Fertil 1993; 99(2):609–15
Sharkey AM, Cooper JC, Balmforth JR, McLaren J, Clark DE, Charnock-Jones DS, Morris NH, Smith SK. Maternal plasma levels of vascular endothelial growth factor in normotensive pregnancies and in pregnancies complicated by pre-eclampsia. Eur J Clin Invest 1996; 26(12):1182–5
Shiraishi S, Nakagawa K, Kinukawa N, Nakano H, Sueishi K. Immunohistochemical localization of vascular endothelial growth factor in the human placenta. Placenta 1996; 17(2–3):111–21
Sierra-Honigmann MR, Nath AK, Murakami C, Garcia-Cardena G, Papapetropoulos A, Sessa WC, Madge LA, Schechner JS, Schwabb MB, Polverini PJ, Flores-Riveros JR. Biological action of leptin as an angiogenic factor. Science 1998; 281(5383):1683–6
Smith K, Fox SB, Whitehouse R, Taylor M, Greenall M, Clarke J, Harris AL. Upregulation of basic fibroblast growth factor in breast carcinoma and itsrelationship to vascular density, oestrogen receptor, epidermal growth factor receptor and survival. Ann Oncol 1999; Jun.10(6):707–13
Soker S, Takashima S, Miao HQ, Neufeld G, Klagsbrun M. Neuropilin-1 is expressed by endothelial and tumor cells as an isoform-specific receptor for vascular endothelial growth factor. Cell 1998; 92(6):735–45
Srivastava RK, Gu Y, Ayloo S, Zilberstein M, Gibori G. Developmental expression and regulation of basic fibroblast growth factor and vascular endothelial growth factor in rat decidua and in a decidual cell line. J Mol Endocrinol 1998; 21(3):355–62
Stoz F, Schuhmann RA, Schmid A. Morphometric investigations of terminal villi of diabetic placentas in relation to the White classification of diabetes mellitus. J Perinat Med 1987; 15(2):193–8
Suri C, McClain J, Thurston G, McDonald DM, Zhou H, Oldmixon EH, Sato TN, Yancopoulos GD. Increased vascularization in mice overexpressing angiopoietin-1. Science 1998; 282(5388):468–71
Takahashi T, Kalka C, Masuda H, Chen D, Silver M, Kearney M, Magner M, Isner JM, Asahara T. Ischemia- and cytokine-induced mobilization of bone marrow-derived endothelial progenitor cells for neovascularization. Nat Med 1999; 5(4):434–8
Tamura T, Goldenberg RL, Johnston KE, Cliver SP. Serum leptin concentrations during pregnancy and their relationship to fetal growth. Obstet Gynecol 1998; 91(3):389–95
Taylor JS, Tofts PS, Port R, Evelhoch JL, Knopp M, Reddick WE, Runge VM, Mayr N. MR imaging of tumor microcirculation: promise for the new millennium. J Magn Reson Imaging 1999 ;10(6):903–7
te Velde EA, Exalto N, Hesseling P, van der Linden HC. First trimester development of human chorionic villous vascularization studied with CD34 immunohistochemistry. Hum Reprod 1997; 12(7):1577–81
Idiopathic intrauterine growth retardation: histomorphometry of the human placenta. Placenta 1984; 5(1):83–92
Thompson WD, Li WW, Maragoudakis M. The clinical manipulation of angiogenesis: pathology, side effects, surprises, and opportunities with novel human therapies. J Pathol 2000; 190(3):330–7
Todros T, Sciarrone A, Piccoli E, Guiot C, Kaufmann P, Kingdom J. Umbilical Doppler waveforms and placental villous angiogenesis in pregnancies complicated by fetal growth restriction. Obstet Gynecol 1999; 93(4):499–503
Torry DS, Holt VJ, Keenan JA, Harris G, Caudle MR, Torry RJ. Vascular endothelial growth factor expression in cycling human endometrium. Fertil Steril 1996; Jul.66(1):72–80
Torry DS, Wang HS, Wang TH, Caudle MR, Torry RJ. Pre-eclampsia is associated with reduced serum levels of placenta growth factor. Am J Obstet Gynecol 1998; 179(6 Pt 1):1539–44

Torry RJ, Rongish BJ. Angiogenesis in the uterus: potential regulation and relation to tumor angiogenesis. Am J Reprod Immunol 1992; 27(3-4):171–9

Vailhe B, Dietl J, Kapp M, Toth B, Arck P. Increased blood vessel density in decidua parietalis is associated with spontaneous human first trimester abortion. Hum Reprod 1999; 14(6):1628–34

van Beck E, Peeters LL. Pathogenesis of pre-eclampsia: a comprehensive model. Obstet Gynecol Surv 1998; 53(4):233–9

Vuorela P, Carpen O, Tulppala M, Halmesmaki E. VEGF, its receptors and the tie receptors in recurrent miscarriage. Mol Hum Reprod 2000; 6(3):276–82

Vuorela P, Matikainen MT, Kuusela P, Ylikorkala O, Alitalo K, Halmesmaki E. Endothelial tie receptor antigen in maternal and cord blood of healthy and pre-eclamptic subjects. Obstet Gynecol 1998; 92(2):179–83

Wilting J, Christ B. A morphological study of the rabbit corneal assay. Anat Anz 1992; 174(6):549–56

Yagel S, Anteby EY, Shen O, Cohen SM, Friedman Z, Achiron R. Placental blood flow measured by simultaneous multigate spectral Doppler imaging in pregnancies complicated by placental vascular abnormalities. Ultrasound Obstet Gynecol 1999; 14(4):262–6

Yagel S, Anteby EY, Shen O, Cohen SM, Friedman Z, Achiron R. Simultaneous multigate spectral Doppler imaging of the umbilical artery and placental vessels: novel ultrasound technology. Ultrasound Obstet Gynecol 1999 14(4):256–61

Zygmunt M, Hahn D, Munstedt K, Bischof P, Lang U. Invasion of cytotrophoblastic JEG-3 cells is stimulated by hCG in vitro. Placenta 1998; 19(8):587–93

Zygmunt M, Mazzuca D, Han V. Human Chorionic Gonadotropin (hCG) induces VEGF expression in vitro. Placenta 2000 (in press)

21 Trophoblast Implantation Versus Tumor Invasion

Russell Foulk and Olga Genbacev

Introduction

The steps involved in hemochorial placentation bear a striking resemblance to tumor invasion. Interestingly, trophoblast and tumor invasion progress with very little, if any, tissue destruction, hemorrhage or necrosis. Undoubtedly, this is because the tumor cells mimic a physiologic process. The major difference between implantation (physiologic invasion) and tumor invasion (pathologic invasion) is that trophoblast invasion during implantation is spatially and temporally regulated whereas tumor cell invasion is not. The sequence of events leading to invasion is similar: it includes cellular attachment (apposition) to the host tissue, transmigration through a basal lamina, stromal infiltration, and aggressive penetration into blood vessels. The end-points, however, differ drastically.

One of the most important differences between tumor cells and trophoblasts is that tumor cells continue to divide as they invade whereas placental cytotrophoblast cells exit the cell cycle as they differentiate along the invasive pathway. Both tumor cells and trophoblasts invade interstitium and blood vessels (endovascular invasion). Endovascular and interstitial invasion of cytotrophoblasts is limited to the uterus whereas tumor invasion is widespread. This is partially due to the ability of tumor cells to extravasate from blood vessels at sites distant from the initial invasion and continue to proliferate and form new colonies. Invasive cytotrophoblasts are terminally differentiated cells of fetal origin (genetically different from the host cell). In contrast, tumor cells are dedifferentiated mutated cells initially derived from host cells. Tumor cells differ widely depending upon their class of origin. Unlike trophoblasts, which vary according to their stage of differentiation, tumor cells consist of many heterogenous cell populations. Some tumor cells, such as those from the prostate gland, are characterized by indolent growth and invasion; others, like those from choriocarcinoma, rapidly proliferate and invade. Different tumor cells have a plethora of mechanisms responsible for their diverse activity. Because of this extreme variety, only the general biochemical processes of tumor–tissue interactions that occur in invasion will be discussed here.

Much of what is known regarding the human pre-implantation trophoblast was discovered from direct observation following in vitro fertilization (IVF). Information regarding subsequent implantation in humans has been derived from laboratory animal data and available specimens of early implantation (Hustin and Franchimont 1992), including the Carnegie collections (O'Rahilly 1973). In addition, several human in vitro culture systems have been developed to investigate both individual trophoblast and villous trophoblast activities (Genbacev 1993b). Tumor cell biology has been studied by direct observation of the behavior of individual cancers in humans and animal models, extraction and purification of proteins produced by tumor cells, and isolation of genes expressed in cells with metastatic activity (Lawrence and Steeg 1997). This chapter will review the similarities and differences between the physiology of trophoblast implantation leading to the development of the fetoplacental unit and the pathophysiology of tumor invasion.

Mechanisms of Trophoblast and Tumor Invasion

Apposition

The blastocyst first initiates implantation through attachment of its outer shell of trophoectoderm to the uterine epithelium. This interaction has not been described in humans, but is assumed to involve cell-to-cell adhesion between the apical uterine epithelial cell and the epithelial-like trophoblast.

In contrast to tumor cells that can potentially infringe upon any tissue of the body, trophoblasts primarily attach to the prepared uterine decidualized endometrium. Prior to attachment, the endometrium undergoes profound synchronous changes. Indeed, there is a precisely controlled time, the "implantation window", in which the blastocyst may implant (Psychoyos and Martel 1985).

The trophoblast–endometrium dialogue is important, but not essential. Human blastocysts occasionally exhibit non-specific implantation in ectopic sites such as the fallopian tube, ovary or peritoneum. The process of trophoblast attachment to these surfaces probably differs from attachment to the uterus, but trophoblasts still differentiate through a coordinated series of events to placenta. Interestingly, the depth of invasion is greater in ectopic sites, suggesting decidual factors might control trophoblast invasion (Enders, Chavez and Schlafke 1981).

The hallmark of tumor spread is by metastasis. Apposition of tumor cells to tissue first requires a "traveling" cell. Metastatic tumor cells originate from a primary colony. Once dislodged, tumor cells typically travel via the lymphatic and/or vascular circulatory systems. Rather than "attach" to a receptive tissue, most tumor cells usually become lodged in a downstream capillary bed or lymph node, where they migrate across the vessel wall into the surrounding tissue. Most tumor cells begin with invasion of tissues anatomically downstream from the primary colony. Some tumor cells survive better in certain organs or tissues where the concentration of a mitogen, growth factor or hormone might attract or promote tumor cell growth. The vast majority of tumor cells do not survive the journey. It is estimated that fewer than one in 10,000 cells that leave the primary colony actually start a new tumor (Liotta 1992).

Invasion

Both trophoblasts and metastatic tumor cells manifest invasive properties. The term invasiveness implies the ability of cells to cross anatomic barriers. An appreciation of these physical barriers is required to understand the mechanisms of invasion. The first barrier, as discussed previously, is the layer of epithelial or endothelial cells through which the invasive cells must pass.

Immediately beneath the epithelial layer of cells is one specialized type of matrix called the basement membrane. The basement membrane is a thin (30–350 nm), continuous layer composed mainly of type IV collagen. The predominant non-collagenous components include heparan sulfate proteoglycan, laminin, tenascin and entactin (Paulsson 1992). The basement membrane functions as an anchor for surface epithelium and a separating layer by ensheathing blood vessels, muscle cells and nervous system. For invasive cells, the basement membrane is a big obstacle that requires great ingenuity to breach.

Beyond the basement membrane lies a highly variable matrix, called the interstitial stroma, which contains other tissue cells, vessels and lymphatic channels. Collagen fibers constitute the main component. Type I collagen combines with type III collagen to form rope-like structures that provide firmness to the matrix structure. Built upon this rope-like scaffold are attached elastin molecules and several glycoproteins that cross-link the meshwork, forming sheets that can stretch and recoil. The "filler" within this meshwork, called ground substance, contains functional molecules like the extremely hydrated glycosaminoglycans and the fibronectins, which are essential for cellular–matrix interactions.

Our knowledge of cytotrophoblast invasion of the uterus is derived from morphological observation of tissue sections of fetal–maternal interface that contain both floating and anchoring villi and the uterine wall (Boyd and Hamilton 1970; Pijnenborg et al. 1980, Fisher et al. 1989, Damsky, Fitzgerald and Fisher 1992). Placental bed biopsy is the only way to obtain anchoring villi, together with cytotrophoblasts involved in interstitial and endovascular invasion. An example of an anchoring villus and its uterine attachment site from a 15-week pregnancy is shown in Fig. 21.1. A second approach to the study of cytotrophoblast invasion is to use in vitro models: cytotrophoblast cell culture (Fisher et al. 1989, Librach et al. 1991), cytotrophoblast co-culture with endometrial tissue explants (Fig. 21.2), and villus explant cultures (Genbacev 1993b, 1996). Using these in vitro systems, it has been shown that removing cytotrophoblast cells from their basement membrane and plating them on extracellular matrix reprograms their fate such that they differentiate along the invasive pathway. It is important to note that in this mode, cytotrophoblasts isolated from term placentas have greatly reduced invasive capacity (Librach et al. 1991). This is analogous to the in vivo situation in which invasion is most active during the first half of pregnancy. The placenta's stage of development is probably important for limiting its tumor-like behavior.

Both the primary tumor and metastatic tumor cell colonies manifest invasive properties. Indeed, the definition of malignancy or cancer is the invasion of tumor cells across the basement membrane. Prior to crossing this barrier, tumor cells are considered dysplastic, but they may or may not have invasive capabilities. As with cytotrophoblasts, the capacity of tumor cells to invade may correlate with their stage of differentiation: however, their invasion and differentiation appear to be under separate control (Hohn 1998). Beyond the basement membrane, the invading cells face the less compact interstitial stroma through which to travel. Tumor cells require mechanisms comparable to those used by invading trophoblasts in order to navigate through this changing landscape.

Liotta describes a three-step process involved in tumor invasion (Liotta 1992). The first is adhesion to the basement membrane by specific receptors. The second step

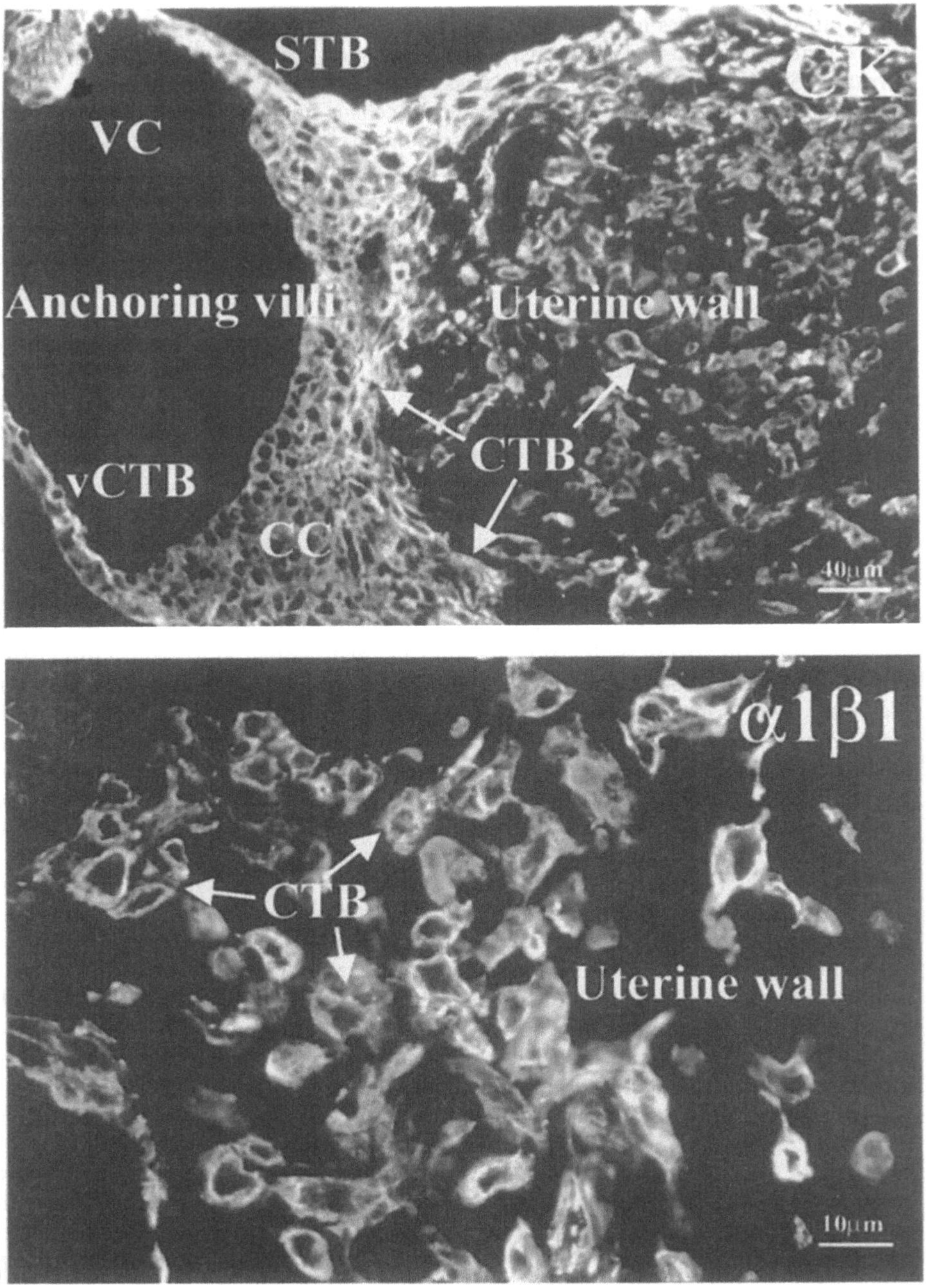

a

b

Figure 21.1 The maternal–fetal interface in the second trimester (15 weeks) of human pregnancy. Tissue section stained with cytokeratin (CK) antibody to detect cytotrophoblasts (CTB), shows a site where cell column (CC) from anchoring villi attaches to the uterine wall. VC–villus core; STB–syncytiotrophoblast. (Top scale 1cm = 40μm; bottom scale 1cm = 10μm)

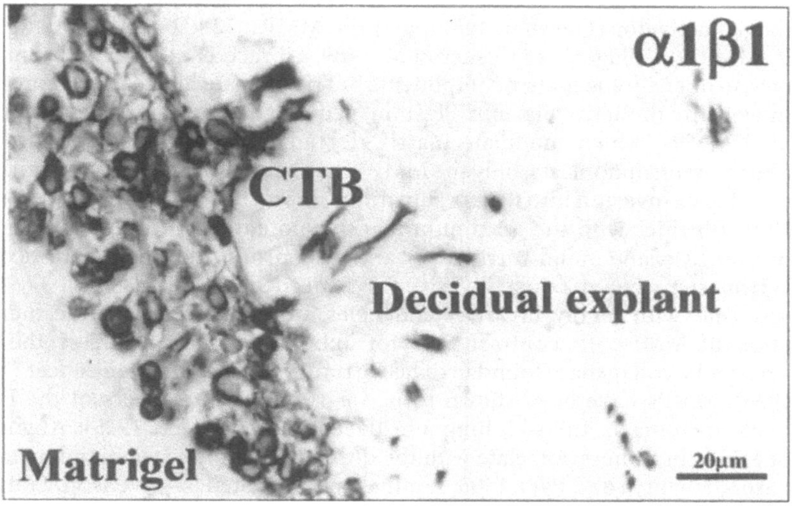

Figure 21.2 Co-culture of decidual explants (8 weeks of gestation) with first trimester (8–18 wks) cytotrophoblasts (CTB). First trimester cytotrophoblasts were co-cultured with decidual explants maintained on Matrigel for 24 hours. After 3 days co-cultures were fixed and frozen sections stained with antibody against integrin α1/β1. Cytotrophoblasts attached to and invaded into decidual tissue. Invasive cytotrophoblasts upregulated the expression of integrin α1/β1 (receptor for collagen I and IV and laminin) at the same pattern of expression as they do in vivo.

requires activation of agents capable of dissolving holes in the fabric of the intercellular matrix, including the basement membrane. The third is cellular transmigration by amoeboid-like motion through the channels. The degree of invasiveness manifested by tumor cells has been shown to correlate with the properties of the second step, namely the ability to lyse the extracellular matrix.

Proteases

Both cytotrophoblasts and tumor cells require the regulated expression of proteases to degrade the extracellular matrix. There are three major classes of matrix-degrading enzymes produced by most invasive cells:

1 serine proteases

2 cysteine proteases

3 matrix metalloproteases (MMPs).

Serine proteases are a class of enzymes that includes plasmin, plasminogen activators, elastases, thrombin and cathepsin G. Plasmin degrades non-collagenous matrix components, such as laminin and fibronectin. Elastases can degrade elastin fibers, which are resistant to most proteinases. Cysteine proteinases, such as cathepsin B, are capable of degrading matrix proteins such as type I collagen, laminin, and proteoglycans. MMPs are a family of three subsets of proteolytic enzymes that require zinc for their catalytic activity. These include collagenases, gelatinases and stromelysins.

The cytotrophoblasts begin to produce different proteases as they differentiate along the invasive pathway, including the serine protease urokinase-type plasminogen activator (Queenan 1987), and the MMPs: 72 kD (MMP-2) and 92 kD type IV (MMP-9) collagenases (Fisher et al. 1989, Librach et al. 1991). Plasminogen activators do not degrade matrix components but participate indirectly by converting plasminogen into the active plasmin. Plasmin mediates fibrinolysis and activates both TGFβ and MMPs, which modulate matrix degradation. Of the several proteases expressed by cytotrophoblasts, only the MMP-9 has been shown to be rate limiting for cytotrophoblasts invasion into matrix substrates (Librach et al. 1991). The expression of MMP-9 coincides with the maximum invasive potential of trophoblasts in mice (Behrendtsen, Alexander and Werb 1992), and peak production in humans occurs in the first trimester when maximal invasiveness is needed (Bass et al.1994).

Cancer cells with highly invasive tendencies are associated with the increased production of MMPs. In contrast to cytotrophoblasts, the MMP-2 is the more common type IV collagenase found in invasive tumors such as ovarian cancer (Young et al. 1996). MMPs have been shown to be instrumental in cancers of the human breast, colon, stomach, thyroid, lung and liver (Sato and Seiki 1996). Augmented levels of MMPs in tumors correlate with the development of invasion and metastasis (Triggvason, Hoyhtya and Pyke 1993; Bonfil et al. 1992; Stetler-Stevenson, Liotta and Kleiner 1993). Blocking antibodies against MMPs can actually abolish the invasive action of the tumor cells in vitro (Liotta 1992). In prostate and breast cancer, the serine protease, urokinase, and its receptor have been strongly implicated in tumor invasion (Rabbani and Xing 1998).

Control of extracellular protease activity is essential in regulating invasive capacity and is critical to the wellbeing of the host organism. The control to cease invasion represents a major difference between cytotrophoblasts and tumor cells. In the physiologic process of implantation several different mechanisms exert stringent control over the degradation of the extracellular matrix by proteinases, particularly MMPs. The control exists at all levels of proteinase production and activity, including transcription, translation, secretion and activation. In tumor cells, high levels of MMP mRNA may be induced by growth factors such as EGF, TGFβ, TNFα, and IL-1 (Matrisian 1993). In cytotrophoblasts, a variety of growth factors, cytokines, oncogenes and tumor promoters regulate transcription of MMPs. Once the MMP is synthesized, it is immediately secreted. This production "on demand" avoids enzyme excess and the need for storage. MMPs are secreted in a non-active form. Activation of most MMPs requires an active serine protease, such as plasmin, kallikrein or cathepsin B. MMP-2 is unique among MMPs in that it is resistant to proteolytic activation by serine proteases, but instead requires a membrane-type MMP. These MMP activators are themselves under separate control, such as plasmin whose activation is under the control of inhibitors PAI_1, PAI_2 and broad-spectrum proteinase inhibitors.

Decidualized endometrium is capable of controlling the invasive property of cytotrophoblasts. In an important demonstration of the cytotrophoblast–endometrium dialogue, trophoblast protease action is regulated by the concomitant uterine production of protease inhibitors. One mechanism of control is the coordinated expression of MMP-9 by cytotrophoblasts with endometrial expression of tissue inhibitors of metalloproteases, TIMP-1 and TIMP-2. For example, TIMP-3 is upregulated in parallel with MMP-9. A balance between the expression of proteinases and their inhibitors regulates cytotrophoblast invasion. This balance is controlled in part by cytokines and growth factors. TGFβ has been shown to exert regulatory control by induction of TIMP-1 in both decidua and cytotrophoblasts (Graham et al. 1992). In conditions where the endometrium is compromised, such as over a previous Cesarean scar, a higher degree of cytotrophoblast invasion is seen, creating a placenta accreta. Where the endometrium is absent, as in an ectopic pregnancy, cytotrophoblast invasion again exceeds physiologic depths.

Tumor cells also express TIMPs to a varying degree. These inhibit MMP action as they do in cytotrophoblasts. Many tumor cells secrete TIMP-2. Several laboratories have demonstrated a loss of tumor cell invasion with the addition of TIMPs to cell culture. The inhibition occurs by non-covalent binding of MMPs in a 1:1 molar ratio. Tumor cell protease activity is subjected to the balance of both positive and negative regulatory proteins, but the greater expression of protease molecules tilts the balance toward unchecked secretion and tumor cell invasion.

Cell Adhesion Molecules

Parallel with the expression of proteases, the invasive capacity of cytotrophoblasts is tightly correlated with the expression of integrin adhesion molecules. Integrins are heterodimers of α/β subunits that mediate cell–cell and cell–matrix interactions. In human melanoma, the αV integrin family is upregulated and highly associated with tumorigenic potential (Felding-Habermann et al. 1992). As cytotrophoblasts invade, dramatic alterations occur in the repertoire of these extracellular matrix receptors (Damsky, Fitzgerald and Fisher 1992). The cytotrophoblasts in the most proximal portion of the anchoring villus column express the epithelial integrin α6/β4. As the cells differentiate along the invasive pathway, the α5/β1 integrin receptor for fibronectin is expressed. Further into the maternal tissue, they begin to express the laminin and collagen type IV receptor, integrin α1/β1, but stop the expression of integrin α6/β4. Functional invasive assays indicate that the invasiveness of these cells is regulated by the balance between α5/β1 and α1/β1 interactions with their respective substrates. Interrupting the interaction of the α5/β1 integrin with fibronectin by antibodies increases the invasive capacity of cytotrophoblasts, whereas disturbing the interaction of the α1/β1 integrin with its substrate inhibits invasion. In other words, interaction of the α5/β1 integrin with fibronectin restrains invasion, and interaction of the α1/β1 integrin with collagen type IV and laminin promotes invasion. Modulation of the β1-integrin subunit contributes to the development of invasiveness by differentiating cytotrophoblasts. Integrin switching may help regulate the depth to which these cells invade into the uterus (Damsky et al. 1994).

Cytotrophoblasts also modulate cadherins expression as they differentiate along the invasive pathway. Cadherins are a ubiquitous class of adhesion molecules. Function- pertubation studies indicate that the epithelial (E) cadherin restrains invasion, while vascular endothelial (VE) cadherin promotes it (Zhou, Damsky and Fisher 1997). The E-cadherin is expressed in the proximal column of the anchoring villous. As the cytotrophoblast invades, the expression of VE-cadherin increases as the cell approximates blood vessels.

Deeply invasive cytotrophoblasts breach maternal spiral arterioles and transform their phenotype to resemble that of the endothelial cells they ultimately replace. They express the αV/β3 integrin, VE-cadherin, platelet endothelial cell adhesion molecule-1 (PECAM-1) and vascular cell adhesion molecule (VCAM-1). This comprehensive switch of adhesion molecule expression mimics the adhesion phenotype of endothelial cells (Zhou, Damsky and Fisher 1997). In melanoma cells, the αV/β3 integrin has also been implicated in endothelial cell migration to angiogenic stimuli (Brooks, Clark and Cheresh 1994) and the transition to an invasive phenotype (Albelda et al. 1990). This remarkable alteration of phenotype probably plays a role in the immunologic tolerance by the mother or host tissue.

Tumor cells also must have considerable flexibility in adhesive properties to migrate through the extracellular matrix. Indeed, prior to any migration, tumor cells must first disassociate from neighboring tumor cells in order to metastasize. During subsequent invasion into extracellular tissue, a complex and dynamic expression of adhesion molecules has been demonstrated, including integrins and cadherins (Bussemakers and Schalken 1996). Alterations of expression and hyperphosphorylation of these molecules by oncogene products are essential for invasion by some tumor cells (Rovensky 1998). The mechanisms of invasion used by cytotrophoblasts and tumor cells are similar, but the poorly understood attributes of control undoubtedly differ.

Conclusion

Trophoblasts and tumor cells use similar tools to invade tissues. Comparable mechanisms are exhibited during intercellular penetration, extracellular matrix dissolution by proteases, and migration by adhesive molecules. Tumor-specific differences exist, but the general mechanisms are analogous. The defining difference between trophoblast and tumor cells is that trophoblast invasion is polarized and self-limiting, whereas tumor cell invasion is not. An informative model to compare physiologic and pathologic trophoblast cell behavior is gestational trophoblastic disease (GTD). This represents a spectrum of trophoblastic neoplasia, including molar pregnancy, invasive mole, placental site tumor and choriocarcinoma. Molar pregnancies comprise trophoblastic hyperplasia of chorionic villi. Invasive moles consist of non-metastatic trophoblast invasion through the myometrial wall. Placental site tumors are rare cases of malignant transformation of interstitial cytotrophoblasts. Gestational choriocarcinomas are highly invasive, metastatic tumors of trophoblastic cells. This spectrum of disease demonstrates an increasing depth of trophoblast invasion, or conversely a decreasing control of limited invasion.

Gestational choriocarcinoma is the most malignant tumor of the female reproductive tract, and until recently, it was fatal in the majority of cases. It can arise following any pregnancy, including first trimester miscarriages, ectopic pregnancy, or a normal term delivery. Histologically, the trophoblasts show various degrees of dedifferentiation. Groups of malignant trophoblastic cells closely resemble a normal early implantation site, except for the lack of direction that is always present in the normally invading trophoblast (Deligdisch 1991).

Cellular invasion involves a complex series of events. The regulation of the process determines the outcome of the individual invading cells. Implantation operates under a delicately balanced mechanism of control at the maternal–trophoblast interface. Failure of this balanced relationship contributes to GTD and ultimately may result in dedifferentiated choriocarcinoma cells. These, like all invading tumor cells, lack regulation for the creation of organized, life-sustaining tissue and instead result in metastatic cancer.

References

Albelda SM, Mette SA, Elder DE, Stewaart R, Damjanovich L, Herlyn M, et al. (1990) Integrin distribution in malignant melanoma: association of the beta 3 subunit with tumor progression. Cancer Research 50:6757–64.

Bass KE, Morrish D, Roth I, Bhardwaj D, Taylor R, Zhou Y, et al. (1994) Human cytotrophoblast invasion is upregulated by epidermal growth factor: evidence that paracrine factors modify this process. Developmental Biology 164:554–61

Behrendtsen O, Alexander CM, Werb A (1992) Metalloproteinases mediate extracellular matrix degradation by cells from mouse blastocyst outgrowths. Development 114:447–56

Bonfil RD, Medina PA, Gomez DE, Farias E, Lazarowski A, Lucero, MF, et al. (1992) Expression of gelatinase/type IV collagenase in tumor necrosis correlates with cell detachment and tumor invasion. Clinical Experimental Metastasis 10:211–20

Boyd JD and Hamilton WJ (1970) The Human Placenta. W Heffer and Son, Cambridge

Brooks PC, Clark RAF, Cheresh DA (1994) Requirement of integrin $\alpha V/\beta 3$ for angiogenesis. Science 264:567–71

Bussemakers MJ, Schalken JA (1996) The role of cell adhesion molecules and proteases in tumor invasion and metastasis. World J Urol 14:3:151–6

Damsky CH, Fitzgerald ML, Fisher SJ (1992) Distribution patterns of extracellular matrix components and adhesion receptors are intricately modulated during first trimester cytotrophoblast differentiation along the invasive pathway, in vivo. J of Clin Invest 89:210–22

Damsky CH, Librach C, Lim KH, Fitzgerald ML, McMaster MT, Janatpour M, et al. (1994) Integrin switching regulates normal trophoblast invasion. Development 120:3657–66

Deligdisch L (1991) General Aspects of Gestational Trophoblastic Diseases. In: Cherry SH, Merkatz IR, Complications of Pregnancy: Medical Surgical, Gynecologic, Psychosocial, and Perinatal. Williams & Wilkins, Baltimore, MD

Enders AC, Chavez DJ, Schlafke S (1981) In: Glasser SR, Bullock DW (eds), Cellular and Molecular Aspects of Implantation. Plenum, New York: 365–82

Felding-Habermann B, Mueller BM, Romerdahl CA, Cheresh DA (1992) Involvement of integrin alpha V gene expression in human melanoma tumorgenicity. J Clin Invest 89:2018–22

Fisher SJ, Cui T-Y, Zhang L, Hartman L, Grahl KT, Zhang G-Y, Tarpey JF, Damsky CF (1989) Adhesive and invasive properties of human placental cytotrophoblast cells in vitro. J Cell Biol 109:891–902

Genbacev O., Jensen, K.D., Powlin, S.S. and Miller, R.K. (1993a) In vitro differentiation and ultrastructure of human extravillous trophoblast (EVT) cells. Placenta, 14: 463–475.

Genbacev O, Joslin RJ, Damsky CH, Polliotti BM, Fisher SJ (1996) Hypoxia alters early gestation human cytotrophoblast differentiation invasion in vitro and models the placental defects that occur in preeclampsia. J Clin Invests 97:540–50.

Genbacev O, White TEK, Gavin CE, Miller RK (1993b) Human trophoblast cultures: models for implantation and peri-implantation toxicology. Reprod Toxicol 7:75–94

Graham CH, Lysiak JJ, McCrae KR, Lala PK (1992) Localization of transforming growth factor-beta at the human fetal–maternal interface: role in trophoblast growth and differentiation. Biol Reprod 46:561–72

Hohn HP, Linke M, Ugele, B, Denker HW (1998) Differentiation markers and invasiveness: discordant regulation in normal trophoblast and choriocarcinoma cells. Exper Cell Res 244:249–58

Hustin J and Franchimont P (1992) The endometrium and implantation. In: Barnea ER, Hustin J, Jauniaux E (eds), The First Twelve Weeks of Gestation. Springer, New York: 26–42

Lawrence JA, Steeg PS (1997) Mechanisms of tumor invasion and metastasis. World J Urol 14:3:124–30

Librach CL, Werb Z, Fitzgerald ML, Chiu K, Corwin NM, Esteves RA, et al. (1991) 92-kD type IV collagenase mediates invasion of human cytotrophoblasts. J Cell Biol 113:437–49

Liotta L (1992) Cancer cell invasion and metastasis. Scientific American Feb:54–63

Matrisian LM (1993) Matrix metalloproteinase gene expression Ann NY Acad Sci 732:42–50

O'Rahilly R (1973) Developmental stages in human embryos. Part A: embryos of the first three weeks gestation (stages 1 to 9). Carnegie Institute of Washington Publication, Washington, DC

Paulsson M (1992) Basement membrane proteins: structure, assembly, and cellular interactions. Criti Rev Biochem Mol Biol 27:93–127

Pijnenborg R, Dixon G, Robertson WB, Brosens I (1980) Trophoblast invasion of human decidua from 8 to 18 weeks of pregnancy. Placenta 1:3–19

Psychoyos A, Martel D (1985) Embryo–endometrial interactions at implantation. In: Edwards RG, Purdy JM, Steptoe PC (eds), Implantation of the Human Embryo. Academic Press, London: 195

Queenan JT Jr, Kao LC, Arboleda CE, Ulloa Aguirre A, Golos TG, Cines DB, Strauss JF (1987) Regulation of urokinase-type plasminogen activator production by cultured human cytotrophoblasts. J Biol Chem 262:10903–906

Rabbani SA, Xing RH (1998) Role of urokinase (uPA) and its receptor (uPAR) in invasion and metastasis of hormone-dependent malignancies. Internat J Onc 12;4:911–20

Rovensky YA (1998) Cellular and molecular mechanisms of tumor invasion. Biochem 63;9:1029–43

Sato H, Seiki M (1996) Membrane-type metalloproteinases in tumor metastasis. J Biochem 119:209–15

Stetler-Stevenson WG, Liotta LA, Kleiner DE (1993) Extracellular matrix 6: role of matrix metalloproteinases in tumor invasion and metastasis. FASEB J 7:1434–41
Triggvason K, Hoyhtya M, Pyke C (1993) Type IV collagenase in invasive tumors. Breast Cancer Res Treat 24:209–18
Young TN, Rodriguez GC, Rinehart AR, Bast RC, Pizzo SV, Stack MS (1996) Characterization of gelatinases linked to extracellular matrix invasion in ovarian adenocarcinoma: purification of matrix metalloproteinase-2. Gynecol Oncol 62:89–99
Zhou Y, Damsky CH, Fisher SJ (1997) Pre-eclampsia is associated with failure of human cytotrophoblasts to mimic a vascular adhesion phenotype: one cause of defective endovascular invasion in this syndrome? J Clin Invest 99:2152–64

22 Pregnancy Derived Compounds that Control Proliferation

Eytan R. Barnea, George Aboagye-Mathiesen, William C. Hatch, and Paul C. Leavis

Introduction

Pregnancy appears to protect against cancer development, and mitigates the effects of cancer once it coexists during pregnancy. Also, epidemiological observations suggest that the protection induced by a previous pregnancy against cancer is long-term. Moreover, recent data emerges to show that these protective mechanisms may be related to a highly complex environment induced by pregnancy and that specific conceptus derived compounds may play a significant role in achieving this protection. Finally, such a protection may be translated into treatment of malignancy in the non-pregnant state. This chapter reviews current evidence that supports the view that better understanding of pregnancy will lead to better management of cancer.

Pregnancy Protects Against Cancer

Pregnancy confers both a short- and long-term protection against cancer. This is reflected by lower rates of several cancers (breast, endometrium, ovary etc) compared to those expected in women of reproductive age. Such a protection is also evidenced for example by the lower rates of breast cancer later in life for women who have achieved successful pregnancy before reaching the age of thirty. The initial suggestion that abortion leads to increased rates of breast cancer was not confirmed (Michels et al. 1995). In experimental models Kimura et al. (1996) have shown that pregnancy protected against food induced carcinogenesis. Similar protective effects were observed by Grubbs et al. (1986). Injections of a highly potent carcinogen to pregnant mice in one study appeared to accelerate postnatal tumor development (Huynh, Alpert and Pollack 1996). In contrast, using a similar agent Grubbs et al. (1986) have found a marked reduction in cancer formation in a similar model. Moreover, even when the rodents were injected with prolactin, a mammary tumor growth promoting agent, the protective effect of pregnancy was maintained. It is likely that in the case of the breast the protection is induced by an upregulation of *BRCA-1*, a tumor suppressor gene (Marquis et al. 1995). Indeed it was recently found that in rodents with mutated BRCA1 and 2 pregnancy was associated with a higher rate of cancer.

Studies of patients with non-Hodgkin's lymphoma (NHL) found a much lower occurrence of the lymphoma during pregnancy among reproductive age women. No differences in the progression of lymphoma between pregnant and non-pregnant patients were found. When patients diagnosed with both Hodgkin's disease and NHL were studied, results indicated similar outcomes for both pregnant and non-pregnant subjects.

Therefore, based on current epidemiologic data, presence of pregnancy or previous pregnancy appears to have a protective role against cancer. A search to identify the protective mechanisms that are involved is currently being intensely pursued. Insight into the precise mechanisms involved would obviously be very important for understanding issues that are related to both cancer prevention and treatment. The main question remains whether this protection results from the pregnant state itself, inducing both long-term and short-term changes in the mother, or it is imparted by pregnancy-specific compounds that are eliminated following the delivery of the fetus, or both. In both instances the unique condition that pregnancy brings on leads to anticancer effects.

Reflections on the Immune System

In general the body defends itself against cancer by the presence of a competent immune system, combined with proper control of cell proliferation through mitosis, differentiation and apoptosis through the action of positive and negative growth regulators, and repair mechanisms of damaged DNA. During pregnancy changes in the immune system do take place. There is also great increase in the expression of growth factors, mitogens and cytokines. Also the trophoblast has a malignant potential which is especially prominent early in the first trimester. In spite of the altered immune state, pregnancy in several instances does actually protect against cancer. These protective influences could result from alterations that are induced in the mother and/or conceptus that affect the cellular or humoral immune system. Obviously, any of those alone or in combination may take place as well. That the immune system is not weakened by pregnancy but is rather uniquely altered on both a cellular and humoral levels was shown in a number of studies. An indirect demonstration was shown in studies of cancer patients with and without concurrent pregnancy. If pregnancy contributes to a diminished immune function, one could expect a less favorable prognosis for those who already have cancer while pregnant. Also a suppressed immune system would likely translate into a heightened rate of cancer development during pregnancy, or even following pregnancy later in life, with disastrous consequences. Fortunately, this is not the case. The similarities between the immune response in pregnancy as compared to non-pregnant subjects provide evidence for a largely maintained defense mechanism. The subject was recently described in detail (Barnea and Levine 1999). The status of the immune system has a strong correlation with the prevalence of cancer. Indeed, it is believed to play a major role in the development of malignancy in the non-pregnant subject. Actually, tumor frequency is increased during stages of life when the immune system is reduced, for example such as the neonatal period which follows pregnancy. The possibility cannot be excluded, however, that somehow the altered immune system that is present during pregnancy may also contribute to a relative protection against malignancy (see Ch. 16).

Biology of Early Pregnancy Placed in Context

The immune system doesn't appear likely to play a major role in protecting against malignancy during pregnancy, which leaves two other possibilities as sources of protection. The maternal system may change in pregnancy and release compounds that are not pregnancy-specific but are in the right combination and concentration. Alternatively, the protective compounds are pregnancy-specific and derive from the conceptus. In our view both arguments may be correct. As seen below, certain pregnancy-specific conditions, but not compounds e.g. using estrogen/ progesterone, may have a protective effect against a number of cancers. On the other hand several pregnancy-derived compounds may play also an important role as well in protecting against malignancy, while having an important role in the development of the fetus.

Previously we have described the concept of the embryo-trophoblastic paradox (Barnea and Barnea 1997). Briefly, it states that the beginning of pregnancy is associated with several malignant-like features. These include implantation of a partial allograft following alteration of the immune system, invasion of the trophoblast into the maternal endometrium reaching the maternal blood vessels, and metastasis of trophoblastic cells into the maternal circulation. However, contrary to what would be expected, the analogy stops here and in general pregnancy does not acquire features of a frank malignancy. Consequently, later in pregnancy the task of the trophoblast is to support the fetus by becoming a functional placenta. The argument was that the presence of the embryo has a mitigating effect on the trophoblast and that based on the theory of complexity, more complex systems which are also highly differentiated (i.e. the embryo) will be controlling less differentiated entities which is the trophoblast (Barnea and Shoefield 1997). The further view was that the role of the embryo is to propagate the maternal genome and the interaction with the paternal genome during fertilization is aimed to facilitate this process. Also since the trophoblast in its majority is due to the paternal genomic contribution (associated with invasivity) a protective system would be built in pregnancy to protect the maternal host against the possibility of abnormal proliferation. If the abnormal proliferation starts very early, a miscarriage (either preclinical or clinical) will ensue. Actually, most abnormal embryos will be eliminated spontaneously. The embryo rapidy becomes integrated as various organs develop. That of the trophoblast, once malignant-like features have been mitigated, is to allow maternal genome derived genes to develop the trophoblastic stroma needed for placental vascularization. Such a dramatic change is necessary in order to facilitate exchange of nutrients and oxygen between the mother and the fetus. Earlier research demonstrated that embryo-derived compounds modulate secretion of hormones (hCG and progesterone) by trophoblastic cells in culture (Barnea, Simon and Kol 1989, Shurtz-Swirsky et al. 1991). Also when the embryo appears to be affected by exposure to teratogens the effect of the embryonal compounds on the trophoblastic hormones is different (Shurtz-Swirsky et al. 1992). Thus the embryo–trophoblastic relationship is being perturbed. It was also shown that if an embryo coexists with a mole then circulating levels of hCG are lower. Also when the embryo is selectively eliminated, trophoblastic function declines (Johnson, Abbas and Nicolaides 1994). Overall, that concept led to the realization that the embryo may contain certain compounds that are involved in controlling abnormal proliferation, since hCG is also considered as a major tumor marker, as well as the trophoblast, which at least in the first trimester has clear malignant-like properties.

Experimental Evidence

Recently, it was shown that teratoma derived from rat embryonal tissues which was engrafted to non-pregnant rats had anticancer properties. Cancer was induced by exposure to chemical agents or to a virus that induced lymphoma. Compared to controls the grafts either partially or totally protected against tumor development. This raises the possibility that embryo-derived factors may control proliferation of abnormal cells (Moroson and Ioachim 1995). In animal studies, 50% of rats inoculated with virally-induced lymphoma during pregnancy did not develop tumors and 35% developed tumors that are only half the size of controls (Ioachim and Moroson 1993). This protection was maximal early in pregnancy, was reduced at term and absent during the lactation period. Earlier workers also have shown that embryo-derived fibroblasts when cultured with cancer cells caused inhibition of the malignant cells (Imanishi et al. 1983). Also neuroblastoma cells' proliferation was inhibited when these malignant cells were incorporated into the neurula stage mouse embryo (Podesta et al. 1984). Evidence for the antitumoral effect of the embryo was shown by Teshima et al. (1983) who were able to induce choriocarcinoma, yolk sac carcinomas, adenocarcinomas and teratomas in rats by simple fetectomy on the twelfth day of gestation.

Embryo-Derived Developmental Proteins

The following is the description of the results obtained by our laboratory when the embryo-derived antiproliferative factors (previously shown by us to control placental hormonal secretion) were investigated in detail as to their identity, effects and characteristics.

As earlier reported (Barnea, Barnea and Pines 1996, Barnea and Barnea 1997) mammalian porcine and human embryos contain compounds that control proliferation. This would suggest that all mammals might have similar protective mechanisms. Based on recent biochemical data these anti-proliferative developmental compounds are found to be proteins or peptides (DPs). Following detailed chromatographic analysis one of the compounds was isolated; it was a novel heptamer. The other is currently in the last stages of characterization and appears to be a 30–40 kDa size protein(s). With respect to the anti-proliferative activity, as earlier reported DPs control proliferation of numerous cancer cell lines, in monolayer culture and also in tissue culture. We found effects against a wide variety of cell types, including those of epithelial origin (breast, uterine cervix, colon, and lung), mesnechymal cells (osteo- and fibrosarcoma), leukemias, melanoma, and brain cancer cell lines. Also preliminary studies showed that DPs prevent cancer development in vivo in mice.

The effects noted were time- and dose-dependent and the effect appeared to be permanent after the compounds were removed from culture. In addition, these DPs also control abnormal cell proliferation caused by viruses, chemical agents, or those induced by ionizing radiation. With respect to viruses, DPs were shown to inhibit viral replication and infection of cells by viruses by all genomic families, single and double stranded DNA and RNA. Those findings are not totally unexpected if one considers the rationale for these compounds' action within the embryo. The task of DPs in our view is to protect the embryo from allowing abnormal cells' proliferation to take place. The offending agent that leads to the abnormal cell proliferation can be practically any mutagen or carcinogen.

In that respect we hypothesize that DPs are secreted by differentiating cells that release these compounds into their immediate surroundings. Those cells that have lost their ability to differentiate along the predetermined developmental lines are stopped in their proliferation, and consequently the embryo is spared from replication of abnormal cells. The known mechanism that the embryo applies in order to eliminate unwanted cells is through induction of apoptosis. We have preliminary data showing that DPs block the cell cycle at the G0–G1 phase, stop DNA synthesis and cause apoptosis. In our view such a gentle but effective approach in eliminating abnormal cells would assure that the cells that are incorporated into embryonal organs are mostly normal with a limited life span, and not immortal which is a feature of malignant cells.

We have also found that control of proliferation by DPs is also exerted on immortalized cells and as well as embryonal cell lines. These cells have lost their ability to die and therefore, following the same argument, it would be counterproductive for the embryo for abnormal cells to be incorporated into the rapidly developing tissues. We have evidence showing that DP compounds do not affect normal cells proliferation and exert only minimal or no toxicity. Therefore, based on recent data, DPs have the ability within minutes to distinguish between normal and abnormal cell proliferation. DPs' rapidity and specificity of action makes it likely that DPs act by binding to a specific receptor which through second messenger action stops DNA synthesis almost completely within 24 hours, leading to cell death within 48 hours. Based on these characteristics we are currently aiming to develop non-animal derived DP compounds (using solid synthesis or recombinant methods) to use for combating abnormal proliferation due to cancer and virally induced damage.

Placental Interferons

The regulation of normal cell growth and differentiation is controlled by the interaction of growth factors and cytokines produced by the cells or neighboring tissues and their cellular receptors. Interferons (IFNs), which are cytokines, are produced by the trophoblast in the human (Bulmer et al. 1990; Tóth et al. 1990; Aboagye-Mathiesen et al. 1993a) as well as in other species (Imakawa et al. 1989; Lefèvre and Boulay 1993). Apart from the classical IFNs (alpha, beta and gamma) the trophoblast also produces the recently identified IFN-w (Adolf 1987, Aboagye-Mathiesen et al. 1997) in humans and IFN-t (Imakawa et al. 1989) in ruminants.

Interferons, produced by the human placenta, can be detected in the maternal and fetal blood (Zdravkovic et al. 1997). Human trophoblast-derived IFNs inhibit the proliferation of normal and trophoblast-derived malignant cell lines (Aboagye-Mathiesen et al. 1994) without toxicity. The anti-proliferative activity of INFs was much more pronounced on trophoblast-derived malignant cells compared with normal trophoblastic cells. The role of placental INFs may be to inhibit the proliferation of trophoblastic cell populations during their interaction with maternal cells. The growth, differentiation and invasion of normal invasive and non-invasive trophoblast has been reported to be regulated by EGF (Genbacev, Powlin and Miller 1994) and CSF-1 (Saito et al. 1993, 1994). We have demonstrated that human trophoblast IFNs inhibit the expression of proto-oncogenes (egf-r, c-fms, and c-erbB2 proteins) in normal invasive and non-invasive trophoblast cells (Aboagye-Mathiesen et al. 1997). EGF induces biochemical and morphological differentiation in non-invasive villous trophoblast (Morrish et al. 1987) whereas it enhances the invasion of the extravillous trophoblast (Bass et al. 1994). Therefore, the inhibition of EGF-R by trophoblast-induced IFNs suggest it may be one of the mechanisms that are involved in the regulation of normal trophoblast differentiation. The cytostatic activity of the trophoblast-derived IFNs on normal and neoplastic trophoblast cells without exerting toxicity suggests their possible clinical application as antineoplastic agents.

The invasion of normal trophoblast is under strict control. This control limits invasion both in a spatial and a temporal manner, a characteristic different from tumor cells. Several in vitro and in vivo studies show that IFNs inhibit or enhance the invasive and metastatic potential of a number of different tumor cells, depending on the duration of the IFN treatment (Hujanen and Turpenniemi-Hujanen 1991).

In order to develop effective cancer treatments using these IFNs, several in vitro and in vivo experiments as well as clinical trials have been carried out. These families of IFNs modify a large number of biochemical and immunological properties of both normal and cancer cells. Other IFNs were shown to suppress cancer cells' proliferation both in vitro and in vivo (Gresser and Tovey 1978; Aboagye-Mathiesen et al. 1996). They modulate several programs of cellular differentiation (Aboagye-Mathiesen et al. 1997) and modify various immunological properties of cells including augmentation of natural killer cell activity (Herbermann et al. 1979, Aboagye-Mathiesen et al. 1994). INFs increase expression and shedding of histocompatibility antigens and b2-microglobulin (Herbermann et al. 1979; Heron, Hokland and Berg 1978), and enhance expression of tumor associated antigens (TAA) on human breast, colon, melanoma and myeloma cells (Giacomini et al. 1984). These biological effects of IFNs have made this cytokine an attractive tool for use in clinical trials.

The treatment of cancers with IFNs utilizes physiological mechanisms as an aim partially to replace more invasive therapeutic measures such as chemotherapy, surgery or radiation. However, the use of the classical IFNs in sufficient dosages to yield efficacy is usually associated with significant side effects characterized by fever, chills, headache, lethargy, arthalgia and myalgia.

In a recent study we have shown that INFgamma derived from placental tissues and produced in a recombinant manner modified the expression of bladder cancer proteins' expression (Aboagye-Mathiesen et al. 1999). IFN-w produced by trophoblast and the trophoblast-specific IFN-t has, however, lower toxicity as compared to the classical IFNs and therefore may provide a safer and more effective therapy to treat diseases requiring higher doses of IFNs.

Other Pregnancy-derived Compounds

Several other factors have been described that are products of pregnancy and may contribute to cancer protection during or following pregnancy. Multiparous women generate MHC-restricted cytotoxic activity against MUC1-bearing breast tumor cells (Agrawal et al. 1995). T cells from parous women, but not from nulliparous women or men, specifically proliferated in response to core peptide sequences of MUC1. Two of the nulliparous women were retested during the first trimester of their first pregnancy, and their T cells proliferated specifically in response to MUC1. These observations support the hypothesis that immunization against MUC1 peptide epitopes during pregnancy may protect against breast cancer and such antibodies may a have a therapeutic role.

The placental hormone hCG has been described in several capacities as an inhibitor or suppressor of tumor proliferation. It protects the mammary gland in rats from carcinogenesis through an ovary-mediated hormonal effect. This involves increased production of inhibin; data indicates that hCG inhibits cell proliferation, which might be modulated through the induction of inhibin synthesis (other data on the possible role of hCG is described in Ch. 17). However, recent evidence points to the fact that hCG or its derivatives, as initially reported, may not be the agent that controls Kaposi's sarcoma, an HIV associated malignancy. According toLunardi-Iskandar et al. the antiviral/tumoral effect is due to as yet unidentified hCG associated factors in the size ranges 15–30 kDa and 2–4 kDa (Lunardi-Iskandar et al. 1998).

Another possible inhibitor of breast cancer MCF-7 cells is human alpha-fetoprotein (AFP). High doses of purified human AFP have been shown strongly to inhibit, in a dose dependent manner, the growth of human hepatoma HepG2 cells, human lymphoblastoma MT4 cells, lymphoma Jurkat cells, murine fibroblastoma L929 cells, and to a lesser extent MCF-7 cells. Lower concentrations of AFP actually induced a slight stimulatory effect, indicating the stimulatory or inhibitory growth effects of AFP depend upon its relative concentration. Also contributing to these disparate effects are exogenous or endogenous growth factors and cytokines present in the cell culture medium (Dudich et al. 1998).

Two mouse embryo-derived factors may also provide insight into mechanisms of tumor growth and suppression. A product of mutant S1 genes may be involved in the suppressive activity of WCB6F1-S1/S1d mouse embryo-derived 3T3 cells on mast cells. Close cell-to-cell contact was necessary for this suppression (Onoue et al. 1989). In contrast, cellular extracts and culture medium of the embryonic mouse cell line BALB/c-3T3 were shown, 9 days after culture, to provoke an intense proliferative effect on human T-47D breast cancer cells. This factor(s) was also shown to antagonize the anti-proliferative effect of anti-estrogen ICI 164,384 (Chetrite and Pasqualini 1992). Recently Zhang et al. (1995) reported that the fetal liver contains antitumoral agent identified as 7-ketocholesterol.

Protection of Pregnancy-like State Against Cancer

Estradiol and progesterone (E&P) provide virgin rats protection from mammary carcinogenesis as effectively as pregnancy. Data further suggests that E&P treatment is a non-toxic means of mimicking the protective effect of pregnancy against mammary cancer and that pregnancy or hormonal treatments may achieve this prophylaxis through a differentiation mechanism. Several similar strategies are being considered as well, for example, hCG injection appeared to have a similar protective effect (Russo and Russo 1994). It was suggested that the protective effects were induced by rising levels of E&P. The chemoprotective effects appeared to be induced by structural changes that take place in the breast tissue. In a retrospective clinical study there was a trend towards lower rates of breast cancer in those women who had previous exposure to injections of hCG as a part of infertility treatment regimens (Bernstein et al. 1995). Another alternative was suggested by using a GnRH agonist combined with low dose estrogen replacement, mimicking the non-cycling status of pregnancy (Spicer and Pike 1994).

Summary

Insight into mechanisms involving allowance for pregnancy, apparent protection of the pregnant subject during and after pregnancy and precise identification of compounds that are pregnancy-derived and identification of their mechanism of action, may help to make major inroads for the prevention and treatment of neoplastic disorders.

References

Aaronson S A (1991) Growth factors and cancer. Science 254:1146–52

Aboagye-Mathiesen G, Tòth F D, Juhl C, et al. (1991) Characterization of Sendai virus-induced human placental interferons. J Gen Virol 72:1871–16

Aboagye-Mathiesen G, Tòth FD, Juhl C, et al. (1991) Purification of human placental trophoblast interferon by two-dimensional high performance liquid chromatography. Pre. Biochem 22:105–21

Aboagye-Mathiesen G, Toth FD, Hager H, et al. (1993) Human trophoblast interferons. Antiviral Research 658:1–15

Aboagye-Mathiesen G, Tòth FD, Pedersen, N, et al. (1993). Differential interferon production in human first and third trimester trophoblast cultures stimulated with viruses. Placenta 14:225–34

Aboagye-Mathiesen G, Tòth FD, Zdravkovic M, Ebbesen P. (1994) Production of interferons in human placental trophoblast subpopulations and their possible roles in pregnancy. Clin Diagn Lab Immunol 1:650–59

Aboagye-Mathiesen G, Tòth FD, Zdravkovic M, Ebbesen P. (1996) Functional characteristics of human trophoblast interferons. Am J Reprod Immunol 35:309–17

Aboagye-Mathiesen G, Zdravkovic M, Toth FD, et al. (1996) Altered expression of the tumor suppressor/oncoprotein p53 in SV40 Tag-transformed human placental trophoblast and malignant trophoblast cell lines. Early Pregnancy: Biology and Medicine 2:102–12

Aboagye-Mathiesen G, Tòth FD, Zdravkovic M, and Ebbesen P. (1997) Effects of human trophoblast-induced interferons on the expression of proto-oncogenes c-fms/CSF-1R, EGF-R and c-erbB2 in invasive and non-invasive trophoblast. Placenta 18:155–61

Aboagye-Mathiesen G, Ebessen P, Van Der Masse H, et al. (1999) Interferon gamma regulates a unique set of proteins in fresh human bladder transitional cell carcinomas. Electrophoresis 20:344–8

Adolf GA. (1987) Antigenic structure of human interferon w1 (interferon aii1): comparison with other human interferons. J Gen Virol 68:1669–76

Agrawal B, Reddish MA, Krantz MJ, Longenecker BM. (1995) Does pregnancy immunize against breast cancer? Cancer Res 55: 2257–61

Barnea ER, Barnea JD, Pines M. (1996) Control of cell proliferation by embryonal-origin factors. Amer J Reprod Immunol 35: 318–24

Barnea ER, Simon RJ, Kol S. (1989) Human embryonal extracts modulate placental function in the first trimester: effects of visceral tissues upon chorionic gonadotropin and progesterone secretion. Placenta 10:331–44.

Barnea ER, Shoefield PN. (1996) Reflections on early pregnancy: organizing chaos or organized chaos? Early Pregnancy 1, 169–70

Barnea ER, Barnea JD. (1997) The Embryo/Trophoblastic Paradox. In: Jauniaux, Barnea and Edwards (eds), Embryonic Medicine and Therapy, Oxford Medical Publishers: 256–79

Barnea ER, Levine SP. (1999) Maternal Response to the Trophoblast GTD and Cancer. In: Y Shoenfeld (ed), The Decade of Autoimmunity, Elsever Science: 309–16

Bass KE, Morrish D, Roth I, Bhardwaj D, Taylor R, Zhou Y, Fisher SJ. (1994) Human cytotrophoblast invasion is upregulated by epidermal growth factor: evidence that paracrine factors modify this process. Develop Biol 164:550–61

Bernstein L, Hanisch R, Sullivan-Halley J, Ross RK. (1995) Treatment with human chorionic gonadotropin and risk of breast cancer. Cancer Epidemiol Biomarkers Prev 4:437–40

Bulmer JN, Morrison L, Johnson PM, Meager A. (1990) Immunohistochemical localization of interferons in human placenta tissue in normal, ectopic and molar pregnancy. Amer J Reprod Immunol 22:109–16

Chetrite G, Pasqualini JR. (1992) Effect of embryonic mouse cells BALB/c-3T3 on the proliferation of the human mammary cancer cell line T-47D. J Steroid Biochem Mol Biol 41:553–6

Dalsgaard AM, Aboagye-Mathiesen G, Justesen J, Zdravkovic M, Ebbesen P. (1995) Basal and interferon-induced 2',5'-oligoadenylate synthetase activity in human placental trophoblast and trophoblast-derived malignant cell lines. Placenta 16:137–46

Dudich E, Semenkova L, Gorbatova E, Dudich I, Khromykh L, Tatulov E, Grechko G, Sukhikh G. (1998) Growth-regulative activity of human alpha-fetoprotein for different types of tumor and normal cells. Tumour Biol 19:30–40

Filla MS, Kaul KL. (1997) Relative expression of epidermal growth factor receptor in placental cytotrophoblasts and choriocarcinoma cell lines. Placenta 18:17–27

Genbacev O, Powlin SS, Miller RK. (1994) Regulation of human extravillous trophoblast (EVT) cell differentiation and proliferation in vitro: role of epidermal growth factor (EGF). Trophoblast Res 8:427–42

Giacomini P, Aguzzi A, Pestka S, Fisher PB, Ferrone S (1984) Modulation by recombinant DNA leukocyte (alpha) and fibroblast (beta) interferons of the expression and shedding of HLA- and tumor-associated antigens by human melanoma cells. J Immunol 133:1649–55

Gill PS, Lunardi-Ishkandar Y, Louie S, Tulpule A, Zheng T, Espina BM, Besnier JM, Hermans P, Levine AM, Bryant JL, Gallo RC. (1996) The effects of preparations of human chorionic gonadotropin on AIDS-related Kaposi's sarcoma. N Engl J Med 335:1261–9

Greiner JW, Hand PH, Noguchi P et al. (1984) Enhanced expression of surface tumor-associated antigens on human breast and colon tumor cells after recombinant human leukocyte alpha-interferon treatment. Cancer Res. 44:3208–14

Gresser I, Tovey M. (1978) Antitumor effects of interferon. Biochem Biophys Acta 516:231–47

Grubbs CJ, Juliana MM, Hill DL, Whitaker LM. (1986) Suppression by pregnancy of chemically induced preneoplastic cells of the rat mammary gland. Anticancer Res 6:1395–400

Herbermann RB, Djeu JY, Kay HD et al. (1979) Natural killer cell: characteristics and regulation of activity. Immunol Rev 44: 439–70

Heron IM, Hokland M, Berg K. (1978) Enhanced expression of beta2-microglobulin and HLA antigens on human lymphoid cells by interferon. Proc Natl Acad Sci USA 75:6215–9

Hujanen ES, Turpenniemi-Hujanen. (1991) Recombinant interferon alpha and gamma modulate the invasive potential of human melanoma in vitro. Int J Cancer 47:576–81

Huynh H, Alpert L, Pollak M. (1996) Pregnancy-dependent growth of mammary tumors is associated with overexpression of insulin-like growth factor II. Cancer Res 56: 3651–4

Imakawa K, Hansen TR, Malathy P-V, Anthony RV, Polites HG, Marotti KR, Roberts RM. (1989) Molecular cloning and characterization of complementary deoxyribonucleic acids corresponding to bovine trophoblast protein–1; a comparison with ovine trophoblast protein–1 and bovine interferon a-ii. Molec Endocrinol 3:127–39

Imanishi J, Hoshino S, Matsuoka H, Uemura H, Imanishi T, Tanaka A, Nishino H, Kishida T. (1983) Tumor degeneration by human embryonic fibroblasts and its enhancement by interferon. Cancer Res 43:4323–6

Ioachim HL, Moroson H. (1993) Lymphoma and pregnancy: clinical and experimental observations (Meeting abstract). International Association for Comparative Research on Leukemia and Related Diseases, 16th Symposium (A46)

Johnson MR, Abbas A, Nicolaides KH. (1994) Maternal plasma levels of human chorionic gonadotrophin, oestradiol and progesterone in multifetal pregnancies before and after fetal reduction. J of Endocrinol 143:309–12

Kimura J, Hasegawa R, Yaono M, Kato T, Wakabayashi K, Sugimura T, Ito N, Shirai T. (1996) Inhibitory potential of pregnancy and lactation on mammary carcinogenesis induced by a food-derived carcinogen, 2-amino-1-methyl-6-phenylimidazo[4, 5-b]pyridine, in Sprague-Dawley rats. Cancer Lett 101:73–8

Lefèvre F, Boulay V. (1993) A novel and atypical type one interferon gene expressed by trophoblast during early pregnancy. J Biol Chem 268:19760–68

Lunardi-Iskandar Y, Bryant JL, Zeman RA, et al. (1995) Tumorigenesis and metastasis of neoplastic Kaposi's sarcoma cell line in immunodeficient mice blocked by a human pregnancy hormone. Nature 375:64–8

Lunardi-Iskandar Y, Bryant JL, Blattner WA, et al. (1998) Effects of a urinary factor from women in early pregnancy on HIV–1, SIV and associated disease. Nat Med 4: 428–34.

Marquis ST, Rajan JV, Wynshaw-Boris A, Xu J, Yin GY, Abel KJ, Weber BL, Chodosh LA. (1995) The developmental pattern of Brca1 expression implies a role in differentiation of the breast and other tissues. Nat Genet 11:17–26

Mattsson R, Mattsson A, Holmdahl R, Scheynius A, Van der Meide PH. (1992) In vivo treatment with interferon-gamma during early pregnancy in mice induces strong expression of major histocompatibility complex class I and II molecules in uterus and decidua but not in extra-embryonic tissues. Biol Reprod 46:1176–86

Michels KB, Hsieh CC, Trichopoulos D, Willett WC. (1995) Abortion and breast cancer risk in seven countries. Cancer Causes Control 6:75–82

Moroson H, Ioachim HL (1995) Protection by grafts of embryonal rat tissues (teratomas) against induction and transplantation of malignant tumors. Cancer Res 55:3664–8

Morrish DW, Bhardwaj D, Dabbagh LK, Marusyk H, Siy O. (1987) Epidermal growth factor induces differentiation and secretion of human chorionic gonadotropin and placental lactogen in human placenta. J Clin Endocrinol Metab 65:1285–90

Nomura S, Goto S, Ino K, Nakanishi T, Okamoto T, Mano H, Kurauchi O, Mizutani S, Tomoda Y. (1996) Autocrine mechanism of epidermal growth factor in choriocarcinoma cell proliferation. Mol Cell Endocrinol 124:63–9

Onoue H, Ebi Y, Nakayama H, Ru XM, Kitamura Y, Fujita J. (1989) Suppressive effect of Sl/Sld mouse embryo-derived fibroblast cell lines on diffusible factor-dependent proliferation of mast cells. Blood 74:1557–62

Podesta AH, Mullins J, Pierce GB, Wells RS. (1984) The neurula stage mouse embryo in control of neuroblastoma. Proc Natl Acad Sci USA 81:7608–11

Russo J, Russo IH. (1994) Toward a physiological approach to breast cancer prevention. Cancer Epidemiol Biomarkers Prev 3:353–64

Saito S, Saito M, Enomoto M. et al. (1993) Human macrophage colony-stimulating factor induces the differentiation of trophoblast. Growth Factors 9:11–19

Saito S, Ibaraki T, Enomoto M, Ichijo M, Motoyoshi K. (1994) Macrophage colony-stimulation factor induces the growth and differentiation of normal pregnancy human cytotrophoblast cells and hydatidiform moles but does not induce the growth and differentiation of choriocarcinoma cells. Japan J Cancer Res 85:245–52

Shurtz-Swirski R, Cohen Y, Barnea ER. (1992) Patterns of secretion of human chorionic gonadotrophin by superfused placental explants and the embryo–placental relationship following maternal use of medications. Hum Reprod 7:300–304

Shurtz-Swirski R, Simon RJ, Cohen Y, Barnea ER. (1991) Human embryo modulates placental function in the first trimester; effects of neural tissues upon chorionic gonadotropin and progesterone secretion. Placenta 12:521–31

Spicer DV, Pike MC. (1994) Sex steroids and breast cancer prevention. J Natl Cancer Inst Monogr 16:139–47

Teshima S, Shimosato Y, Koide T. et al. (1983) Transplantable choriocarcinoma of rats induced by fetectomy and its biological activities. Gann 74, 205–12

Tòth FD, Juhl C, Nørskov-Lauritsen N, Mosborg-Pedersen P, Ebbesen P. (1990) Interferon production by cultured human trophoblast induced with double stranded polyribonucleotide. J Reprod Immunol 17:217–27

Zdravkovic M, Knudsen HJ, Liu X, Hager H, Zachar V, Aboagye-Mathiesen G, Ebbesen P. (1997) High interferon alpha levels in placenta, maternal and cord blood suggest a protective effect against intrauterine herpes simplex virus infection. J Med Virol 51:210 –18

Zhang QL, Wu CT. (1995) Isolation, purification and structure identification of a low molecular tumor suppressor of human fetal liver origin. Anticancer Res 15:1632–3

23 Cancer and Pregnancy: Bioethical and Legal Dilemmas

Frank A. Chervenak and Laurence B. McCullough

Ethics is an essential dimension of the management of cancer in pregnancy.[1] In this chapter we define ethics, medical ethics and two basic ethical principles, and develop the concept of the fetus as a patient. We then apply these concepts to the clinical issues of counseling and advance directives in the care of prepared patients with cancer.[2]

Ethics, Medical Ethics, and Ethical Principles

Ethics has been understood for centuries to be the disciplined study of morality, based on the disciplines of the humanities, especially philosophy. Medical ethics is the disciplined study of morality in medicine. Medical ethics therefore addresses the obligations of physicians and health care organizations to patients, as well as the obligations of patients.

It is important not to confuse ethics with the many sources of morality in a pluralistic society.[3] These include, but are not limited to, law, our political heritage as a free people, the world's religions, ethnic and cultural traditions, families, the traditions and practices of medicine (including medical education and training), and personal experience. These sources of morality are useful reference points for ethical inquiry but must be subject to critical scrutiny, especially when they are in conflict, which they often are.

The traditions and practices of medicine, including education and training, provide an important source of morality for physicians and therefore provide the starting point for ethics in medicine: the obligation of the physician as moral fiduciary of the patient to protect and promote the interests of the patient.[1,4] This obligation tells physicians what morality in medicine ought to be in a very general, abstract fashion. Providing a more concrete account of that obligation and its application in clinical practice is the central task of medical ethics.

To accomplish this important clinical task, medical ethics focuses on the question of "How *ought* the physician to conduct himself or herself with patients?" Relevant tools of ethics for answering this question include ethical principles, because they help the physician to interpret and implement his or her general moral obligation to protect and promote the interests of the patient, which has been the traditional moral foundation of the physician–patient relationship.[1,4] We will consider two medical ethical principles, beneficence and respect for autonomy, and then apply them to clinical judgement and decision making about the fetal patient. Doing so will lay the foundation for discussing ethical issues concerning cancer and pregnancy.

The Principle of Beneficence

In general, the ethical principle of beneficence requires us to act in ways that are reliably expected to produce the greater balance of goods over harms in the lives of others.[1,4,5] To put this principle into clinical practice requires a reliable account of the goods and harms relevant to the care of the patient and of how those goods and harms should be reasonably balanced against each other when not all of them can be achieved in a particular clinical case. In medicine, the principle of beneficence requires the physician to act in ways that are reliably expected to produce the greater balance of clinical goods over harms for the patient.

Beneficence-based clinical judgement has an ancient pedigree in the history of western medical ethics, dating back at least to the Hippocratic Oath and accompanying texts.[1,5] Beneficence-based clinical judgement makes the following crucial claim: To interpret reliably the interests of the patient from medicine's perspective,[1] which, in turn, appeals to accumulated scientific research, clinical experience, and reasoned responses to clinical and scientific uncertainty. This perspective is thus not the function of the individual clinical perspective of a particular physician and therefore should not be based merely on the clinical impression or intuition of an individual physician.

On the basis of this rigorous, clinical perspective, beneficence-based clinical judgement identifies the goods that can be achieved for the patient in clinical practice based on the competencies of medicine. The goods that medicine is competent to seek for patients are the prevention and management of disease, injury, handicap, and unnecessary pain and suffering and the prevention of premature or unnecessary death.[1] Pain and suffering become unnecessary when they do not result in achieving the other goods of medical care. Death is unnecessary when it can be prevented at reasonable costs of iatrogenic harm, loss of functional status, and loss of quality of life.[1]

There is an inherent risk of paternalism in beneficence-based clinical judgement. If beneficence-based clinical judgement is, *mistakenly*, taken by the physician to be the sole source of moral responsibility and therefore moral authority in medical care, the unwary physician could conclude that beneficence-based judgements can be imposed on the patient in violation of her autonomy.[1,4,5] Paternalism is a dehumanizing response to the patient, and therefore should be avoided in the care of pregnant women with cancer.

The Principle of Respect for Autonomy

In addition to the principle of beneficence, there has been increasing – even dominant – emphasis in the literature of Western medical ethics on the principle of respect for autonomy.[3,5] This principle requires one always to acknowledge and carry out the value-based preferences of others, irrespective of what one might think the consequences for them of doing so might be.

The female or pregnant patient increasingly brings to her medical care her own perspective on what is in her interest. The principle of respect for autonomy translates this fact into autonomy-based clinical judgement. Autonomy-based clinical judgement owes a debt to the common law of informed consent, starting in the second decade of our century, and then in ethics, starting three decades ago.[3,6] Because each patient's perspective on her interests is a function of her values and beliefs, it is impossible to specify the goods and harms of autonomy-based clinical judgement in advance. Indeed, it would be inappropriate to do so, because the definition of her goods and harms and their balancing are the prerogative of the patient. Autonomy-based clinical judgement is intentionally antipaternalistic in nature.

To understand the moral demands of this principle, physicians require an operational account of autonomy, to make it applicable to clinical practice. We therefore identify three sequential autonomy-related behaviors on the part of the patient:

1 absorbing and retaining information about her condition and alternative diagnostic and therapeutic responses to it

2 understanding that information, that is, evaluating and rank-ordering those responses

3 expressing a value-based preference for a particular response.

The physician has a role to play in each of these. They are, respectively:

1 to recognize the capacity of each patient to deal with medical information (and not to underestimate that capacity), provide information, i.e. disclosure, and explain all alternatives supported in beneficence-based clinical judgement, disclose and explain the alternatives of nonintervention, and recognize the validity of the values and beliefs of the patient

2 not to interfere with but, when necessary, to assist the patient in her evaluation and ranking of diagnostic and therapeutic alternatives to her condition

3 to elicit, and

4 implement the patient's value-based preference, unless there is some overriding ethical justification for not doing so.[1,5]

The legal obligations of the physician regarding informed consent were established in a series of cases during the twentieth century.[6] *Schloendorff vs The Society of The New York Hospital* established the concept of simple consent, i.e. whether the patient says "yes" or "no" to medical intervention. "Every human being of adult years and sound mind has the right to determine what shall be done with his body, and a surgeon who performs an operation without his patient's consent commits an assault for which he is liable in damages."[6] The legal requirement of consent further evolved to include disclosure of information sufficient to enable patients to make informed decisions about whether to say "yes" or "no" to medical intervention.

There are two legal standards for such disclosure. The professional community standard defines adequate disclosure in the context of what the relevantly trained and experienced physician tells patients. The reasonable person standard goes further and requires the physician to disclose "material" information, what the lay person of average sophistication should not be expected to know. This second standard has emerged as the ethical standard[14] and we therefore urge obstetrician–gynecologists to adopt it. It is also the dominant legal standard among the United States of America. On this standard the physician should disclose to the patient her or the fetus' diagnosis (including differential diagnosis that that is all that is known), the medically reasonable alternatives to the management of the patient's condition, and the short term and long term benefits and harms of each alternative for both the woman and her fetus.

The Interaction of Beneficence and Respect for Autonomy in Obstetric Clinical Judgement and Practice

The ethical principles of beneficence and respect for autonomy play a complex role in obstetric clinical judgement and practice. There are obviously beneficence-based and autonomy-based obligations to the pregnant patient.[1] The physician's perspective on the pregnant woman's interests provides the basis for the physician's beneficence-based obligations to her. Because of an insufficiently developed central nervous system, the fetus cannot meaningfully be said to possess values and beliefs. Thus, there is no basis for saying that a fetus has a perspective on its interests. There can therefore be no autonomy-based obligations to any fetus.[1] Hence the language of fetal rights has no clinical application or relevance to the fetus in obstetric clinical judgement and practice, despite its popularity in public and political discourse in the United States and other countries. Obviously, the physician has a perspective on the fetus' health-related interests and the physician can have beneficence-based obligations to the fetus, *but only when the fetus is a patient.*

Two Senses of the Concept of the Fetus as a Patient

Developments in fetal diagnosis and management strategies to optimize fetal outcome have become widely accepted, encouraging the development of the concept of the fetus as a patient.[1] This concept has considerable clinical significance because, when the fetus is a patient, directive counseling, i.e. recommending a form of management for fetal benefit and recommending against a form of management that could be harmful to the fetus is appropriate. When the fetus is not a patient, non-directive counseling, i.e. offering but not recommending a form of management, is appropriate. However, these apparently straightforward roles for directive and non-directive counseling are often difficult to apply in actual perinatal practice because of uncertainty about when the fetus is a patient. One approach to resolving this uncertainty would be to argue that the fetus is or is not a patient in virtue of personhood[3,7] or some other form of independent moral status.[18,11] We now show that this approach fails to resolve the uncertainty and we therefore defend an alternative approach that does resolve the uncertainty.[1]

The Independent Moral Status of the Fetus

One approach for establishing whether or not the fetus is a patient has involved attempts to show whether or not the fetus has independent moral status. Independent moral status for the fetus means that one or more characteristics that the fetus possesses in and of itself and, therefore, independently of the pregnant woman or any other factor, generates and therefore ground obligations to the fetus on the part of the pregnant woman and her physician.

Many characteristics have been nominated for this role, e.g. moment of conception, implantation, central nervous system development, quickening and the moment of birth.[12-14] Given the considerable variability of these proposed characteristics, there is considerable variation among ethical arguments about when the fetus acquires independent moral status. Some take the view that the fetus has independent moral status from the moment of conception or implantation.[15-17] Others argue that independent moral status is acquired in degrees, thus resulting in "graded" moral status.[7,8,10] Still others hold, at least by implication, that the fetus never has independent moral status so long as it is in utero.[9]

Despite ever-expanding theological and philosophical literature on this subject, there has been no closure on a single authoritative account of the independent moral status of the fetus.[18,19] Moreover, given the absence of a single method that would be authoritative for all of the markedly diverse theological and philosophical schools of thought involved in this endless debate, closure is impossible, because authority within and between theological and philosophical traditions would have to be resolved in a way satisfactory to all, an inconceivable intellectual and cultural event. We therefore abandon the futile attempt to understand the fetus as a patient in terms of independent moral status and turn to an alternative approach.[5]

The Dependent Moral Status of the Fetus

Our account of the concept of the fetus as a patient begins with the recognition that being a patient does not require that one possesses independent moral status.[11] Instead, being a patient means that one can benefit from the applications of the clinical knowledge and skills of the physician. Put more precisely, a human being without independent moral status is properly regarded as a patient when two conditions are met: first, that a human being is presented to the physician, and second that there exist clinical interventions that are reliably expected to be efficacious, in that they are reliably expected to result in a greater balance of clinical goods over harms for the human being in question.[20] We call this the dependent moral status of the fetus.

The authors have argued elsewhere that beneficence-based obligations to the fetus exist when the fetus is reliably expected *later* to achieve independent moral status (sometime during the second year postpartum).[1] That is, the fetus is a patient when the fetus is presented for medical interventions, whether diagnostic or therapeutic, that reasonably can be expected to result in a greater balance of goods over harms for the child or person the fetus can later become during early childhood. The ethical significance of the concept of the fetus as a patient, therefore, depends on links that can be established between the fetus and its *later* achieving independent moral status.

The Viable Fetal Patient

One such link is viability. Viability must be understood in terms of both biological and technological factors,[19,21,22] because it is only in virtue of both factors that a viable fetus can exist ex utero and thus achieve independent moral status. Moreover, these two factors do not exist as a function of the autonomy of the pregnant woman. When a fetus is viable, i.e. when it is of sufficient maturity so that it can survive into the neonatal period and achieve independent moral status given the availability of the requisite technological support, and when it is presented to the physician, the fetus is a patient.

Viability exists as a function of biomedical and technological capacities, which are different in different parts of the world. As a consequence there is, at the present time, no worldwide, uniform gestational age to define viability. In the USA, the authors believe, viability presently occurs at approximately 24 weeks of gestational age.[23,24]

When the fetus is a patient, directive counseling for fetal benefit is ethically justified. In clinical practice directive counseling for fetal benefit involves one or more of the following: recommending against termination of pregnancy; recommending against non-aggressive management; or recommending aggressive management. Aggressive obstetric management includes interventions such as fetal surveillance, tocolysis, Cesarean delivery, or delivery in a tertiary-care center when indicated. Non-aggressive obstetric management excludes such interventions. Directive counseling also includes recommending against clinical management that could, on balance, be harmful to the fetal patient. Directive counseling for fetal benefit, however, must take account of the presence and severity of fetal anomalies, extreme prematurity, and obligations to the pregnant woman.

Any directive counseling for fetal benefit or against fetal harm must occur in the context of balancing beneficence-based obligations to the fetus against beneficence-based and autonomy-based obligations to the pregnant woman.[1,25] Any such balancing must recognize that a pregnant woman is obligated only to take reasonable risks of medical interventions that are reliably expected to benefit the viable fetus or child later. The unique feature of obstetric ethics is that whether, in a particular case, the viable fetus ought to be regarded as presented to the physician is, in part, a function of the pregnant woman's autonomy.

Obviously, any strategy for directive counseling for fetal benefit or avoiding fetal harm that takes account of obligations to the pregnant woman must be open to the possibility of conflict between the physician's recommendation and a pregnant woman's autonomous decision to the contrary. Such conflict is best managed preventively through informed consent as an ongoing dialogue throughout the pregnancy, augmented as necessary by negotiation and respectful persuasion.[1,26]

The Previable Fetal Patient

The only link between the previable fetus and the child it can become is the pregnant woman's autonomy. This is because technological factors cannot result in the previable fetus becoming a child. This is simply what previable means. The link, therefore, between a fetus and the child it can become, when the fetus is previable, can be established only by the pregnant woman's decision to confer the status of being a patient on her previable fetus. The previable fetus, therefore, has no claim to the status of being a patient independently of the pregnant woman's autonomy. The pregnant woman, according to her own values and beliefs, is free to withhold, confer, or, having once conferred, withdraw the status of being a patient on or from her previable fetus. The previable fetus is presented to the physician solely as a function of the pregnant woman's autonomy.[1]

Counseling the pregnant woman regarding the management of her pregnancy when the fetus is previable should be non-directive in terms of continuing the pregnancy or having an abortion, if she refuses to confer the status of being a patient on her fetus. If she does confer such status in a settled way, at that point beneficence-based obligations to her fetus come into existence and directive counseling for fetal benefit becomes appropriate for these previable fetuses. Just as for viable fetuses, such counseling must take account of the presence and severity of fetal anomalies, extreme prematurity, and obligations owed to the pregnant woman.

For pregnancies in which the woman is uncertain about whether to confer such status, the authors propose that the fetus be *provisionally* regarded as a patient.[1] This justifies directive counseling against behavior that can harm a fetus in significant and irreversible ways, e.g. substance abuse, until the woman settles on whether to confer the status of being a patient on the fetus.

In particular, non-directive counseling is appropriate in cases of what we term near-viable fetuses,[5] i.e., those which are 22–23 weeks gestational age for which there are anecdotal reports of survival.[1] In the authors' view, aggressive obstetric and neonatal management should be regarded as clinical investigation, i.e. a form of medical experimentation – not a standard of care.[27] There is no obligation on the part of a pregnant woman to confer the status of being a patient on a near-viable fetus, because the efficacy of aggressive obstetric and neonatal management has yet to be proven.

The Care of Pregnant Patients with Cancer

Cancer and pregnancy are two words fraught with potential ethical conflict.[2] Perhaps a woman knew she was pregnant and then discovered she had cancer; perhaps it was the other way around. Maybe she already had children; maybe not. Treatment decisions may confront her with decisions about abortion as an option to protect her own life, but that consideration and action may come at the expense of treasured religious, spiritual, and other moral values.

Under these circumstances, the goal of protecting and promoting the interests of the woman and the fetus may not be achievable. The ethical challenge to physicians is to create an environment of "preventive ethics" in which the woman's values and beliefs are taken into account and strongly shape the process of and decision-making about her care. This environment should seek and support the patient's autonomy, coupled with beneficence-based clinical judgements that include opportunities for emotional and spiritual support. In this section of this chapter we address counseling regarding management of cancer when the fetus is previable and when the fetus is viable, as well as advance directives.

Counseling Regarding Management of Cancer when the Fetus Is Previable

Counseling regarding the previable fetus should be non-directive. For the previable fetus, the woman is free to confer, withhold, or having once conferred, withdraw the moral status of patient from the fetus. Consequently, the decision to continue pregnancy of a previable fetus is for the woman to decide on the basis of her values and beliefs. Her choice may create conflict within her family, friends, or faith group, and therefore, one preventive ethical obligation of the health care professional is to protect the woman from undue, potentially coercive, influence from family members and others.

When the woman confers the status of patient on the previable fetus, there is a beneficence-based obligation to the fetal patient to prevent serious, far-reaching and irreversible harm. A crucial issue becomes whether the risks involved in therapies are documented or theoretical.

If serious harm to the fetus is documented and the woman has not conferred the status of being a patient on the previable fetus, counseling should be non-directive, taking the form of offering a choice between termination of the pregnancy (that is, withdrawing or withholding the status of patient from the fetus) or forgoing treatment of the cancer until delivery (conferring the status of patient on the fetus). In the case of documented, serious harm to the fetal patient, the pregnant woman and those caring for her have a beneficence-based obligation to prevent such harm. Counseling should involve a recommendation to forgo intervention until it is safe to deliver the fetus.

For theoretical risk of serious harm and for documented and theoretical risk of lesser harm, beneficence-based judgement offers more options because of the variability of beneficence-based judgement. In these situations, whether the fetus is a patient or not, counseling takes the form of offering a choice among termination of pregnancy, forgoing treatment of cancer until early delivery is consistent with beneficence-based obligations to protect a fetal patient, or treatment of the cancer.

Potential ethical conflict in favoring the pregnant woman or fetus can be prevented by avoiding a "default" position of managing the ethical dilemma. A default position manages ethical conflict in favor of either the pregnant woman or the fetus. A default position also assumes competence of beneficence-based clinical judgement to say with intellectual and therefore moral authority which of the two lives is more worth saving. Physicians have no such competence; such competence rests with the patient.

Counseling Regarding the Management of Cancer when the Fetus Is Viable

Counseling regarding the viable fetal patient should be directive. The pregnant woman, her health care professionals, and her family have beneficence-based obligations to protect and promote the viable fetal patient's interests. Those obligations must be balanced in clinical judgement against autonomy-based and beneficence-based obligations to the pregnant woman. The pregnant woman is not obligated to take any risk to protect the viable fetal patient, although a beneficence-based obligation exists to the viable fetal patient to prevent serious, far-reaching, and irreversible harm.

As with the previable fetus, documented vs theoretical risk to the viable fetus is a matter to be weighed in clinical judgement and discussions with the pregnant woman. When serious harm to the viable fetus is documented, counseling should be directive in recommending to forgo treatment of cancer until early delivery is consistent with beneficence-based obligation to protect the fetal patient.

Accurate medical assessment of the clinical consequences for the fetal patient of cancer management is crucial to the decision-making process at this juncture. The choice to have an abortion, start treatment, or delay treatment may require a negotiated settlement. The physician has an obligation to inform the patient as clearly as possible about the health risks and harm to the woman and the fetal patient of each of the possible choices. Given the emotionally charged nature of such situations, the physician may be placed in the difficult role of respectfully persuading the woman, based on values which can be reasonably assumed she ought to want to hold regarding protection of the fetal patient's interest, e.g., being protected against serious insult or death. However, as earlier observed, the physician should avoid a default position of managing ethical conflict in favor of the pregnant woman. Such a default position incorrectly assumes that beneficence-based clinical judgement always favors a woman's interests over those of the viable fetal patient. In addition, such a default position incorrectly assumes the woman's autonomy regarding the management of her now-viable pregnancy is unconstrained by beneficence-based obligations to the fetal patient.

When theoretical risks exist of serious, far-reaching, and irreversible harm to the viable fetal patient, the question of whether to apply directive counseling is open. The risks to the woman may be less serious but documented, and it is not a settled matter that she is obligated to take such risks to prevent theoretical serious harm to the fetal patient. Prudential, beneficence-based clinical judgement about such matters by clinicians will justifiably vary and, therefore, such judgements by pregnant women will justifiably vary. Counseling should be non-directive in the sense of helping the woman draw distinctions between documented risks to herself and theoretical risks to the fetal patient. Risk can be assessed by considering the probable incidence of the occurrence of a foreseen harm coupled with consideration of the quality of the outcome. For the reasons stated earlier, a default position of managing ethical conflict should be avoided.

Advance Directives

The introduction of "advance directives" was spurred by the case of Karen Quinlan in New Jersey in 1976. Legislatures have enacted "living will" legislation and there is legislative or common law authority for durable power of attorney for health care in all states of the USA.[1]

The basic idea of an advance directive is that a patient, when autonomous, can make decisions regarding her medical management in advance of a time during which she becomes incapable of making health care decisions. The ethical dimensions of autonomy that are relevant here are the following:

1. A patient may exercise her autonomy now in the form of a refusal of life-prolonging interventions
2. autonomy-based refusal, expressed in the past and left unchanged, remains in effect for any future time during which the patient becomes non-autonomous
3. that past autonomy-based refusal should therefore translate into physician obligations at the time the patient becomes unable to participate in the informed consent process
4. in particular, refusal of life-prolonging medical intervention should translate into the withholding or withdrawal of such interventions.

The living will is a type of advance directive that permits the patient to make a decision to refuse life-prolonging medical intervention in the future. The living will typically becomes effective when the patient is a "qualified patient," i.e. terminally or irreversibly ill as defined in the applicable statute, and is also not able to participate in the informed consent process. Obviously, terminally or irreversibly ill patients who are able to participate in the informed consent process retain their autonomy to make their own decisions. Some states prescribe the wording of the living will, while others do not. The physician should become familiar with the legal requirements in the physician's particular jurisdiction, especially the fact that some states do not allow implementation of a living will for pregnant patients. A living will, to be useful and effective, should be as explicit as possible. The legal basis for the living will is the legal right of self-determination, the right of any competent adult to determine what shall be done to her body. Statutes and state courts have made it clear that this right extends to the refusal of both hydration and nutrition. The recent US Supreme Court ruling in the famous *Uzan* case assumes that there is such a right based in the US Constitution.[1] Physicians should be familiar with hospital, clinic, and managed care organizations' policies and practices on documentation of a patient's living will.

The concept of a durable[6] power of attorney for health care (sometimes called medical power of attorney) is that any autonomous adult, in the event that that person later becomes unable to participate in the informed consent process, can assign decision making authority to another person. The advantage of the durable power of attorney for health care is that it applies only when the patient becomes incapable of decision making. It does *not*, as does the living will, also require that the patient also be terminally or irreversibly ill. However, unlike the living will, the durable power of attorney does not necessarily provide explicit direction, only the explicit assignment of decision making authority to an identified individual or "agent." Obviously, any patient who assigns durable power of attorney for health care to someone else has an interest in communicating her values, beliefs, and preferences to that person. The physician should play a facilitating role in this process. Indeed, in order to protect the patient's autonomy, the physician should play an active role in encouraging this communication process, so that there will be minimal doubt about whether the person holding durable power of attorney is faithfully representing the wishes of the patient. Some states exclude implementation of a durable power of attorney for withdrawal of treatment or abortion when the patient is pregnant. The reader should consult appropriate institutional management to identify legal required formats of a durable power of attorney for health care.

The main clinical advantages of these two forms of advance directive are that they encourage patients to think carefully in advance about the refusal of medical intervention, and that these directives, therefore, help to prevent ethical conflicts and crises in the management of nonferrous patients and nonferrous terminally or irreversibly ill patients. Unfortunately, the use of advance directives is not as widespread as it should be. The physician should regard advance directives as powerful, practical strategies for preventive ethics and encourage patients to consider them carefully, especially patients with gynecological diseases – particularly gynecological cancers – that could become or are life threatening.

References

1. McCullough LB, Chervenak FA. Ethics in Obstetrics and Gynecology. New York, Oxford University Press, 1994
2. Thorny S, McCullough LB, Chervenak FA. # Cancer Bull 1994; 5:391–94

3. Englehardt, Jr, HT. The Foundations of Bioethics, 2nd edn. New York, Oxford University Press, 1996
4. Beauchamp TL, McCullough LB. Medical Ethics: The Moral Responsibilities of Physicians. England Cliffs, Prentice-Hall, 1984
5. Beauchamp TL, Childress JF. Principles of Biomedical Ethics, 4th edn. New York, Oxford University Press, 1994
6. Faden RR, Beauchamp TL. A History and Theory of Informed Consent. New York, Oxford University Press, 1986
7. Strong C. Ethics in Reproductive Medicine: A New Framework. New Haven, Yale University Press, 1997
8. Dustan GR. The moral status of the human embryo. A tradition recalled. J Med Ethics 1984; 10:38–44
9. Elias S, Annas GJ. Reproductive Genetics and the Law. Chicago, Year Book Medical Publishers, 1987
10. Evans MI, Fletcher JC, Zador IE, et al. Selective first-trimester termination in octuplet and quadruplet pregnancies: Clinical and ethical issues. Obstet Gynecol 1988; 71:289–96
11. Ruddick W, Wilcox W. Operating on the fetus. Hastings Cent Report 1982; 12:10–14
12. Macklin R. Abortion: Contemporary Ethical and Legal Aspects. In: Reich WT (ed.) Encyclopedia of Bioethics, 2nd edn. New York, Macmillan, 1995: 6–16
13. Hellegers AE. Fetal development. Theological Studies 1970; 31:3–9
14. Noonan JT (ed.) The Morality of Abortion. Cambridge, Harvard University Press, 1970
15. Bopp J (ed.) Restoring the Right to Life: The Human Life Amendment. Provo, Brigham Young University, 1984
16. Bopp J (ed.) Human Life and Health Care Ethics. Frederick, University Publications of America, 1985
17. Noonan JT. A Private Choice. Abortion in America in the Seventies. New York, The Free Press, 1979
18. Callahan S, Callahan D (eds.) Abortion: Understanding Differences. New York, Plenum Press, 1984
19. *Roe v. Wade*, 410 US 113 (1973)
20. Chervenak FA, McCullough LB. What is obstetric ethics? J Perinat Med 1996; 3:331–41
21. Fost N, Chudwin D, Wikker D. The limited moral significance of fetal viability. Hastings Cent Rep 1980; 10;10–13
22. Mahowald M. Beyond abortion: Refusal of Cesarean section. Bioethics 1989; 3:106–121
23. Hack M, Fanaroff AA. Outcomes of extremely-low-birth-weight infants between 1982 and 1988. N Engl J Med 1989; 321:1642–7
24. Whyte HE, Fitzhardinge PM, et al. External immaturity: outline of 568 pregnancies of 23–26 weeks' gestation. Obstet Gynecol 1993; 82:1–7
25. Chervenak FA, McCullough LB. Perinatal ethics: A practical method of analysis of obligations to mother and fetus. Obstet Gynecol 1985; 66:442–6
26. Chervenak FA, McCullough LB. Clinical guides to preventing ethical conflicts between pregnant women and their physicians. Am J Obstet Gynecol 1990; 162:303–307
27. Chervenak FA, McCullough LB. The limits of viability. J Perinat Med 1997; 25:418–20

Epilogue
Cancer and Pregnancy: A Reason for Hope

Eytan R. Barnea

The progress that we have achieved in the last decade both in early pregnancy investigation and in understanding of cancer has led to this text. There is an obvious need to deal with the dark side of cancer and pregnancy – patients who face the serious threat of having cancer during pregnancy. However, the discussion would clearly be incomplete if we did not also look at the brighter side of the equation: that patients can and will benefit from our understanding of the similarities and differences between the unique biological phenomena of pregnancy and cancer. This understanding could become very useful in both diagnosing and treating cancer in pregnant and non-pregnant patients.

Cancer During Pregnancy

In this epilogue both clinical and basic biological issues are discussed. On the clinical side, the major difficulties that exist in both diagnosis and management of the patient will be discussed. On the other hand, recent progress in understanding of the biological analogy between and cancer and pregnancy will be examined as well.

Although the incidence of cancer during pregnancy is low, when it occurs it presents a serious challenge for both patients and physicians alike. This is due to the fact that in most instances our knowledge comes mostly from individual case reports, and therefore management also has frequently to be applied on an individual basis.

Cancer diagnosis and therapy during pregnancy are rather complicated. Certain diagnostic and treatment modalities that are readily used in non-pregnant patients may be limited or avoided altogether because of the side effects that they may have on the pregnant woman and fetus (e.g. X-rays, angiography). In addition, since more than one biological entity is involved (mother and fetus), clinical decisions must take into account both entities, and frequently complex sensitive decisions and choices have to be made. This requires the involvement of an interdisciplinary team, to include perinatologists, oncologists, gynecological oncologists, specialists in internal medicine, and often, general surgeons. Patients may also consult social workers, clinical psychologists, and bio-ethicists, in cases when decisions are particularly thorny, or clergy, in the case of religious patients. Despite the multidisciplinary input, patients, families and treating physicians often still face difficult and uncomfortable choices.

In non-pregnant subjects cancer treatment is aggressive and invasive, e.g. surgery, radiation therapy, and chemotherapy; it is also associated with serious side effects. Such approaches are normally justified since the patient's life is in the balance. However, the presence of the fetus and the unique maternal physiological status make the use of such approaches much more problematic. Care providers must find a balance between allowing the fetus to reach viability and avoiding immediate and/or long-term damage to the maternal host. When this is not possible, then one entity may be sacrificed so that the other may survive. This may involve elective pregnancy termination or postponement of therapy until after delivery, both being difficult decisions. The latter approach can involve avoiding therapy altogether or alternatively limiting treatment to those modalities that pose only minimal risks to the fetus, which may be inadequate for achieving total remission from the malignancy.

When cancer is present during pregnancy, multiple and complex interacting physiological systems have to be taken into account: the maternal organism, the fetus, and the placenta and the amnion/chorion. Furthermore, since cancer can involve any organ or system in the body and may affect any function, it can cause both direct and indirect damage throughout the maternal and fetal systems. This is doubly important since pregnancy itself already tests the maternal physiological limits: in the third trimester, for example, pregnancy burdens the woman's cardiovascular, respiratory, digestive and genitourinary systems, and labor exerts an even higher burden. In some cases, therefore, pregnancy termination, induction of premature delivery, or elective Caesarean section may be performed.

These difficulties do not end after delivery since the patient may still need to fight her malignancy and its consequences, especially if therapy was limited or postponed because of the pregnancy. The newborn may also experience problems requiring further medical attention, due to the intrauterine exposure to chemotherapeutic agents, for example. Furthermore, even if the cancer is in complete remission, questions remain as to future pregnancies.

Ultimately, as the age at which women become pregnant continues to rise, and cancers that only rarely occurred during pregnancy are becoming more common, the importance of increasing our understanding of cancer during pregnancy will need to rise accordingly.

Insight into Biology of Cancer and that of Pregnancy: A Reason for Hope

Cancer in Pregnancy

It is rather remarkable that despite the fact that cells of the developing fetus and placenta do proliferate rapidly and that the early trophoblast has invasive properties, metastasis of maternal derived cancer to the placenta or fetus occurs very rarely. This apparent paradox is sharpened by the observation that gestational tissues, specifically the embryo that grows at a faster pace, appear to be the least vulnerable to becoming malignant. This raises intriguing questions regarding the protective mechanisms that may be involved in creating such a delicate balance. We know, for example, that pregnancy protects against several types of cancer, including those of the breast, brain, colon, ovaries, and endometrium, and perhaps others. In addition, pregnancy does not affect cancer prognosis when compared stage for stage to non-pregnant subjects. In addition presence of choriocarcinoma during pregnancy is frequently associated with a very high cure rate. In contrast, the prognosis of the same malignancy is dismal when it is present in a non-pregnant state. Actually, gestational choriocarcinoma is almost the only cancer that with proper management with surgery and chemotherapy is close to 100% curable.

Pregnancy that occurs before the age of thirty appears to be one of the favorable prognostic criteria that are associated with lower rates of future development of breast cancer. Thus, the pregnancy experience present or past must provide a unique form of protection that is rather significant. Because of these clinical observations there are also ongoing efforts to create pregnancy-like conditions in order to reduce, for example, the rate of breast cancer in high-risk subjects. On a closer view, such clinical observations would appear clearly counterintuitive. Moreover, if the profound pregnancy related changes were to occur in a non-pregnant subject with cancer that would most likely lead towards a very unfavorable outcome. The reasons behind such an apparent protection just recently started to be elucidated. What follows is a description of the analogies and differences between cancer and pregnancy that may explain such a remarkable protection.

Cancer

It is established that similar basic mechanisms are involved both in cancer and in pregnancy, albeit in a greatly altered form. Cancer involves changes in cellular proliferation rate, reduction in cell differentiation, reduction in programmed cell death, an increase in tumor invasiveness, and cell migration leading to metastasis. Furthermore, most tumors are monoclonal, deriving from only one abnormal cell that has acquired a growth advantage resembling the fertilized egg that from the beginning has a growth advantage within the maternal organism. In addition cancer disrupts the host's function, changes its metabolism, reduces the immune system and if left untreated may lead to the death of the host. How cancer develops remains to be fully elucidated. Some argue that cancer reflects a progressive regression in cellular differentiation. Recently certain key changes that lead to the transformation of normal to malignant cells were reported. They involve inhibition of tumor suppressor genes, stimulation of oncogenes, and modulation of telomerase activity. Malignant cells become less functional and acquire an end of their own to proliferate at the expense of the host using all possible resources to their advantage.

Unlike pregnancy (except for early embryonal development), as it progresses, cancer requires a less favorable environment, low oxygen tension, poor vascularization, and a reduced dependence on growth factors. This actually reflects a move from a well-organized organism to a stage of an almost complete self-sufficiency, where chaos reigns. Most tumor markers are actually fetal antigens and their re-expression in malignancy reflects a return to a dedifferentiated stage of the cells. Such re-expression may be a generalized phenomenon, a genomic de-repression, but it may serve another purpose, the recreation of an embryo-like environment, thereby conferring immune protection and preferential nutrient supply for the tumor.

Pregnancy

On the other hand pregnancy associated changes also involve rapid cell proliferation, cellular migration, trophoblastic invasiveness, and spread of trophoblastic cells through a metastatic like process into the maternal peripheral circulation. However, in a normal pregnancy all these changes are actually beneficial adaptive systems allowing the woman to carry the pregnancy safely to term.

As pregnancy develops, cell proliferation is tightly associated with cellular differentiation; thereby from a raw structure a highly coordinated functional entity results which is the embryo, further specializing through fetal development, creating a functional fetal unit together with the placenta, amniotic fluid and chorion. Fetal development also progresses from a low to a high oxygen environment required for postnatal life. Within the maternal system there are also major adaptive physiological changes in every function. Of great relevance is hypertrophy of major maternal organs that include the uterus, breast, and the subcutaneous tissue as well as formation of new blood vessels. Levels of compounds promoting proliferation also greatly increase in the maternal system. These involve growth factors, sex steroids, placental proteins like hPL and hCG, just to mention a few.

From the major changes earlier described it would appear that in the pregnant subject the body should be the most prone to rapidly becoming affected in case cancer should develop. This could be magnified by the changes within the maternal immune system that would even further diminish the protection against malignancy. However this is clearly not the case.

Therefore, it appears that when cancer is compared to pregnancy there are major changes that may explain the radically opposite outcomes associated with the two conditions. In cancer there is a shift from a beneficial proliferation and differentiation towards blastic primitive cells' proliferation. There is a decrease in conditions that are required for cancer development, namely reduced oxygen tension, nutrients, and dependence on growth factors. In contrast, as a pregnancy progresses all these elements increase in importance. Cancer growth is actually a destructive process, while pregnancy, in contrast, reflects a major effort in building an independent entity. In cancer the host is destroyed, while in pregnancy the symbiosis is very successful, with almost no delayed consequences beyond delivery. In cancer suppression of the immune system takes place which seriously affects the host, while in pregnancy the immune system in general is well preserved.

Consequently, drawing a parallel between conditions and specific compounds that are present during pregnancy and those present in cancer becomes very important. They provide a great opportunity to better understand the disorder, and derive lessons both with respect to diagnostic and even therapeutic standpoints. Some compounds like hCG and some specific hCG antibodies for the same show some clinical promise as well as some other trophoblastic derived agents. This may occur also through the expression of conceptus derived factors that control proliferation in a non-toxic manner. The author is currently investigating a potentially novel class of proteins derived from early gestation, which control abnormal proliferation such as in cancer and due to the action of viruses without associated toxicity or interference with normal cells' proliferation.

Thus, in the relationship between cancer and pregnancy we envision shifting from the scary scenario viewed earlier, of the need to sacrifice the fetus for preserving maternal wellbeing, to the realization that the presence of cancer during pregnancy may allow in certain instances the saving of both entities. Facing a difficult disease such as cancer with hope, and the encouragement of a better understanding of the unique processes that are ongoing during pregnancy together with specific products that can be derived from it to control abnormal proliferation, are steps in the right direction. If the reader goes away from reading this text with a sense of hope and a better understanding of possible cancer control then our task has been accomplished.

Index

C

O

P

R

S

T

U

V

X

Z

MIX
Papier aus verantwortungsvollen Quellen
Paper from responsible sources
FSC® C105338

If you have any concerns about our products,
you can contact us on
ProductSafety@springernature.com

In case Publisher is established outside the EU,
the EU authorized representative is:
Springer Nature Customer Service Center GmbH
Europaplatz 3, 69115 Heidelberg, Germany

Printed by Libri Plureos GmbH
in Hamburg, Germany